D0198692

THE NEW GUIDE TO
REMEDIES

HOMEOPATHY · ESSENTIAL OILS · CRYSTALS · HOME REMEDIES

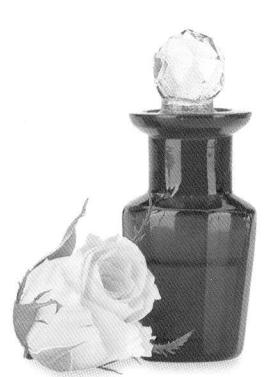

p

This is a Parragon Book

First published in 2002

Parragon

Queen Street House

4 Queen Street

Bath BA1 1HE, UK

Hardback ISBN: 0–75258–521–5

Paperback ISBN: 0–75258–522–3

Printed in Indonesia.

Designed and created with the Bridgewater Book Company Ltd.

NOTE

Any information given in this book
is not intended to be taken as a
replacement for medical advice. Any person
with a condition requiring medical attention
should consult a qualified medical practitioner
or therapist before taking any of the remedies
described in this book.

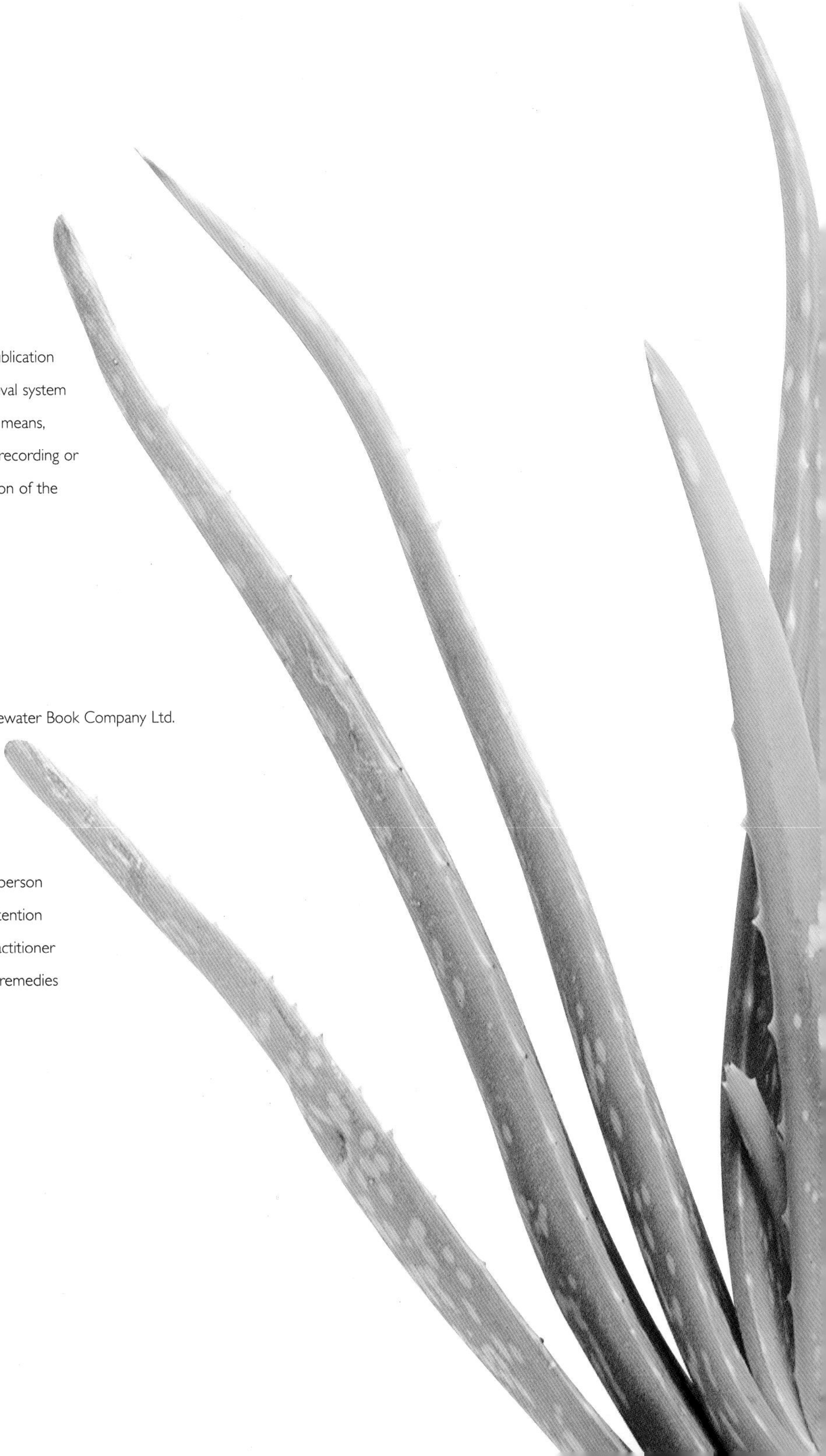

contents

Introduction

Today, many of us are interested in finding alternative ways of staying healthy that do not rely on conventional medicine. This book offers a collection of traditional, natural remedies that can be used to treat everyday complaints without the need to turn to the modern medicine cabinet. The remedies suggested here are suitable for young and old alike. They can be used to ease specific symptoms or to enhance general well-being.

The first section deals with homeopathy, which can be used to self-treat many common ailments, as well as to complement conventional medicine. Homeopathy considers every aspect of a person – physical, emotional and mental – before a treatment is proposed. Two people with the same symptoms will not necessarily be prescribed the same remedy. Homeopathy is based on the principle of treating like with like. Medicines are made from flowers, plants, roots, trees, poisons, minerals, metals and even from certain insects. The current popularity of homeopathy means that qualified practitioners are easy to find and that remedies are widely available.

The use of essential oils is an accessible form of complementary treatment which has also become more widespread. It is a well-known fact that scents and aromas can affect our mood, helping us to relax or lifting our spirits. Aromatherapy takes this idea one step

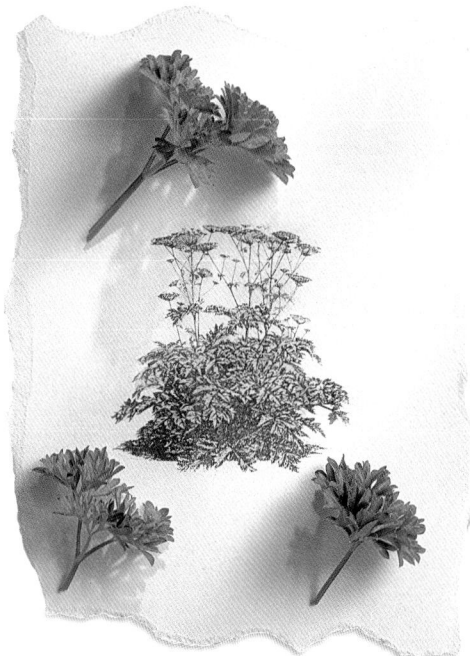

Traditional remedies are made from natural sources such as flowers, plants, roots, minerals and metals.

further, using particular oils to treat specific conditions, either by inhaling them, or by applying them to the skin. Essential oils produced from roots, wood, resins, leaves, berries, seeds and fruit can have gentle, nurturing effects on body and mind.

The beautiful, natural minerals we call crystals can be used not only to enhance our environment, but also as powerful healing tools. This section links 32 precious stones to their different colours. It looks at their geology and history and teaches us how to share the positive energies of their light, colour and beauty. The role of crystals in balancing the chakras (the body's seven energy centres) is also explained.

Finally, we turn to the kitchen for traditional home remedies that date back many years. No longer dismissed as old wives' tales, the treatments in this section are effective for first-aid uses as well as for many general ailments. Everyday natural ingredients can be used in all kinds of forms such as poultices, drinks or rubs for immediate relief, or added to your diet for long-term benefit. From healing burns, bites and bruises to soothing arthritis, eczema and even hangovers, home remedies have the answer.

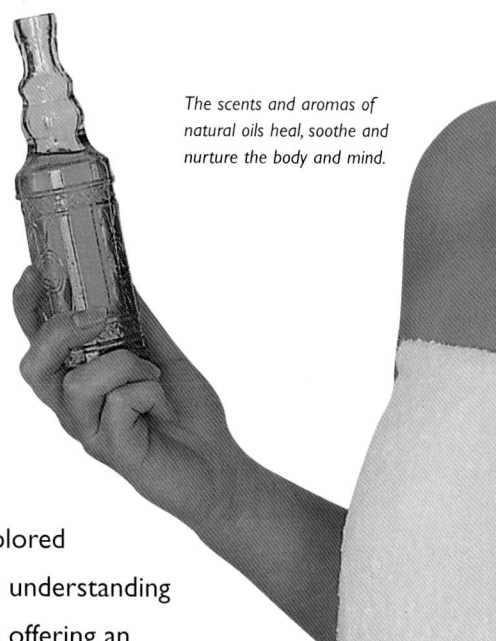

The scents and aromas of natural oils heal, soothe and nurture the body and mind.

Serious medical conditions should always be treated by a professional and the information given in this book is not intended to replace the advice of your doctor. Nevertheless, any of the four branches of complementary remedies explored here can lead you towards an understanding of how to heal yourself, while offering an excellent source of front-line treatment.

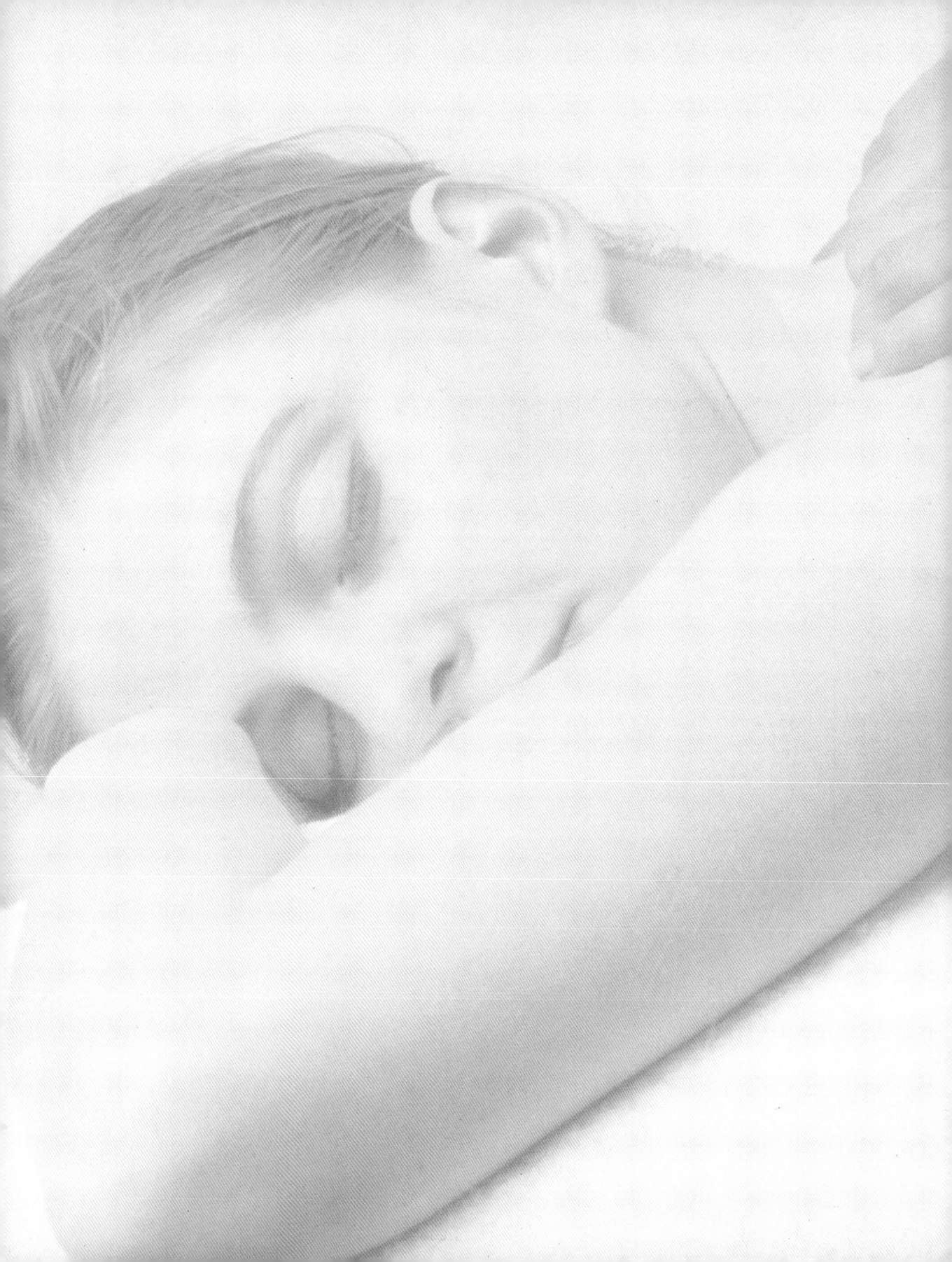

homeopathy

Introduction

Homeopathy is one of many alternative and complementary therapies available today. Such therapies take a 'holistic' approach to the treatment of patients. The word 'holistic' is taken from the Greek word for 'holos' meaning 'whole'. The idea is that the person is treated as a whole, with every aspect of them – physical, emotional and mental – being taken into account when selecting a remedy.

The purpose of this section is to introduce and describe the effects of the most common homeopathic remedies, enabling the reader to choose a remedy for the

Your doctor can refer you to a trained homeopath or another medical doctor who uses homeopathic treatments.

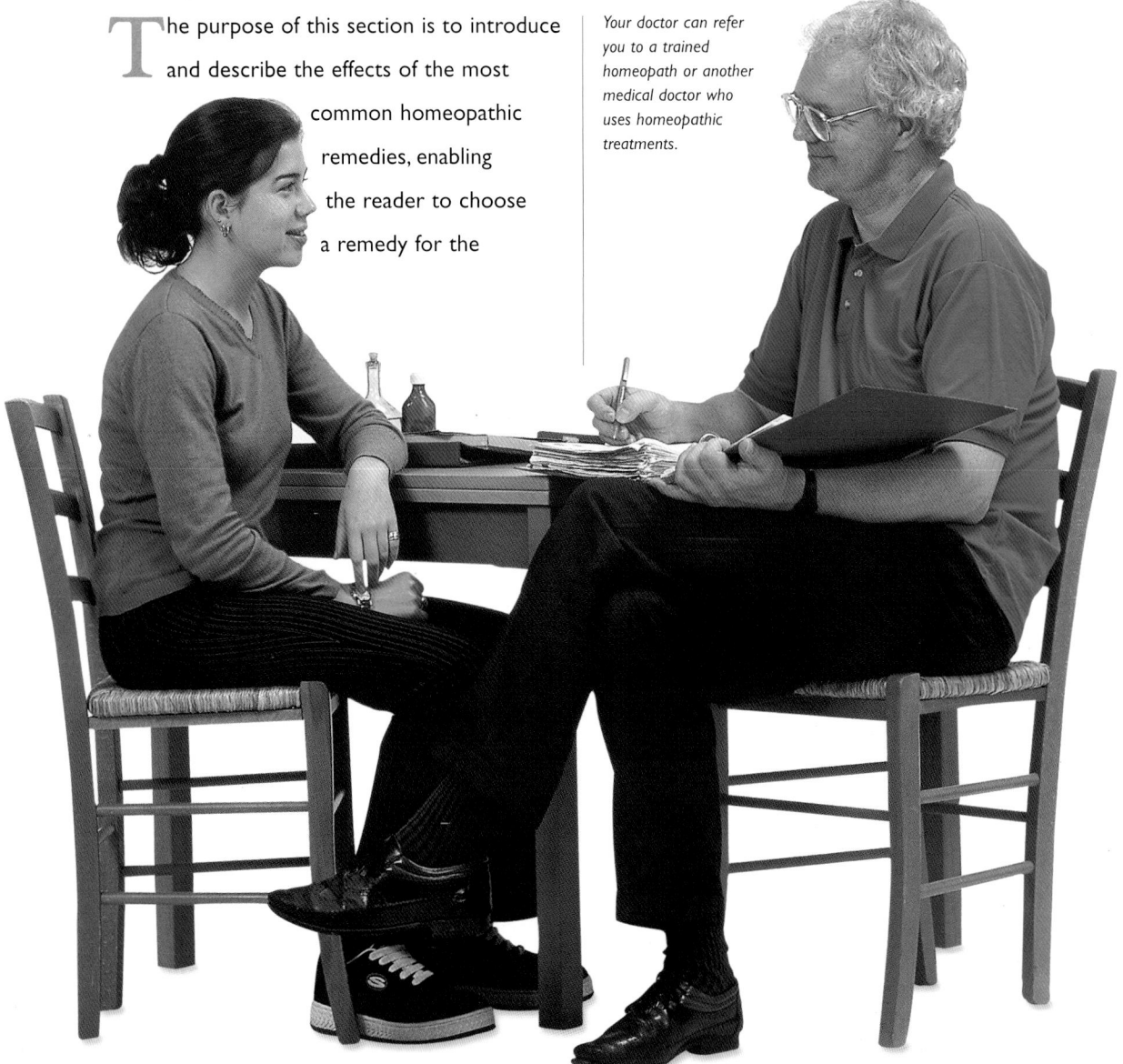

self-treatment of many common ailments, or to use them to complement conventional treatment. It should be stressed, however, that using this book for self-treatment should not replace conventional medicine. If you are concerned about your health, you should visit your doctor for a diagnosis before prescribing yourself any of the remedies. If you are currently under medical supervision, or are on a prescribed course of treatment, then check with your doctor or consultant before self-treating.

Although this book is a good way to begin self-treatment with homeopathy, it is worth noting that other forms of homeopathic treatment are also available. There are several National Health Service homeopathic hospitals in the UK, with treatments available from medically qualified doctors. Access to these facilities can be obtained by referral from your doctor. There are also medical doctors who are trained homeopaths who work in the private sector. Non-medically qualified homeopaths also work in private practices. Several health insurance companies now include homeopathic referral and treatment within their cover.

Homeopathy has grown in popularity in recent years, and high street pharmacies now sell a large selection of homeopathic medicines. Some pharmacists are also trained

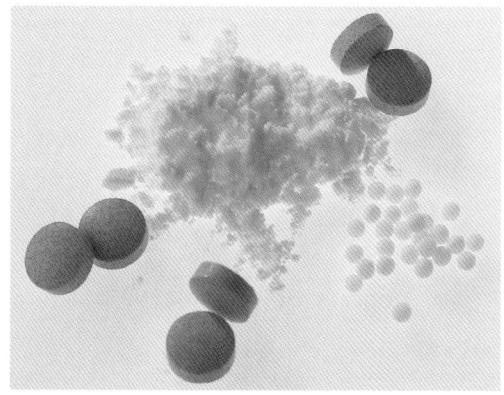

Today, homeopathic remedies are widely available. Many high street pharmacies stock a range of homeopathic medicines.

in homeopathic pharmacy, so they may be able to help you choose a remedy. Supermarkets, health food stores, mail order and internet companies also stock many of the most common remedies, so your chosen remedy should be easy to obtain.

Minor ailments such as colds can be successfully treated using homeopathy at home.

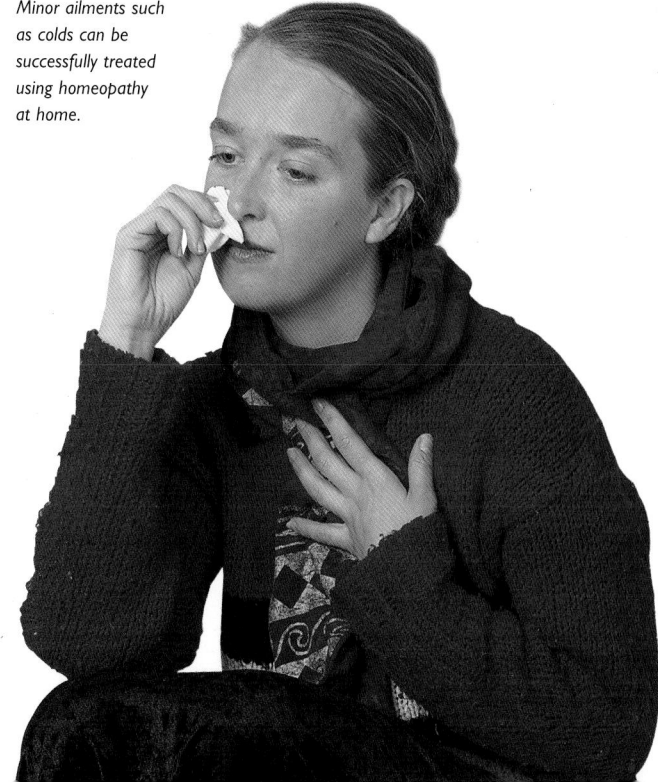

What is Homeopathy?

Homeopathy uses very dilute substances to stimulate the body's healing power. Its basic principle is treat 'like with like'. This involves treating a patient's symptoms with minute amounts of a substance that would cause similar symptoms in a healthy person. This practice contrasts with conventional allopathic medicine, in which treating 'like with opposite' prevails; that is, a disease is treated with a substance that opposes it.

The first person to practise the healing principle of treating 'like with like' was Greek physician Hippocrates (c.460–377BCE). His method went against the thinking of the time, which held that the gods were the main force behind a disease, and that a cure could be found by treating with a substance that had an opposite effect in a healthy person.

German doctor Samuel Hahnemann (1755–1843) was the modern-day founder of homeopathy. He proved the principle of 'like curing like' with his experiments with quinine, known to be an effective treatment for malaria. He found he developed malarial symptoms after taking doses of quinine (he was otherwise in good health). These effects lasted hours after each dose.

Samuel Hahnemann devised the system of homeopathy.

He tested other substances in the same way, in a process known as 'proving'. He 'proved' more than 100 homeopathic remedies in his lifetime, publishing his findings in 'The Organon of Rational Medicine' in 1811. He believed that the remedies worked by activating a person's 'vital force', that is, the body's own healing potential. Having conducted tests on many volunteers, he came to realise the importance of taking into account the personality traits of each person receiving the treatment. He found that particular 'types' of people manifested different symptoms to the same disease and so required treatment with different remedies in accordance with their 'type'.

American doctor James Tyler Kent (1849–1943) furthered Hahnemann's work on the different 'types' of people and the matching of a remedy to their emotional and physical characteristics. These 'types' became known as 'constitutional types'.

Remedy Dilution and Potentisation

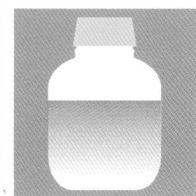
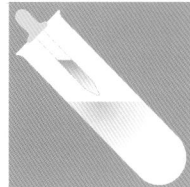
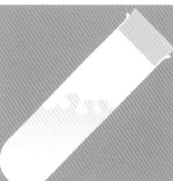
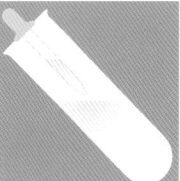
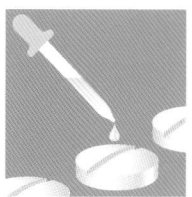

The mother tincture is prepared from the source material.

One drop of the tincture is diluted with 99 drops of alcohol and water.

The remedy is then succussed. This makes the 1c potency.

Using the 1c potency, the process is then repeated to reach the required potency.

A few drops are added to lactose tablets.

Homeopathic remedies

Remedies can be made from many different substances. The most common sources are flowers, plants, roots, trees, poisons, minerals and metals. Certain insects are also used.

Hahnemann used the smallest possible amount of a substance to trigger a healing effect. This was to minimise side effects. He realised that the more a substance was diluted, the better the results, provided it was also vigorously shaken (in a process known as succussion) at each stage of dilution. Counterintuitive though it seems, the less of the original substance that remained in the remedy, the greater its potency and effectiveness.

The process of diluting a remedy to render it effective is called potentisation. First an alcohol/water extract is made from the substance. This is the mother tincture. The extract is diluted to the required potency. The main potencies are denoted by x, c and m: x means the remedy has been diluted one part

mother tincture in 9 drops of water; c means one part of mother tincture in 99 drops of water; and m means one part of mother tincture in 999 drops of water. A 1c potency is one part in 99 parts of water. A 2c potency is created by taking one part of the previous dilution (i.e., the 1c potency) and diluting it in 99 parts of water. The most common potencies used are 6c, 12c and 30c.

Once the required potency is reached, a few drops of the substance are applied to lactose (milk sugar) tablets. The tablets must be kept dry and away from direct sunlight.

For the purposes of self-treatment as detailed here, it is suggested that the 30c potencies are used, as these are commonly available. To obtain the best results, consult a homeopath. They may prescribe higher potencies depending on the initial consultation and the presenting problem. This is particularly the case if the ailment has a strong emotional or mental aspect.

Using the Remedies

When taking the remedies orally it is possible to choose from several mediums that are available from a homeopathic pharmacy or supplier. The tablets also can often be found in a high street pharmacy or health shop.

Tablets

These are the most readily available form. The tablets should be sucked or lightly chewed until they dissolve completely. This usually takes several minutes. Tablets are ideal for adults and older children.

Soft Tablets

These dissolve instantly on the tongue. They are ideal for young children, babies and for adults who are impatient and do not want to spend time sucking or chewing.

Pillules

These are small, round, hard pills. They can take longer to dissolve in the mouth than ordinary tablets. This form is often found in homeopathic first aid kits because they are smaller than the tablets and fit easily into a smaller container.

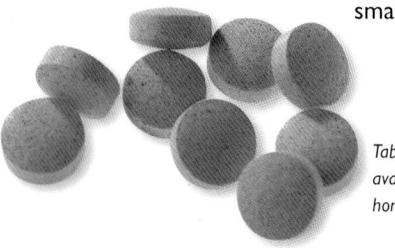

Tablets are the most readily available form of homeopathic remedies.

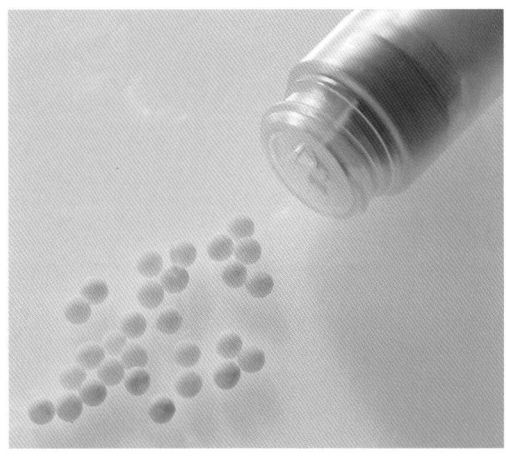

Pillules are small tablets that are dissolved slowly in the mouth. They are useful for homeopathic first-aid kits.

Powders

Powders are usually prescribed by homeopaths for a single dose or several-dose treatment of a higher potency remedy (e.g. 200c or over, or 1m and over). They are supplied wrapped in paper and, like soft tablets, dissolve instantly on the tongue. It is possible simply to crush a tablet to make a powder by folding it in paper and hitting it with the back of a metal spoon. The powder can then be held in the paper, made into a funnel shape and placed in the mouth for

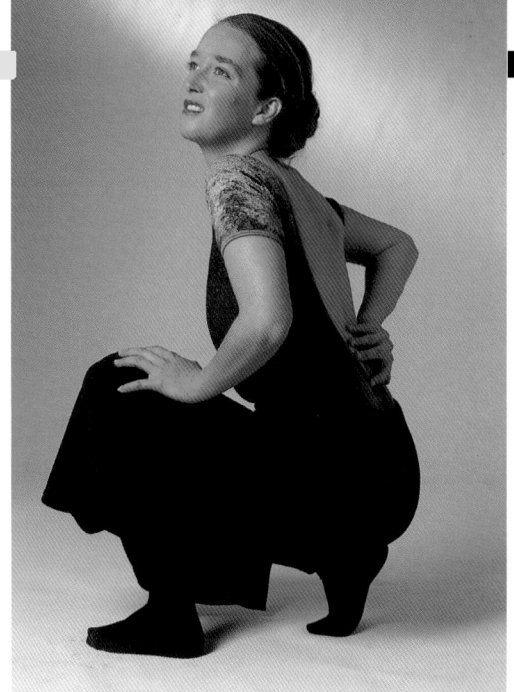

Back pain is a chronic condition that can be treated by taking several tablets a day.

quick absorption. This method can be used in a first-aid situation to administer a dose to young children or babies, or to children who refuse to take the tablets.

Frequency of Treatment

Once you have chosen a remedy, the next consideration is how often to take it. The main distinction is between acute and chronic conditions (acute illnesses have a rapid onset and short duration, whereas chronic conditions are of long duration and often gradual onset). For an acute condition such as an injury or a stomach upset, take one tablet every one to two hours for the first six doses (you can take fewer if the condition is relieved before this). If the condition does not improve

after six doses, continue with one tablet two or three times a day until the symptoms are relieved. Once there is improvement, stop taking the remedy immediately.

If the condition is chronic, such as irritable bowel syndrome, chronic fatigue syndrome, arthritis or depression, then one tablet should be taken twice a day until the condition has improved. Once the condition is relieved, stop the treatment immediately.

Stopping the treatment as soon as the condition improves may seem strange, as conventional medicines, such as antibiotics, often require the whole course to be completed. However, in homeopathy, it is of no benefit to continue a treatment once the condition improves.

If you notice no improvement from a remedy after giving it sufficient time to work, or notice only a very minor improvement, it is worth trying another remedy. Always take into account your constitutional remedy, if possible. The selection of remedies often involves some trial and error.

A bad cold is an acute condition that can be treated by taking a tablet every 1–2 hours.

Constitutional Types

Homeopathy treats the individual as a whole, taking into account physical, emotional and mental states as well as disease or ailment. Knowing a person's constitutional type offers insight into the best remedy for them. This is particularly important, as two people suffering from the same problem may have different symptoms. They may find that different modalities (influences) improve or worsen their condition. Therefore, they may need to be treated with different remedies, despite having the same illness.

Mental and emotional factors of constitutional types are taken into consideration when prescribing. These include such matters as the individual's fears and anxieties — for example, whether they have a fear of animals, spiders, the dark, thunderstorms, loneliness, robbery, attack, failure, death or poisoning. It also takes into account an individual's temperament — whether they tend to be tearful, happy, sad, confident, lazy, perfectionist, mild, gentle, caring, optimistic, irritable, aggressive or spiteful. Then we need to examine whether certain factors affect the

Knowing a person's constitutional type can provide a valuable insight into their problem.

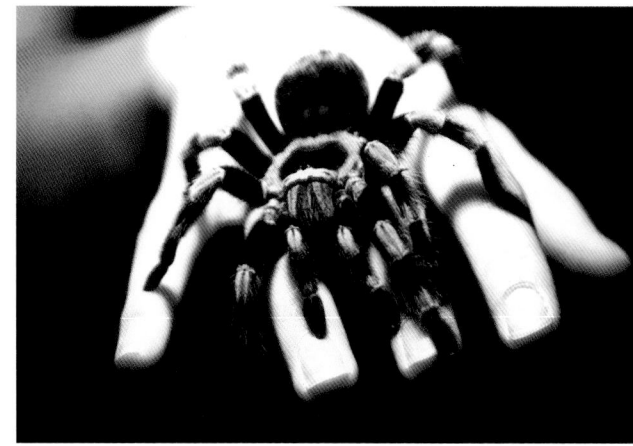

Knowing a person's fears and anxieties helps to reveal the emotional and mental state of the individual.

individual and whether they have an effect on the condition itself. For example, how do they respond to noise? Does music bring on emotional reactions? Are they bright and alert in the morning or dull and unresponsive? Do they like their own company or prefer to be with others? Do they prefer hot or cold weather? Do they prefer dry or wet atmospheres? Do they talk to others about problems or keep themselves to themselves? Do they have strong likes and dislikes for food and drinks?

Physical factors are also important. These aspects include whether the patient is tall or short; fat or thin; long-limbed; under or overweight. Do they have dark rings under the eyes? What is their hair and eye colour? Do they have thick, curly or thin hair? What is their skin texture? Preferred type of clothing? Is their manner of dress formal or casual? Do they have frown lines?

Once you have discerned someone's constitutional type, it is easier to select the most appropriate remedy. For example, consider a person who is suffering from a sore throat and cold. The best remedy for the physical symptoms of a sore throat and cold is remedy A, B or C. The best remedy for the emotional aspects of the person with the sore throat and cold is either remedy B or C. The best remedy according to the person's constitution is remedy B. Therefore, remedy B is likely to be most effective.

It is not essential to calculate the remedy in this way – prescribing remedy A based on the physical symptoms only will have some effect – but the best effect would be remedy B, as it fits all aspects for that individual.

Some of the main constitutional types are outlined on the next few pages.

The Argent. Nit. Type

Appearance: Pale complexion. Looks older than actual age, due to worry and tension.

Mental and emotional aspects: Cheerful and impressionable. Often anxious and worried. Always in a hurry and can be impulsive. Finds it difficult to control emotions. Readily laughs, cries and loses temper. Quick-thinking and good at solving problems. Tends to be extraverted in order to hide true feelings.

Physical weaknesses: Nervous system. Digestive system. Eyes. Ailments tend to be left-sided.

Dietary factors: Likes chocolates, sweets, salt and cheese. Dislikes chilled foods.

The Argent. nit. child: Always moving around and never wants to sit still. Prone to nervousness and can experience upset stomach when stressed. May react badly to new situations such as moving school. Can be prone to insomnia due to anxiety. Prone to bedwetting.

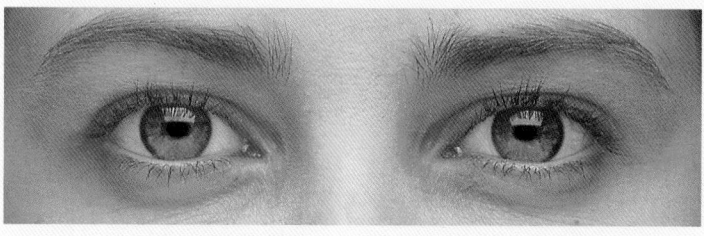

Argent. nit. types tend to have weak mucous membranes in their eyes.

The Arsen. Alb. Type

Appearance: Usually thin or slim. Often well groomed and 'stylish'. Fine facial features with delicate, sensitive skin. Frown lines can appear on the forehead.

Mental and emotional aspects: Restless person. Perfectionist at work and at home. Can be critical and intolerant. Strong opinions. Can have a deep fear of being alone. Obsessive-compulsive behaviour, in particular involving cleanliness and 'tidying up'; this can hide a hoarding mentality. Can pull out of plans and projects early if they think it is not going to work out 100%.

Warm drinks and sweet foods are favoured by the Arsen. alb. type.

Pessimistic in nature, with a need to receive constant reassurance.

Physical weakness: Digestive system. Skin. Respiratory system (asthma, coughs and colds).

Dietary factors: Likes fatty foods, warm food and drinks, in particular coffee, sweets, alcohol and sour-tasting foods. Dislikes large amount of fluid.

The Arsen. alb. child: Highly sensitive and 'highly strung'. Easily upset by loud noise. Becomes tired and exhausted after periods of exertion. Suffers nightmares due to very active imagination. Increasingly physically and mentally agile with age. Can worry too much about parents' well-being. Keeps room neat and tidy. Does not like mess or getting messy.

The Calc. Carb. Type

Appearance: Overweight or gains weight easily. Sluggish, bloated and tired in appearance. May have poor posture.

Mental and emotional aspects: Impressionable. Sensitive and quiet. May become withdrawn due to a deep fear of failure. Can dwell too much on a particular problem. May be greatly upset by cruelty to animals or children. Needs motivation to succeed in tasks. Can be prone to mild depression when unwell. Reassurance helps to improve condition.

Physical weaknesses: Ears, nose and throat. Skeletal system (may manifest in backache). Digestive system: may be prone to irritable bowel syndrome and bloatedness. Skin. Teeth. Exhaustion; prone to chronic fatigue syndrome. Prone to depression.

Dietary factors: Likes dairy products, eggs, sweets, salt, desserts, chocolate, carbohydrates, iced drinks and ice-cream. Dislikes fatty meat, boiled food and boiled milk.

The Calc. carb. child: Plump and overweight. Placid and calm. Complexion often pale. Slow to walk and talk and teeth are slow to develop. Can fall over easily. Scared of the dark and prone to waking up because of nightmares. Often lazy and may need encouragement with schoolwork as gives up easily.

The ears, nose and throat are all weak areas of the Calc. carb. type.

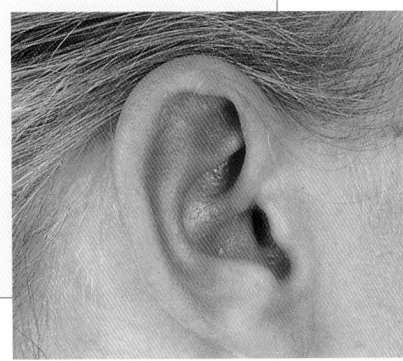

The Graphites Type

Appearance: Prone to being overweight and has a large appetite. Blushes easily. Can have a rugged, windswept appearance. May have rough, dry skin that can crack and flake easily. Dry hair, usually dark in colour. Flaky scalp.

Mental and emotional aspects: A plodder – takes time to work things out and solve problems. Deep concentration on a task can cause irritability. Unwilling to change attitudes and routines. Not best first thing in the morning. Prone to mood swings. Can become tearful and despondent and then impatient.

Physical weaknesses: Skin. Nails. Slow metabolic rate. Common ailments may include soreness in the corners of the mouth, exhaustion, bad breath, nose bleeds, styes and travel sickness.

Dietary factors: Likes sour and savoury foods, cool drinks. Dislikes sweet foods, salt, seafood, hot drinks.

The Graphites child: Feels the cold and gets chilled very quickly. Timid, hesitant and anxious. Does not like long periods of travel, as often suffers from travel sickness.

The Graphites type likes savoury foods, such as salads or vegetables, rather than sweets and desserts.

The Ignatia Type

Appearance: Slim build. Prone to dark circles under the eyes. May have a tired, drawn expression and involuntary twitching of the eyes and mouth. Dry lips. Hair is of a dark to medium colour. Sighs a lot.

Mental and emotional aspects: The most highly strung of the constitutional types. Tendency to rapid and extreme mood swings. Can switch quickly from depression to joy and from tears to laughter. Prone to suppressing grief. May find it difficult to end relationships and perceive this to be a weakness. Addictions to nicotine and caffeine are common.

Physical weaknesses: Nervous system. Emotional trauma may be the cause of any number of physical problems. Common problems include hysterical grief over bereavement, leading to depression, headaches, sore throats, coughs and colds, constipation, twitching, and grinding of teeth.

Dietary factors: Likes coffee (although it may not agree with them), sour and savoury foods, dairy products, carbohydrates. Dislikes sweet foods.

The Ignatia child: Highly strung. Excitable and sensitive. Finds it difficult to perform under stress. Finds separation or divorce of parents very hard to deal with, leading to outbursts of anger, crying and poor performance at school. Prefers company to being alone. May suffer with headaches, coughs, sore throats. Responds well to reassurance.

Dairy foods are popular with the Ignatia type.

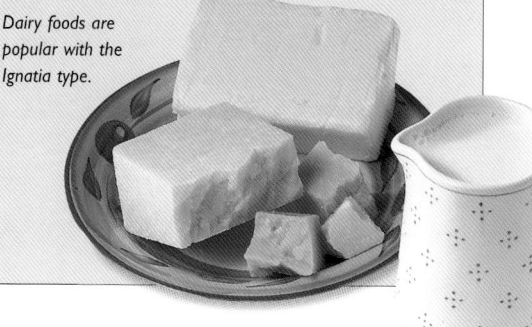

The Lachesis Type

Appearance: May look bloated or lean. Strong, fixed expression. Complexion usually pale and prone to slight freckles. Strong and staring eyes. Can lick the lips a lot.

Mental and emotional aspects: Very ambitious. Highly creative. Mind can become crowded with thoughts. Jealous and possessive. Talkative. Can be sensitive to noise. If religious, is prone to view self as sinful. Can be suspicious of strangers.

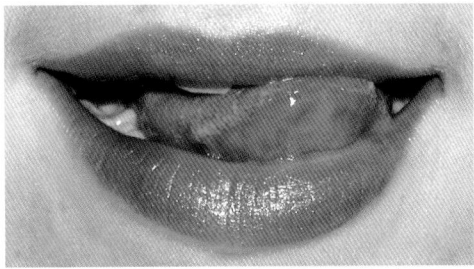

Physical weaknesses: Circulation. Nervous system. Common problems include varicose veins, hyperactivity, menopausal problems, sore throats and asthma, disturbed sleep and insomnia, palpitations and panic attacks. Prone to left-sided problems. Physical problems made worse when trying to sleep or remain still.

Dietary factors: Likes coffee, alcohol, seafood, cool drinks, sour and savoury food and carbohydrates. Dislikes sweet drinks.

The Lachesis child: Spiteful, possessive and can be hurtful to peers. Hyperactive. Jealous of siblings, particularly newly born. Prone to nightmares. May be prone to ADHD (attention deficit and hyperactivity disorder).

Lachesis types have a tendency to lick their top lip.

The Lycopodium Type

Appearance: Tall and lean. Worry and frown lines on the forehead. Can look older than their actual years. Facial twitches. Thinning hair in men. Dislikes wearing tight clothing.

Mental and emotional aspects: Prone to exaggeration. Can create a drama over minor matters. Insecure and hates change. Avoids commitment. Anxious of challenging events. Strong fear of being alone and of the dark. Forgetful. Finds small mistakes disproportionately irritating. Hates being contradicted.

Physical weakness: Common problems include digestive disorders, kidney stones, prostate problems, headaches, sore throats, male-pattern baldness and alopecia. May be prone to chronic fatigue syndrome.

Right-sided problems are more prevalent.

Dietary factors: Likes sweet foods, warm drinks, onions, garlic and seafood. Dislikes cheese and strongly flavoured meats.

The Lycopodium child: Basically insecure and shy, although can be bossy and dominant with other children. Likes to be indoors rather than doing outdoor pursuits. Likes to read and is conscientious and good academically.

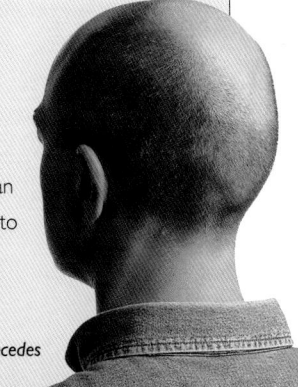

The hairline of Lycopodium men recedes early and they may become prematurely grey or bald.

The Merc. Sol. Type

Appearance: Medium build. Skin on the face may be shiny or moist due to perspiration, with a grey translucent look. Hair colour may be fair to medium.

Mental and emotional aspects: May have an inner battle with emotions. Resentment, anxiety and lack of trust in others may cause feelings of insecurity. Dislikes criticism that is directed at self or taking orders from others. May explode with rage and anger.

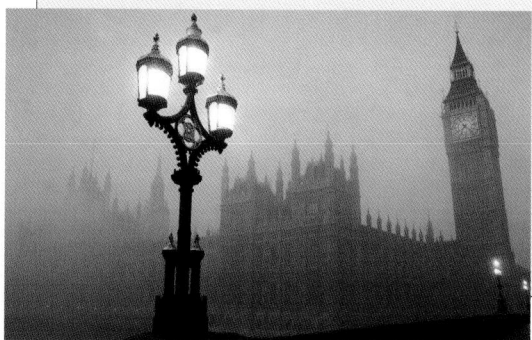

Memory may become poor with age and thought patterns may become muddled later in life.

Physical weaknesses: Common problems include sore throat; swelling of glands; exhaustion. Skin sensitivity and allergies are common. May be prone to chronic fatigue syndrome. May suffer from SAD (seasonal affective disorder).

Dietary factors: Likes cold drinks, carbohydrates and citrus fruits. Dislikes strongly flavoured foods.

The Merc. sol. child: Irritating behaviour. Shy and cautious. May have a tendency to stammer. Susceptible to ear, nose and throat ailments.

The Merc. sol. type may be affected by changes in the weather or may suffer from SAD (seasonal affective disorder).

The Nat. mur. type

Appearance: Pear-shaped build in women. Solid, strong-to-lean build in men. Skin can be oily and puffy with a tendency to swell. Red, watery eyes. Dry cracked lips. Medium to dark hair.

Mental and emotional aspects: Prone to suppressing emotions such as fear, loneliness, guilt and anger, which can lead to depression. Suppressed feelings of grief or loss for a loved one or for the self. Can become very despondent and depressed after relationship break-up. May want to cry but cannot. Prone to suffer in silence and not ask for help when needed. Career-minded and successful with a serious outlook on life.

Physical weaknesses: Nervous system. Common problems include: depression; premenstrual

syndrome; anorexia; skin problems; mouth ulcers and cold sores; palpitations and headaches.

Dietary factors: Likes cool drinks, sour and savoury foods and craves salt and most carbohydrates. Dislikes coffee and bread.

The Nat. mur. child: Small for their age. Slow development. Well-behaved. Loves animals. Excellent academically but if criticised at school can become very hurt. Can be prone to headaches under pressure.

Nat. mur. types are serious and conscientious. They may be professional and career-minded.

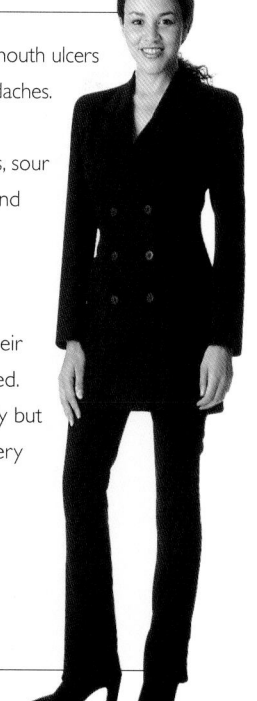

The Nux Vomica Type

Appearance: Slim, particularly when young. Smart appearance. May look stressed and tense. Ages prematurely. Prone to dark circles under the eyes. Face becomes flushed through anger or excitement.

Mental and emotional aspects: Can suffer from addictions and over-indulgence. May have cravings for alcohol, food, and stimulants such as coffee and cigarettes. Can be addicted to sex. Finds it difficult to relax. Can be very ambitious. Impatient. Intolerant

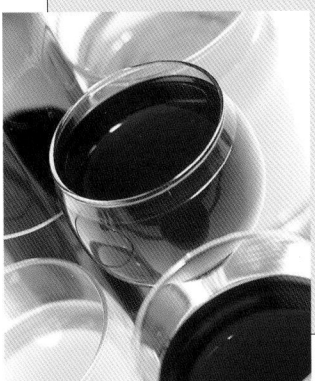

The Nux vomica type may become over-dependent on alcohol or stimulants, which may be craved.

and critical and requires perfection in others. The worst thing that can happen to a Nux vomica type is failure.

Physical weaknesses: Digestive disorders from hangovers and over-indulgence. Migraines and headaches, hernia and hay fever. Feels better for sleep.

Dietary factors: Likes fatty and rich food, cheese and cream, alcohol, coffee and spicy foods. Dislikes the effect of some strong spicy foods (despite enjoying eating them).

The Nux vomica child: Irritable and easily bored. May be prone to hyperactivity and ADHD (attention deficit and hyperactivity disorder). May throw tantrums. Competitive as a teenager. Can become addicted to alcohol and drugs, as likes to be rebellious.

The Phosphorus Type

Appearance: Tall and slim with long limbs. Likes to dress well and look stylish. May be artistic and creative in appearance. Fine skin. Can have fair to dark hair.

Mental and emotional aspects: Needs a lot of love and attention. Good fun to be with but can be needy and demanding. Likes to be the centre of attraction. Enjoys sympathy when upset or unwell. Expressive, affectionate and shows emotions easily. Needs reassurance, in particular with looks and body image. Short attention span. Challenging, particularly towards a partner.

Physical weaknesses: Nervous system – in particular fear and hypersensitivity. Circulation

problems. Vertigo. Coughs and colds. Weakness of the lungs. Headaches. Prone to left-sided problems.

Dietary factors: Likes salt, spicy food, sour and savoury food, carbonated drinks, alcohol, mild cheeses and sweet foods. Dislikes strongly flavoured fish and fruit.

The Phosphorus child: Tall and slim with long legs and arms. Nervous. Likes to be with people and centre of attention. Loves to receive affection. Strong fear of the dark.

Phosphorous types enjoy mild cheeses. They also enjoy spicy, sour and savoury dishes.

The Pulsatilla Type

Appearance: Can be slightly overweight. Gentle and kind in appearance. Can look younger than actual age. Hair is fair and skin has a rosy complexion. Usually has blue eyes. Blushes easily. Often rests with hands behind the head.

Mental and emotional aspects: Shy and easily embarrassed. Kind and gentle and makes friends easily. Likes to be supported by others. Not assertive and can be indecisive. Cries easily, in particular over cruelty to children and animals, tragic news or weepy movies. Also laughs easily. Avoids confrontation. Loves animals.

Pulsatilla types often rest with their hands behind their head.

Can suppress guilt and anger. Occasionally prone to obsessive or compulsive behaviour.

Physical weaknesses: All female reproductive problems. Catarrh. Irritable bowel syndrome. Skin problems. Varicose veins. Styes. Physical symptoms can fluctuate and change rapidly.

Dietary factors: Likes sweet foods, cold foods and cool drinks. Dislikes fatty foods (particularly cream and butter) and very rich, spicy food.

The Pulsatilla child: Fears the dark and dislikes bedtime. Sensitive to changes in the weather. Becomes tearful and weepy when overtired. Prone to coughs and colds.

The Sepia Type

Appearance: Slim and tall. Often sits with legs crossed. Likes to look attractive and elegant. Medium to dark hair, often with brown eyes.

Mental and emotional aspects: Can be irritable and easily offended. Tendency to be aggressive to loved ones. Cannot handle too much stress and tries to escape pressure and deadlines. Can feel better after weeping, but dislikes it when other people are fussing around. Avoids crowds but fears being alone. Hates being contradicted, as holds strong opinions.

Physical weaknesses: These include all menopausal problems. Headaches and migraine. Skin problems. Other common ailments include constipation and haemorrhoids; chronic fatigue syndrome and depression. Conditions usually improve with exertion. Physical problems occur mostly on left side.

Dietary factors: Likes spices, sour and savoury food, citrus fruits, sweet foods and alcohol. Dislikes dairy products, in particular milk, rich and strongly flavoured meats, and fatty foods.

The Sepia child: Greedy. Prone to constipation. Can become a bedwetter. Moody. Feels the cold and becomes tired easily. Does not like being alone.

The Sepia type fears being alone but at the same time does not like to be part of a large crowd.

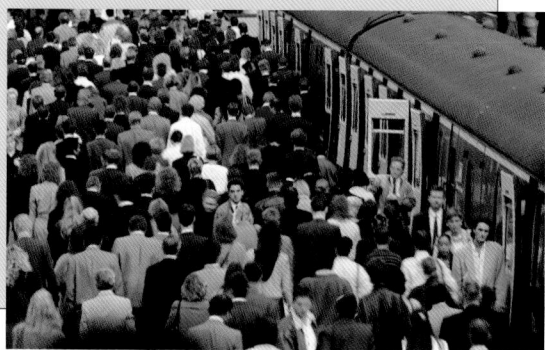

The Silicea Type

Appearance: Often slim or thin, with a large forehead. The head can appear too large for the body. Delicate, fine features – almost doll-like in appearance. The skin of the lips looks grey and can be cracked. The palms of the hand feel sweaty to touch and the nails can be brittle.

Mental and emotional aspects: Appears to have low confidence from a young age. Prone to mental exhaustion. Can become overburdened and overwhelmed. Responsibility weighs heavily upon the Silicea type. Can be indecisive about taking on new projects, moves and new jobs. Fear of failure may manifest itself as workaholism. Fear of failure

The nails of Silicea types may be rough or brittle. If injured, their skin can take a long time to heal.

can also spread into personal relationships. May stubbornly resist advice from loved ones and friends in order to hide true feelings.

Physical weaknesses: Problems with nervous system, in particular burn-out from new ventures. Exhaustion. Slowness in healing and convalescence. Respiratory illnesses and weaknesses including chest infections and low resistance to coughs and colds. Constipation. Skin problems. Headaches. Feels the cold.

Dietary factors: Likes cold food such as salads and raw vegetables. Dislikes meat and dairy products, in particular cheese and milk. Dislikes very hot food.

The Silicea child: Can be smaller than children of a similar age, with a petite appearance, apart from the head, which may look large for the body size. Feels the cold. Not sporty as has little stamina. Can be shy. Usually tidy and well-behaved.

The Sulphur Type

Appearance: May be slim with poor posture. May look untidy. Hair may be coarse, dry. Skin and lips can be prone to redness.

Mental and emotional aspects: Mind can be cluttered. Can be critical. Likes to argue. May lack willpower and self-esteem. Might not complete ideas or projects.

Physical weakness: Prone to: skin and circulation problems; haemorrhoids and constipation; hot, burning feet; body odour.

Dietary factors: Likes sweet foods, fatty foods and stimulants such as coffee and chocolate. Likes alcohol, spicy foods, savoury foods, citrus fruits, salads and seafood. Dislikes dairy foods, in particular milk and eggs. Dislikes most hot drinks.

The Sulphur child:: Untidy looking. Can be hyperactive in the evening. Does not like bathing, showers or washing hands. Has a very healthy appetite.

The Sulphur type enjoys sour foods such as citrus fruits.

Homeopathic Remedies

In the following pages are details of the main remedies: derivation, treatment use and tips. Before continuing, read about modalities and get to know the do's and don'ts.

Modalities

Modalities are influences that worsen or improve the symptoms of the patient. They are an invaluable guide to narrowing down the choice of a homeopathic remedy. These are the main types of modality:

• **Physical modalities:** include how the patient is affected by movement, position of the body, touch, rest, exertion, noise and smells.

• **Temperature:** heat, cold, warmth, wind, damp, and the season of the year may affect the individual's symptoms.

• **Time:** symptoms may be more noticeable in the daytime or at night, or in the morning, afternoon or evening. Symptoms may even change hourly.

• **Diet:** different foods, drinks, stimulants or alcohol may affect the patient and his or her ailment.

• **Localised modalities**: symptoms may be worse on the left or right side of the body. Left-handed and right-handed people may experience symptoms differently.

Do's

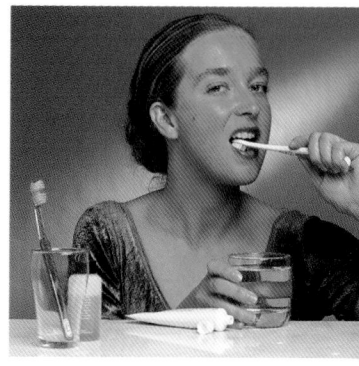

• Leave your mouth free from food and liquid 20–30 minutes each side of taking the remedy.

• Use a homeopathic tooth-paste such as calendula, as this will be free from substances that may antidote the remedy.

• Store the remedy in a dark, cool place.

• Check the expiry date before use.

• Keep tablets out of reach of children and pets.

• Store the remedy away from strong-smelling perfumes or essential oils.

Don'ts

• Don't swallow the tablet; suck it till it dissolves.

• Don't drink coffee or smoke while taking treatment.

• Don't eat mints, peppermints or menthol cough sweets, as this may interfere with the remedy's action. This also means avoiding brushing your teeth with mint or peppermint-flavoured toothpaste.

• Don't use the essential oils of camphor, eucalyptus, menthol, peppermint or rosemary.

• Don't touch the pills directly. Always tap the tablets into the lid, as the sweat from your fingertips or palm may absorb the remedy rather than your mouth.

• Don't apply perfume or aftershave thirty minutes either side of taking the remedy.

Aconite

Aconite is derived from Monkshood, a toxic plant used for centuries to treat infections and also to poison arrows for hunting.

Treatment Use

Aconite is useful when any of the following are indicated:

Mental and emotional aspects

● Anxiety and great fear ● Feelings of doom and gloom, especially when accompanied by illness ● A strong fear of death, the dark and ghosts ● Agoraphobia and panic ● Any form of shock ● Worry and stress about the future ● Nightmares ● Panic attacks ● Vivid imagination ● Unhappiness ● Emotional and physical tension that drain energy from the mind and the body.

Aconite is often used to treat panic attacks. It can also be used when a person is facing any situation that is an ordeal.

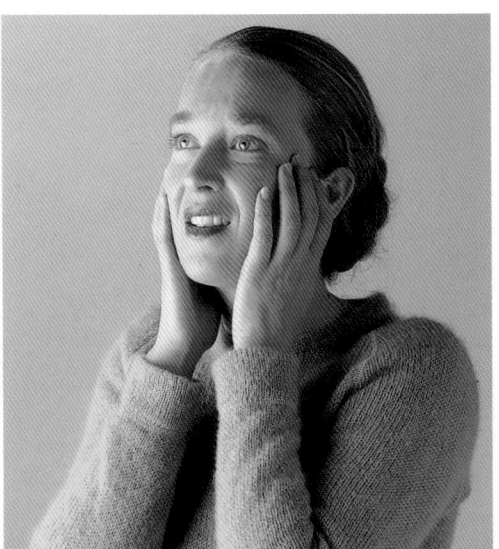

The Monkshood plant (Aconitum napellus) is the source of the remedy Aconite.

Physical aspects

● Headaches with a hot and heavy sensation ● Sore, gritty eyes ● Sore nose, throat or ear problems ● Tightness and pressure around the chest ● Coughs, colds and influenza ● Sleep problems ● Feelings of restlessness ● Palpitations ● Nervous twitching of the eye ● Sunburn, when accompanied by shaking and fever.

Modalities

● **Better:** for fresh air and warmth.
● **Worse:** in the evening and at night.

Treatment Tips

This remedy is useful for treating ailments that develop suddenly.

This remedy is a useful addition to a homeopathic first-aid kit.

Apis Mel.

Apis mel. is derived from the honeybee – the whole bee is used. Propolis, a resin-type substance secreted by bees to repair damage to hive walls, has been used for centuries as a natural antibiotic.

Treatment Use

Apis mel. is useful when any of the following are indicated:

Mental and emotional aspects

● Poor memory ● Feelings of jealousy ● Being hard to please ● Tearfulness ● Apathy and indifference ● Constantly complaining and hard to please ● Fear of death.

Physical aspects

● Clumsiness ● Headaches with a stabbing and stinging pain ● Fever with a lack of thirst accompanied by skin that is sensitive to the touch ● Itchy, stinging skin ● All eye problems that sting and burn ● Arthritis when the pain is burning in sensation ● Cystitis and other urinary tract infections that cause stinging on passing urine

Apis mel. is often used to help overcome tearfulness.

The remedy from the honeybee provides a range of medicinal substances.

● Insect bites and stings ● A constant but spasmodic cough.

Modalities

● **Better:** cool water and a cool room; the application of cold compresses.
● **Worse:** for pressure and touch; heat.

Treatment Tips

Apis mel. is an excellent remedy for treating burning and stinging pain that responds well to being treated with a cool remedy. It is useful for swollen and itchy skin, particularly following insect bites and stings. Useful for any sudden swelling or puffiness of the skin.

This remedy is a useful addition to a homeopathic first-aid kit.

Argent. Nit.

Argent. nit. is derived from silver nitrate (a compound of silver). It is poisonous in large amounts. It has a caustic nature and it was used historically to cauterise wounds.

Treatment Use

Argent. nit. is useful when any of the following are indicated:

Silver nitrate crystals are extracted from the mineral acanthite, the main ore of silver.

Mental and emotional aspects

- Apprehension • Fearfulness
- Nervousness • Overactive imagination
- Stage-fright • Phobias, in particular claustrophobia and fear of spiders and insects
- Feeling stressed and in a hurry • Fear of giving talks or addressing groups • Fear of taking examinations.

Physical aspects

- Diarrhoea caused by anxiety and tension

• Nightmares • Tight, sore muscles due to constant body tension • Headaches caused by concentrating hard • Flatulence • Trembling and weakness in muscles and limbs • Palpitations and tightness in the chest • Aching, tired eyes • Irritable bowel syndrome.

Modalities

- **Better:** for cool, fresh air and pressure.
- **Worse:** when highly emotional; for concentration; for warmth.

Treatment Tips

A remedy that helps to relieve apprehension and anxiety. Useful when there is fear of a forthcoming event, for example an examination or an interview. Helps control nerves both before and during the event.

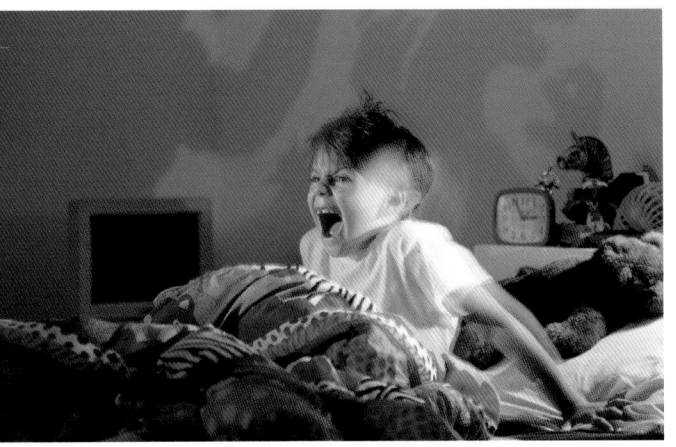

Argent. nit. can be used to help overcome fears and phobias and help with nightmares or an overactive imagination.

Arnica

Arnica is derived from the herb *Arnica montana* (also known as Leopard's Bane, Wolf's Bane or Mountain Arnica), a plant used since the 16th century as a remedy for bruises, muscular aches and pains, and rheumatism.

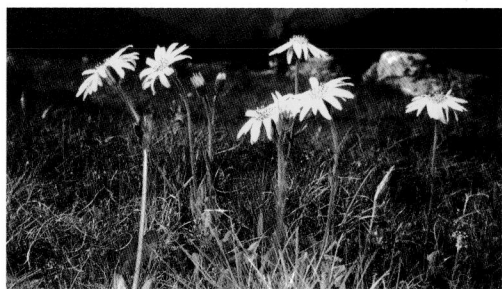

The fresh flowers of the plant Arnica montana *are used to provide a remedy for physical and emotional shock.*

Treatment Use

Arnica is useful when any of the following are indicated:

Mental and emotional aspects

* Irritability * Nervousness and oversensitivity * Inability to focus on a task for long * Forgetfulness and indifference * Agoraphobia * All forms of shock * Bereavement.

Physical aspects

* Post-surgical convalescence * Labour pains and childbirth * Sore muscles * Swelling * Bruising * Backache and joint pain * Sprains * Black eyes * Accidents and falls

* Hot, sensitive, aching headache * Heavy, tired eyes * Concussion * Nosebleeds * Sore muscles in chest following a bad cough * Over-exertion * Vertigo.

Modalities

* **Better:** for lying down.
* **Worse:** for moving; cold, damp weather.

Treatment Tips

Arnica is a key remedy for all forms of muscular pain and bruising. It is also very useful applied topically to unbroken skin in a cream or ointment form or as a compress using the tincture. Arnica is one of the most commonly used remedies and is an over-the-counter bestseller.

This remedy is a useful addition to a homeopathic first-aid kit.

Arnica is a useful remedy for the physical and emotional impact of childbirth.

Arsen. Alb.

Arsen. alb. is derived from arsenic, which is a metallic poison.

Treatment Use

Arsen. alb. is useful when any of the following are indicated:

The arsenic compound arsenic trioxide is used to treat a variety of symptoms.

Mental and emotional aspects

- Restlessness • Anguish and anxiety
- Feelings of hopelessness • Over-reaction to ailments • Agitation • Hypochondria
- Perfectionism demonstrated by obsessive-compulsive behaviour • Inability to cope
- Insecurity • Fear of the dark • Fear of poisoning • Twitches • Fixed ideas • Jealousy
- Addictions, including those to alcohol and tobacco • Fear of being alone • Fear of death
- Fear of suffocation.

Physical aspects

- Skin, hair and scalp problems, such as psoriasis and dandruff • Food poisoning
- Vomiting • Exhaustion • Headaches
- Mouth ulcers • Fluid retention • Mild forms of asthma • Sore throat, particularly if swallowing is difficult • Cramp • Disturbed, restless sleep • Angina pain.

Modalities

- **Better:** for warm drinks; heat; movement.
- **Worse:** for cold, wet weather.

Treatment Tips

A very useful remedy for the treatment of digestive problems. It is also excellent for treating anxiety and restlessness. It acts on every organ and tissue of the body.

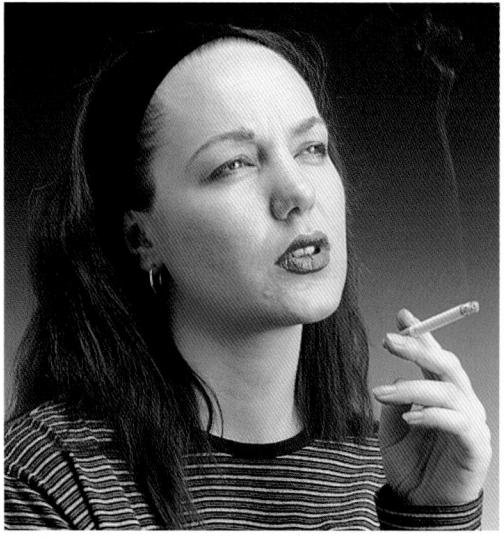

Arsen. alb. acts on the mucous membranes of the digestive tract and respiratory system. It can be used to treat addictions such as smoking.

Aurum Met.

Aurum met. is derived from gold that has first been ground to a powder.

Treatment Use

Aurum met. is useful when any of the following are indicated:

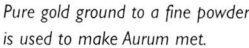

Pure gold ground to a fine powder is used to make Aurum met.

Mental and emotional aspects

● Tendency to become a workaholic ● Prone to perfectionism, leading to dissatisfaction ● Can become deeply upset if criticised ● Extreme unhappiness ● Depression, sometimes leading to suicidal thoughts ● Obsessed with illness and death ● Illness triggered by grief ● Fixed ideas ● Prone to criticise everyone around them ● Cannot always share worries with others, instead brooding on them in isolation ● Prone to nightmares ● Anxiety triggered by loud noises.

Physical aspects

● Illness through depression ● Heart disease, blood and circulatory problems ● Headaches ● Chest pain and breathlessness ● Sinus problems and sinusitis ● Catarrh ● Ear, nose and throat problems ● Joint pain and skin ulcers ● SAD (seasonal affective disorder).

Modalities

● **Better:** for fresh air and movement.

● **Worse:** for emotional stress and tension; at night; in wintertime.

Treatment Tips

A good remedy to try when others have failed, in particular in cases of depression where there appears to be 'no light at the end of the tunnel'.

Overwork and stress can be treated by Aurum met. It is used to help many different problems, from depression to heart disease.

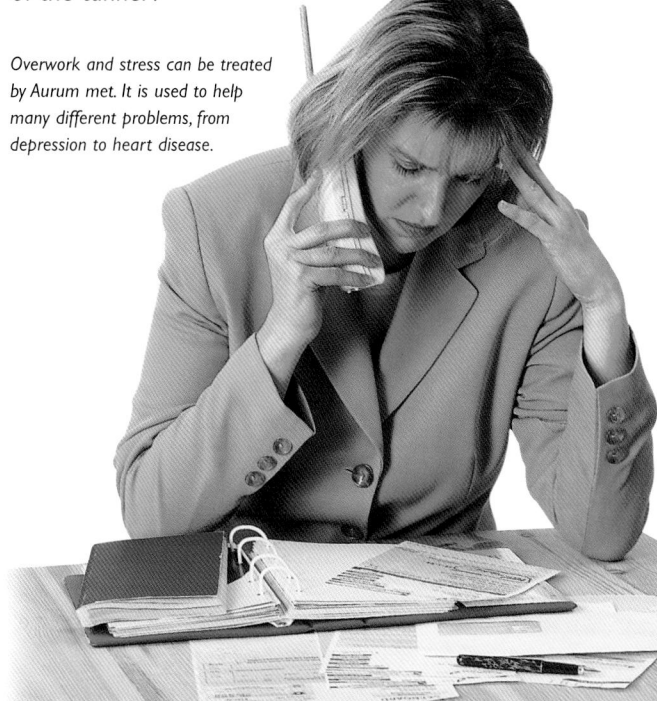

Belladonna

Belladonna is derived from the deadly nightshade plant, which was popular during the Middle Ages for magic rituals.

Treatment Use

Belladonna is useful when any of the following are indicated:

Mental and emotional aspects

• Sudden anger • Feelings of guilt • Stress • Depression triggered by agitation • Sudden temper tantrums and a red face.

Physical aspects

• All pain where there is heat, burning, redness or throbbing • Cold, coughs and influenza • Sore throats • Earache, made

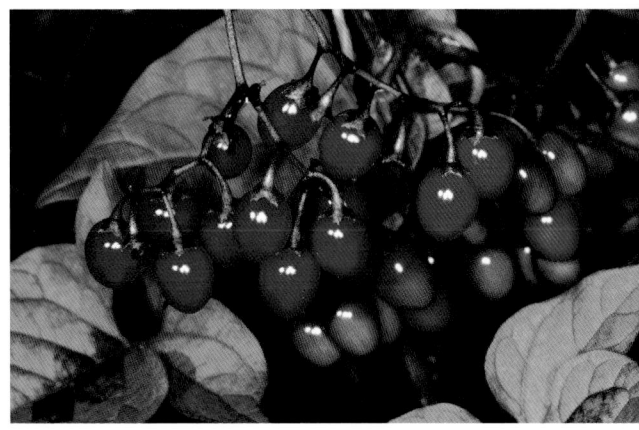

Although every part of the belladonna plant (Atropa belladonna) is poisonous, the leaves and flowers are used in homeopathy.

worse by getting the head wet or cold • Labour pains • Cystitis • All infections that result in inflammation • Teething pain • Boils • Insomnia.

Modalities

• **Better:** for sitting up.
• **Worse:** for noise and movement.

Treatment Tips

An excellent remedy for acute complaints, particularly when accompanied by hot, throbbing sensations.

This remedy is a useful addition to a homeopathic first-aid kit.

The remedy Belladonna is used to control sudden anger and violent outbursts of behaviour.

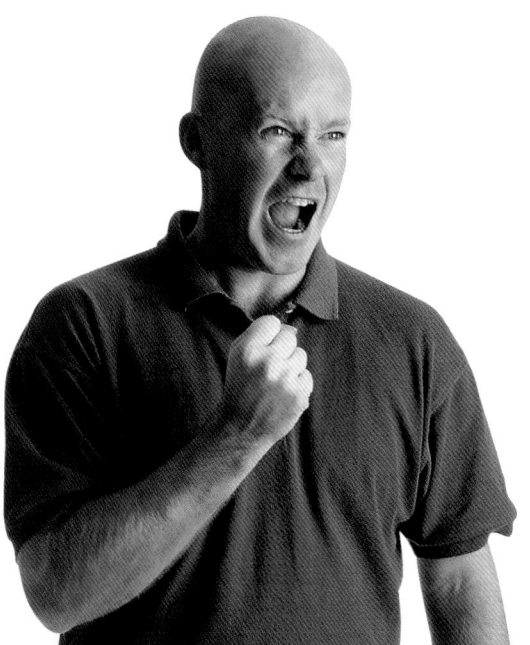

Bryonia

Bryonia is derived from the roots of wild hops grown in central and southern Europe. Bryonia was used by the Romans to treat coughs and wounds.

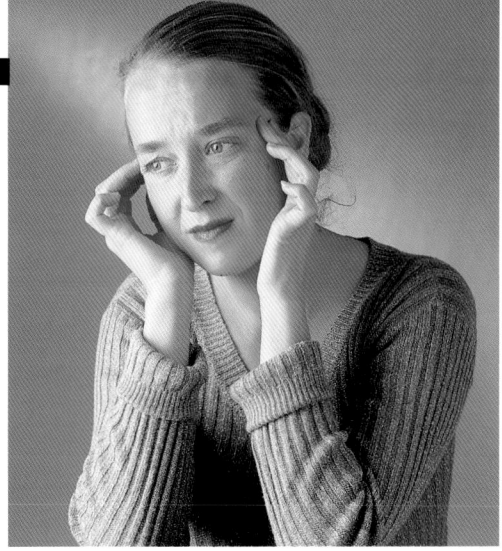

Bryonia is used to treat anger and anxiety, but can also be used as a treatment for violent headaches.

Treatment Use

Bryonia is useful when any of the following are indicated:

Mental and emotional aspects

● Anger, irritability and restlessness ● Poor memory ● Fear of death ● Prefers to be left alone, particularly when unwell.

Physical aspects

● Headaches with a bursting or splitting sensation ● Arthritis and rheumatism ● Dry eyes and lips ● Very dry and sore throat ● Dry, irritating cough ● Constipation ● Influenza ● Pneumonia ● Pleurisy with severe chest pain ● Colic.

Modalities

● **Better:** for rest and stillness; a cold environment.
● **Worse:** with any kind of movement; cold winds.

Treatment Tips

Best used when there is pain on the slightest movement. Most effective when colds are accompanied by a strong thirst and a very dry throat.

The fresh roots of Bryonia (Bryonia alba) are chopped and pounded to make a pulp for the Bryonia remedy.

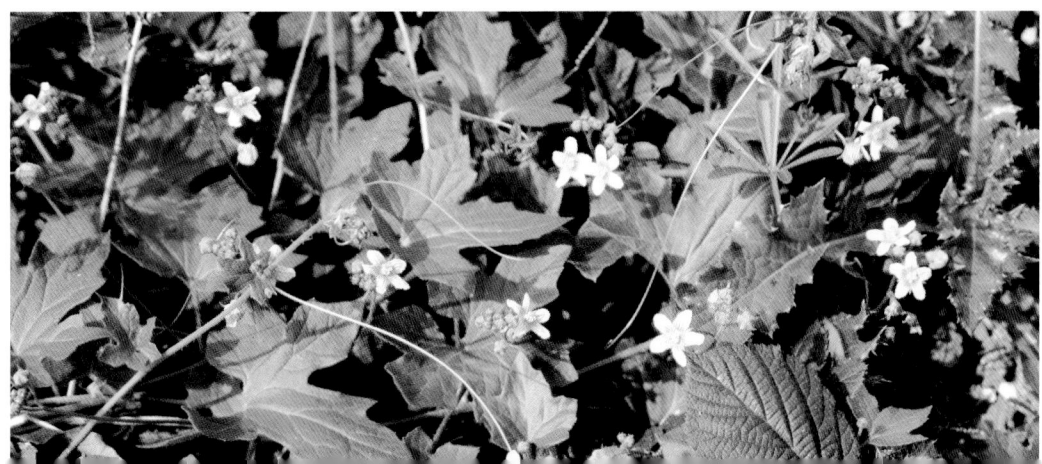

Calc. Carb.

Calc. carb. is derived from calcium carbonate in oyster shells.

Treatment Use

Calc. carb. is useful when any of the following are indicated:

Mental and emotional aspects

● Fear of the dark, death, insanity and impending doom ● In the elderly, fear of a stroke ● Anxiety which can cause palpitations ● Depression with tiredness/lethargy ● Poor memory ● Tiredness and slowness of thought ● Obsession with problems ● Anxiety when criticised ● Hypochondria ● Lowness of spirit ● Jealousy ● Laziness ● Fear of disease.

Physical aspects

● Teeth, joint and bone pain ● Fractures that are slow to heal ● Back pain ● Digestive problems ● Irritable bowel

The Calc. carb. remedy is used to help with anxiety, fear, depression and feelings of extreme helplessness.

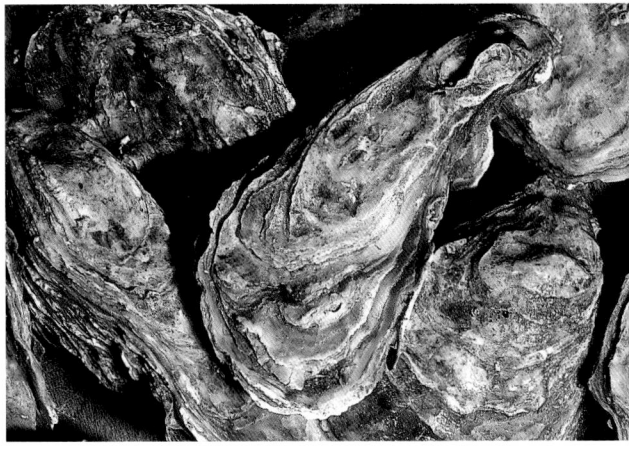

The mother-of-pearl inside oyster shells contains calcium carbonate. This salt is ground to a powder to make this remedy.

syndrome ● Constipation ● Premenstrual syndrome ● Nasal congestion ● Polyps ● Dry, irritating or tickling coughs ● Obesity ● Eating disorders, in particular bulimia ● Chronic fatigue syndrome ● Warts ● Headaches caused by study or when head feels heavy ● Light-sensitive eyes ● Loss of hearing ● Dark rings around the eyes ● Sour taste in the mouth ● Bleeding gums ● Toothache ● Cramp ● Stiff neck ● Weakness in the knees ● Unhealthy looking skin.

Modalities

● **Better:** for warm weather.
● **Worse:** when cold and damp; for exertion.

Treatment Tips

An excellent remedy for when bones are slow to heal.

Calc. Phos.

Calc. phos. is derived from the mineral salt calcium phosphate.

Treatment Use

Calc. phos. is useful when any of the following are indicated:

Mental and emotional aspects

- Unhappiness and discontentment with life, possibly stemming from childhood
- Relationship break-ups may trigger the onset of an illness • Prone to irritability
- Can complain a lot • Tendency to become restless • Difficulty keeping to routines
- In constant need of new things for stimulation • Poor memory.

Physical aspects

- Breaks, fractures and painful joints • Slow bone or tooth growth in children and teenagers • Exhaustion and fatigue
- Digestive disorders
- Recurrent throat problems.

Modalities

- **Better:** for warm, dry, sunny weather.
- **Worse:** in the cold or damp; for stress and worry.

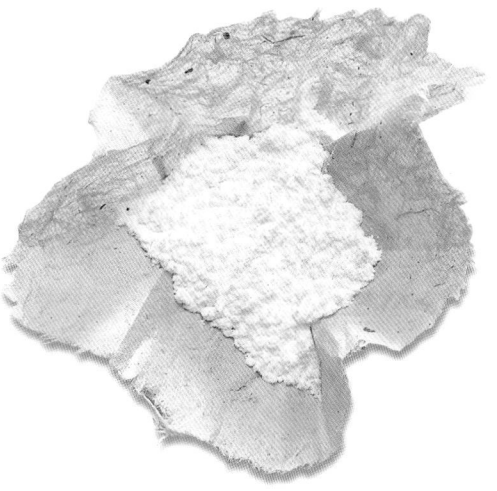

Calc. phos. is made into a powder through a chemical process.

Treatment Tips

A good remedy if healing is slow or for any bone and joint complaints. It can be used to help 'growing pains' in children and adolescents. Good for convalescence.

Calcium phosphate occurs naturally in our teeth, making them hard and rigid. The remedy can be used to treat tooth decay.

Cantharis

Cantharis is derived from a bright green beetle known as the Spanish fly, which has been known for centuries for its poisonous and irritant properties.

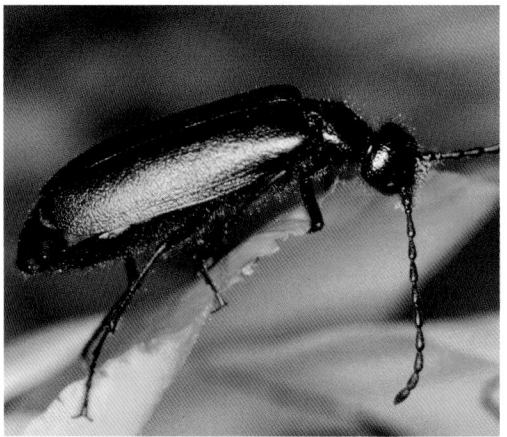

The Spanish fly is the source of the Cantharis remedy. It secretes a substance called cantharidin, which is an irritant.

Treatment Use

Cantharis is useful when any of the following are indicated:

Mental and emotional aspects

● Addiction to sex ● Irritability and anger leading to rage and violence ● Screaming with rage ● Severe anxiety.

Physical aspects

● All conditions where there is stinging, burning, itching and pain ● Cystitis and all urinary tract infections, with pain when urinating ● Burns ● Diarrhoea with burning sensation ● Insect stings and bites ● Burning, sore throat ● Sore, stinging eyes ● Hot, aching sensation in the stomach ● Sunburn and inflammation of the skin.

Modalities

● **Better:** for gentle rubbing.
● **Worse:** for touch and movement.

Treatment Tips

Excellent remedy for treatment of cystitis, especially when the condition worsens without warning.

This remedy is a useful addition to a homeopathic first-aid kit.

The remedy Cantharis can be used to treat ailments that have burning symptoms, including sunburn.

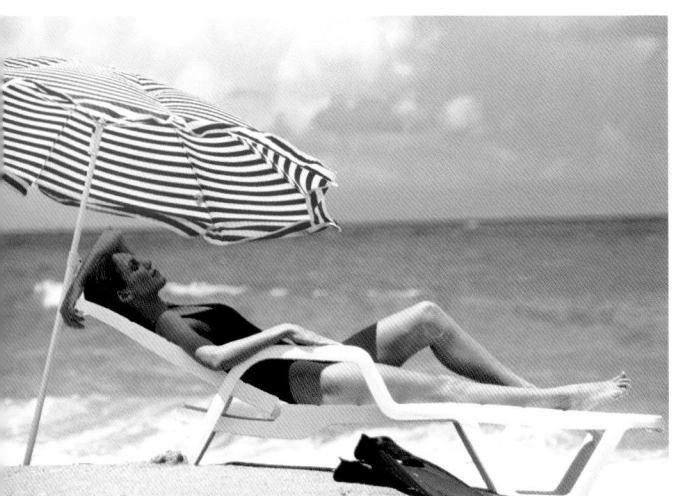

Carbo Veg.

Carbo veg. is derived from vegetable charcoal made from beech, birch or poplar wood. In the past, vegetable charcoal was used to absorb gases to help relieve flatulence.

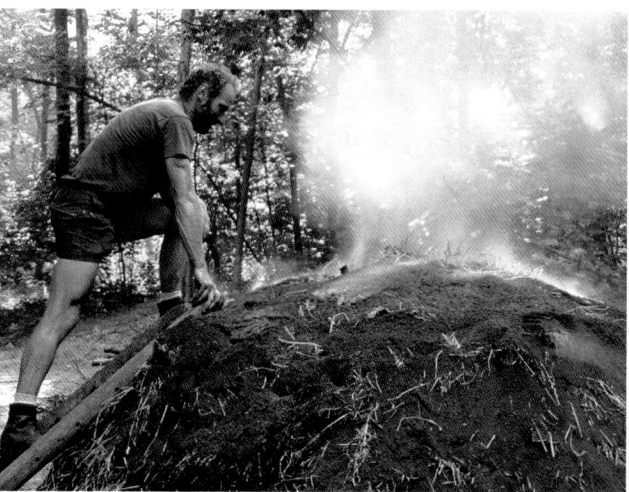

Woods from trees such as beech, birch or poplar are partly burned to make charcoals that have individual properties.

● Indigestion ● Flatulence ● Feelings of abdominal bloating (even after eating only small amounts) ● Headaches after too much food ● Headaches with sickness ● Coughing ● Hoarseness and dryness of the throat ● Nosebleeds ● Prolonged illness, leaving feelings of exhaustion.

Modalities

● **Better:** for cool, fresh air.

● **Worse:** for fatty foods; in the evening; for lying down.

Treatment Use

Carbo veg. is useful when any of the following are indicated:

Mental and emotional aspects

● Loss of memory ● Fear of strangers ● Claustrophobia ● Acute shock ● Extreme mental exhaustion ● Feelings of mental and emotional weakness.

Physical aspects

● Poor circulation ● Varicose veins

Treatment Tips

A very good remedy for feelings of overtiredness and being run down. Useful after any operation or illness. Good for speeding a slow recovery. Good for chronic complaints or conditions.

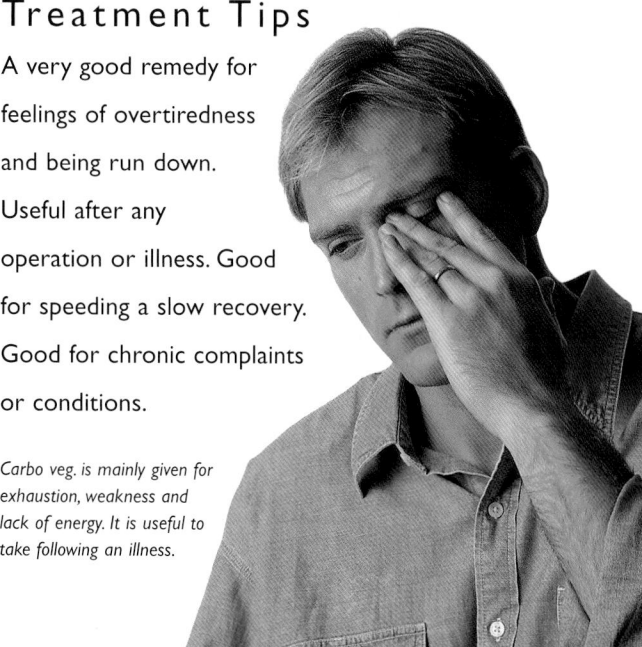

Carbo veg. is mainly given for exhaustion, weakness and lack of energy. It is useful to take following an illness.

Chamomilla

Chamomilla is derived from the whole, fresh chamomile plant. Chamomile has been used for centuries because of its calming, soothing and healing abilities, particularly in the treatment of skin conditions.

Treatment Use

Chamomilla is useful when any of the following are indicated:

Chamomilla is derived from the juices of the whole, fresh plant (Matricaria recutita) in flower.

Mental and emotional aspects

- Bad temper and anger when unwell
- Irritability and whining • Impatience
- Oversensitivity, which can lead to short-tempered behaviour towards loved ones • Difficult to satisfy.

Chamomilla is good for people who suffer from sleeplessness, or who cry out in their sleep because of anxious dreams.

Physical aspects

- Earache • Toothache
- Insomnia • All skin conditions including eczema • Inflamed skin
- Sleeplessness and colic in children
- Diarrhoea • Coughing, particularly at night.

Modalities

- **Better:** for mild weather.
- **Worse:** for heat; for cold winds or fresh air; when angry.

Treatment Tips

Especially good remedy for the treatment of children or babies. Chamomilla is a good bedtime remedy for a baby. Teething problems or colic may cause the baby to cry out and be restless. Chamomilla will help the baby to calm down and sleep.

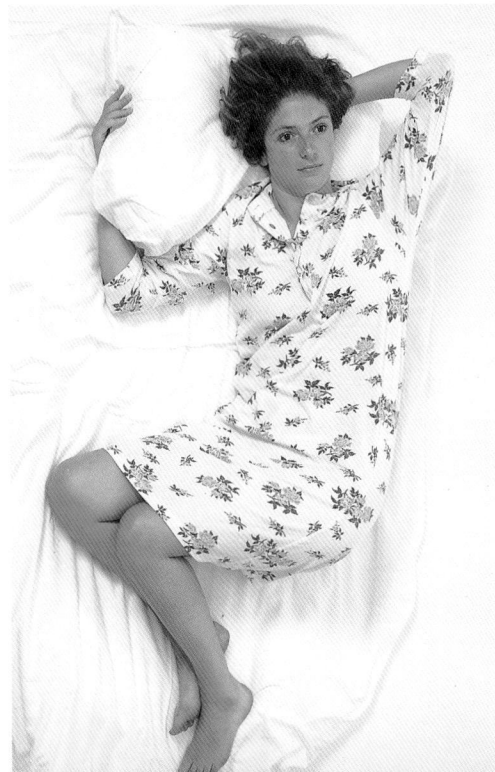

China

China is derived from Peruvian bark, which contains quinine – one of the first remedies investigated by Samuel Hahnemann.

These leaves are from the Cinchona tree, whose bark contains important remedies.

Treatment Use

China is useful when any of the following are indicated:

Mental and emotional aspects

- Indifference and apathy • Nervous exhaustion • Despair • Fear of creeping, crawling creatures • Outbursts of anger • Spitefulness • Sudden tearfulness • Depression • Eating disorders such as anorexia and bulimia • Lack of concentration • Feelings of being on edge • Hypersensitivity • Alcoholism • Difficulty in self-expression.

Physical aspects

- Loss of body fluid through heat-stroke • Heavy sweating • Fluid retention • Swollen ankles • Headaches • Dizziness • Twitches • Nosebleeds • Tinnitus • Digestive problems including diarrhoea and vomiting • Gall bladder complaints

- Feelings of coldness • Shivering • Fatigue, including post-viral exhaustion • Chronic fatigue syndrome • Skin that is sensitive to the touch • Tender scalp.

Modalities

- **Better:** for warmth and sleep.
- **Worse:** for losing bodily fluids; for cold and draughts.

Treatment Tips

A good remedy for burn-out caused by overwork or emotional traumas that produce feelings of exhaustion and weakness. Also a good convalescent remedy.

The China remedy is helpful for irritability and unexpected angry outbursts.

Coffea

Coffea is derived from caffeine: the unroasted coffee bean is used.

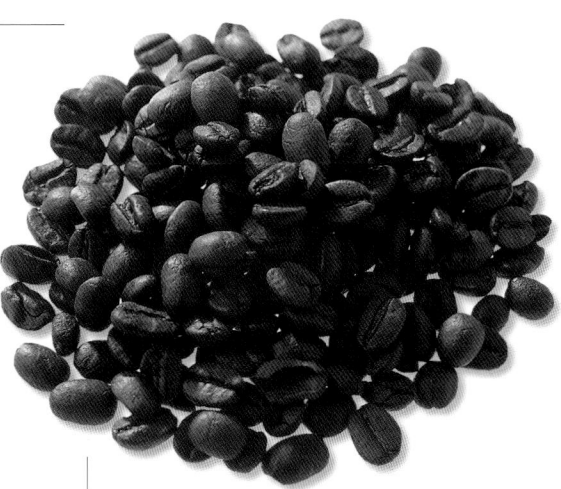

Beans roasted for coffee are derived from ripe berries of the Coffea arabica tree. The berries are also used for the Coffea remedy.

Treatment Use

Coffea is useful when any of the following are indicated:

Mental and emotional aspects

- Hyperactivity and inability to rest the mind
- Insomnia • Over-excitement in children
- Anxiety and feelings of irritability • Sensory overload • Feelings of guilt, particularly over children • Problems in relationships that

Coffea is used to treat overactive mental activity including hyperactivity and over-excitement in children.

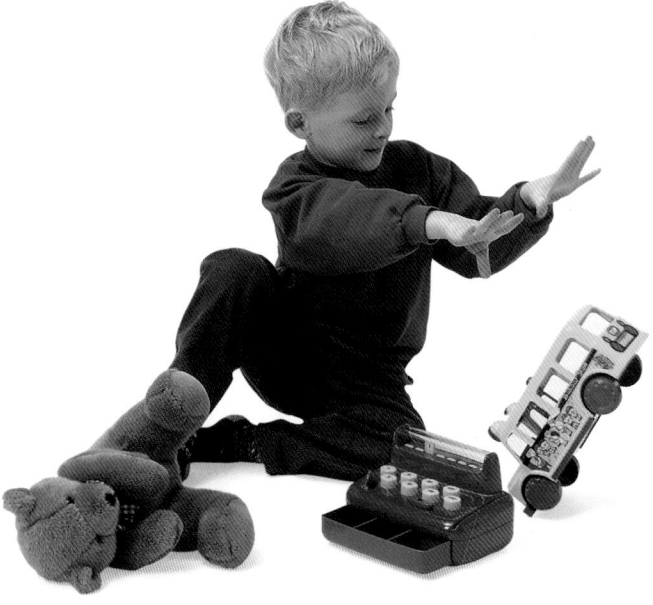

cause physical problems such as headaches and migraines.

Physical aspects

- Sensitive reaction to pain • Headaches
- Facial pain and neuralgia • Palpitations brought on by anger or stress • Skin that reacts in a hypersensitive manner • Migraine.

Modalities

- **Better:** for warmth.
- **Worse:** for the open air and strong smells.

Treatment Tips

A good remedy for insomnia caused by too much mental activity, particularly when combined with an inability to relax.

D r o s e r a

Drosera is derived from a tiny plant that traps insects inside its leaves.

Treatment Use

Drosera is useful when any of the following are indicated:

Mental and emotional aspects

● Feelings of restlessness and anxiety when left alone ● Fear of ghosts ● Difficulty in concentrating ● Sense of persecution ● Prone to talkativeness ● Suspicious of bad or unwelcome news.

Physical aspects

● Colds, especially when accompanied by a violent cough ● Coughs that will not stop and are spasmodic ● Coughs accompanied by nausea or vomiting ● Whooping cough ● Joint pain and growing pains in the legs of teenagers if accompanied by symptoms of stiffness.

Modalities

● **Better:** for being outside in the fresh air and stretching the body and limbs.

● **Worse:** late at night, or lying down for long periods of time; after drinking and eating cold food, after periods of talking.

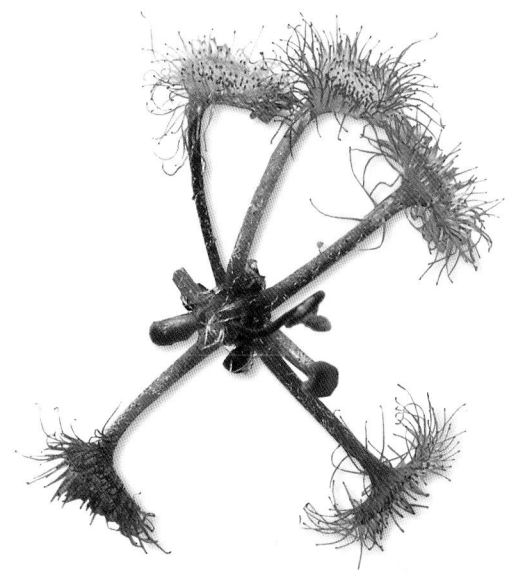

Drosera rotundifolia is a tiny plant found in bogs and heaths. The whole fresh plant in flower is used for the remedy.

Treatment Tips

An excellent remedy for coughs and colds, in particular for a dry, retching cough.

Drosera is good for joint pain and for 'growing pains' of teenagers. The symptoms can be helped by stretching, especially outside.

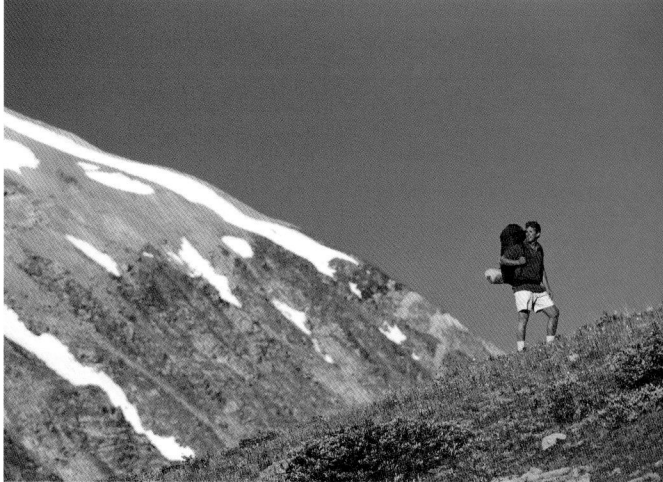

Gelsemium

Gelsemium is derived from the yellow jasmine plant.

Treatment Use

Gelsemium is useful when any of the following are indicated:

Mental and emotional aspects

- Fears and phobias when accompanied by shaking and trembling
- Fear of dentists and doctors • Fear of being left alone • Anxiety about forthcoming events, such as meetings
- Drowsiness and confusion • Panic attacks
- Dislike of insects and creatures that creep and crawl • Difficulty in sleeping.

Physical aspects

- Influenza • Sore throat with red tonsils
- Difficulty swallowing • Fatigue, exhaustion and drowsiness • Coughs and colds
- Shivering • Sneezing with a hot and flushed face • Sore, inflamed eyes • Migraine and headaches, in particular at the base of the skull or the back of the head • Weakness and heaviness in the extremities • Diarrhoea that is made worse when anxious.

The climbing plant Carolina jasmine grows in parts of the United States. Its aromatic fresh roots are used in the remedy.

Modalities

- **Better:** for rest and stillness; after going to the toilet.
- **Worse:** for cold, damp weather.

Treatment Tips

The main remedy for influenza. Also excellent for coughs, colds and sore throats, particularly if accompanied by shivering and fever.

This remedy is a useful addition to a homeopathic first-aid kit.

Gelsemium is used for fears and phobias that cause trembling. The remedy works on the spinal cord and respiratory system.

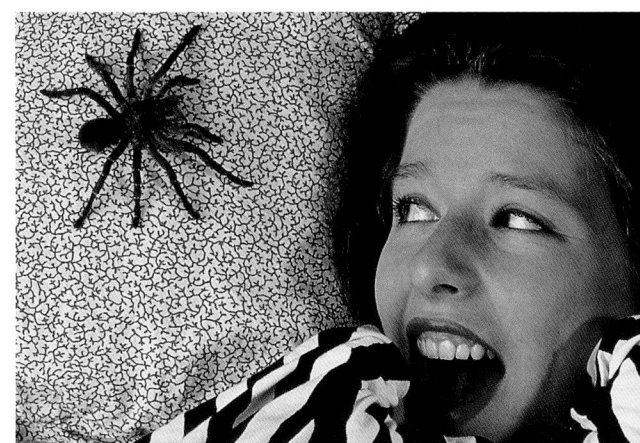

Graphites

Graphites is derived from the mineral graphite or black lead, which is commonly used for pencil leads.

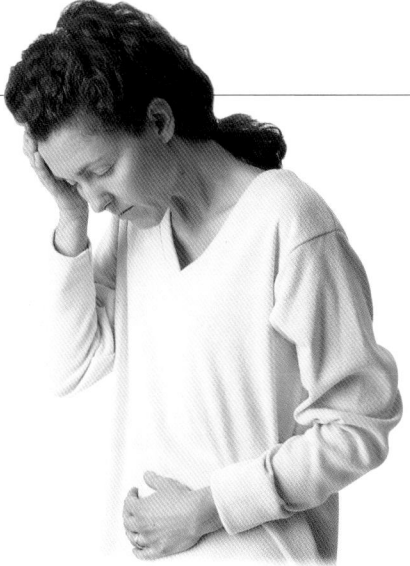

Graphites can be used to a wide range of complaints, including stomach problems and morning headaches.

Treatment Use

Graphites is useful when any of the following are indicated:

Mental and emotional aspects

● Fidgeting, in particular when nervous and anxious ● Easily triggered feelings of guilt ● Depression ● Indecisiveness ● Timidness ● Post-menopausal depression ● Bulimia.

Physical aspects

● Eczema, particularly behind the knees, on the wrist, inside and outside of ears ● Contact dermatitis, particularly on the palms of the hands and between the fingers ● Psoriasis ● Dry, cracked and sore skin ● Itchiness or skin eruptions of the scalp ● Cold sores ● Stomach problems ● Cramp ● Constipation ● Styes ● Nail problems ● Chilblains ● Erratic menstrual cycle ● Morning headaches.

Modalities

● **Better:** for eating.
● **Worse:** for heat.

Treatment Tips

Use to treat the first outbreak of skin complaints – in particular eczema and dermatitis, particularly where there is a discharge. In these cases, the remedy should be supported topically with an application of the homeopathic ointment or cream.

This remedy is a useful addition to a homeopathic first-aid kit.

Graphite is a carbon, the main constituent of pencils. The mineral graphite is ground into a powder to make the Graphites remedy.

Hamamelis

Hamamelis is derived from the witch-hazel plant. The twigs, bark and outer layer of the root are used.

Treatment Use

Hamamelis is useful when any of the following are indicated:

Fresh bark, twigs and the outer root of the witch-hazel plant (Hamamelis virginiana) are ground together and used for the remedy.

Mental and emotional aspects

● Mild depression; the person feels better for being alone ● Irritability and restlessness, particularly in the presence of others.

Physical aspects

● Varicose veins ● Varicocele (varicose veins in the testes) ● Heavy and tired, throbbing and itching, or stinging and aching legs ● Irritated and bloodshot eyes ● Black eyes ● Bruising ● Chilblains ● Nosebleeds ● Mild skin rashes ● Insect bites where accompanied with stinging and aching around the bite ● Mild burns ● Acne and oily skin ● Haemorrhoids.

Modalities

● **Better:** for fresh air; for reading, thinking or talking.

● **Worse:** for warm, damp heat and pressure; for movement.

Treatment Tips

Use at the first sign of varicose veins or haemorrhoids or when these conditions become worse. Treatment can be backed up with a cream or ointment applied directly onto the affected sites.

Hamamelis is excellent for both internal and external bleeding. It can be used to treat bruising of the body caused by injury.

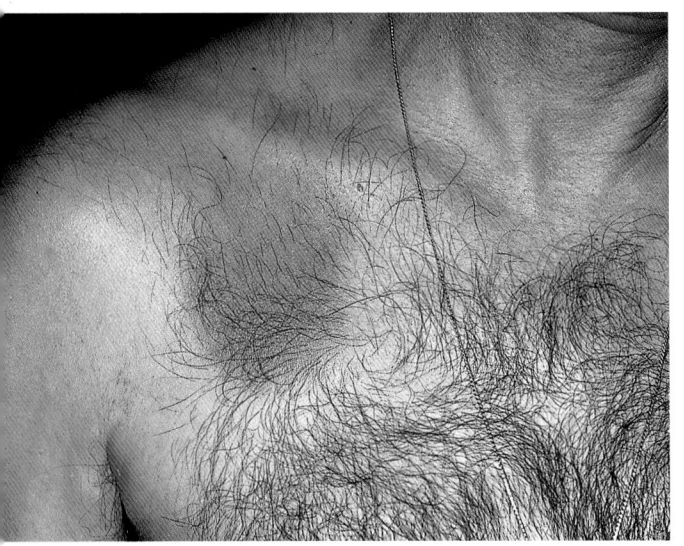

Hepar sulph.

Hepar sulph. is derived from calcium sulphide.

Treatment Use

Hepar sulph. is useful when any of the following are indicated:

Mental and emotional aspects

● Irritation over the slightest matter ● Quick to take offence ● Talks quickly when anxious ● Over-reacts when angry ● Prone to bouts of sadness and depression.

Physical aspects

● All skin problems that gather pus and are slow to heal ● Skin ulcers and bedsores ● Acne and boils ● Earache ● Ear pain with a sore throat ● Catarrh ● Coughs that create a hoarse and dry throat ● Cold sores, particularly around the eyes ● Mouth ulcers ● Influenza with sweating and sneezing ● Cracked dry lips ● Perspiration that causes a bad odour, even when deodorant is used.

Modalities

● **Better:** for warmth and for wrapping up and keeping the head warm.
● **Worse:** for touch and the cold.

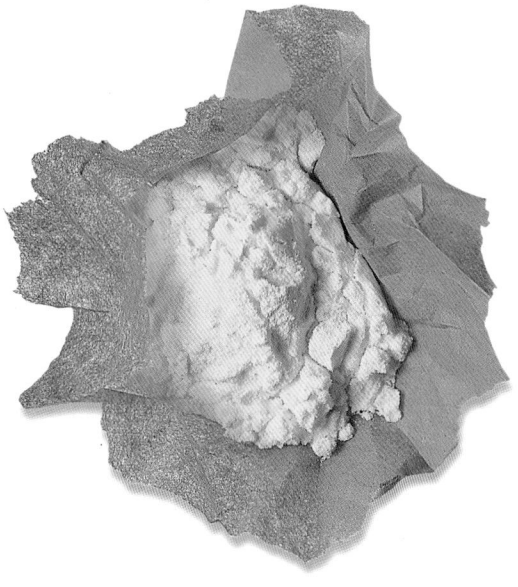

The remedy is prepared chemically by mixing calcium carbonate (derived from oyster shells) together with flowers of sulphur.

Treatment Tips

A good remedy to use when conditions are slow to heal. Good for clearing infection and discharges.

The Hepar sulph. remedy can be used to treat infections that cause earache. It helps to expel the discharge from the site of the infection.

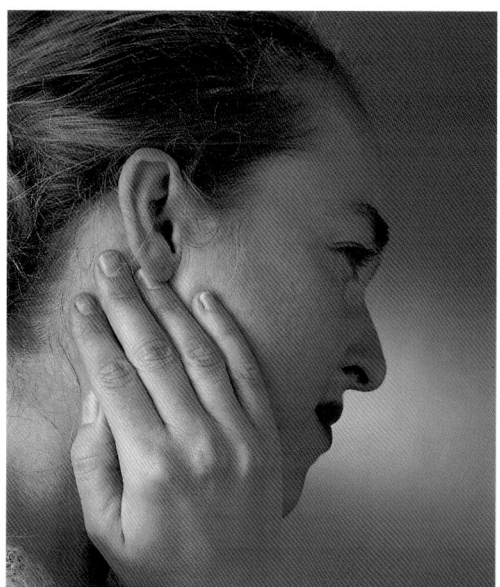

Hypericum

Hypericum is derived from the St John's Wort herb.

Treatment Use

Hypericum is useful when any of the following are indicated:

Mental and emotional aspects

● Depression with tiredness and lethargy

● Depression after surgery or after injury ● Vertigo ● Shock through injury or emotional trauma

● Stress and anxiety that cause spasms and feelings of tightness in the body.

Physical aspects

● Neuralgia ● Puncture wounds received from sharp objects (glass, nails etc) ● Splinters ● All wounds and injuries, in particular if crushing is involved ● Concussion ● Nerve pain or stabbing ● Shooting pains ● Injuries to the feet, hands and spine ● Minor eye injuries ● Chronic back pain, with a sensation of pain travelling up and down the back ● Asthma when in a damp environment

The hypericum plant (Hypericum perforatum) produces a red juice from its flowers and leaves, which are used in the remedy.

● Toothache and pain from dental procedures

● Diarrhoea ● Haemorrhoids with pain and bleeding.

Modalities

● **Better:** for resting the head bent backwards; for gentle massage.

● **Worse:** for cold, damp and foggy weather.

Treatment Tips

A good remedy to use after an injury to the skin, particularly where there is a risk of infection.

This remedy is a useful addition to a homeopathic first-aid kit.

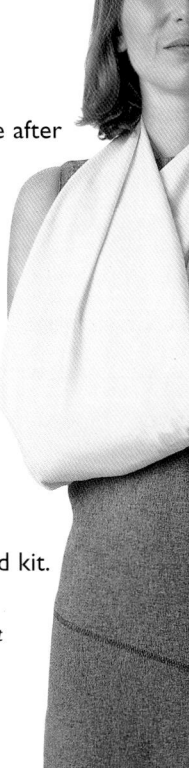

Hypericum can be used to treat nerve pain after injury.

Ignatia

Ignatia is derived from St Ignatius bean, a seedpod from the *Ignatia amara* tree.

Treatment Use

Ignatia is useful when any of the following are indicated:

Mental and emotional aspects

- Highly emotional states • Shock • Anger
- Grief • Inability to express emotions
- Hysteria • Insomnia • Quick, sudden tearfulness • Self-blame and self-pity
- Worry • Sadness over divorce and broken relationships • Sudden, unexpected mood changes • Exhaustion caused by overwork
- Obsessive-compulsive behaviour
- Hypochondria • Jealousy • Fixed ideas.

Physical aspects

- Headaches caused by emotional stress and tension • Coughs and sore throats
- Difficulty in swallowing • Twitching of the face triggered by anxiety • Digestive problems, in particular after shock or grief when accompanied with a sinking sensation • Cravings for odd foods when ill
- Diarrhoea • Disruptive sleep patterns, particularly if grieving.

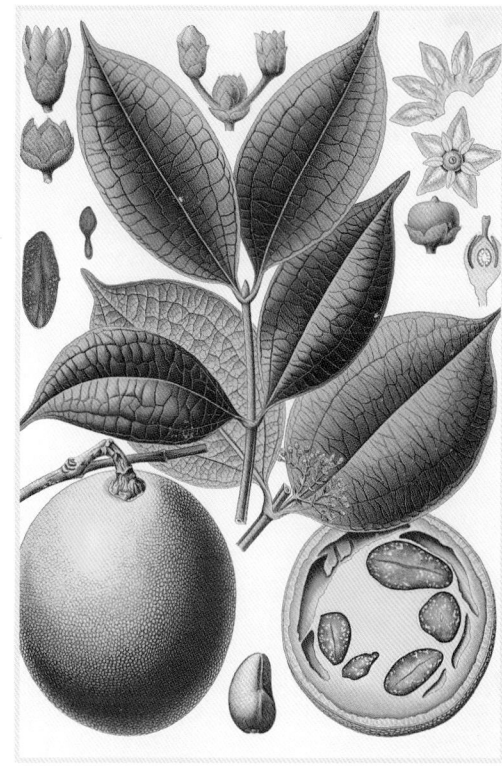

The Ignatia remedy is made from the seeds of the Ignatius amara fruit. The seeds are ground to a powder.

Modalities

- **Better:** for warmth and the sun; change of position.
- **Worse:** in cold air; for emotional upset; in the morning.

Treatment Tips

One of the best remedies for emotional problems. It is good for mood swings, bereavement and any accompanying physical ailments. It is also good if the ailments are very changeable.

Kali phos.

Kali phos. is derived from potassium phosphate.

Treatment Use

Kali phos. is useful when any of the following are indicated:

Mental and emotional aspects

- Complete exhaustion
- Oversensitive reactions and nervousness when stressed
- Frustration due to lack of assertiveness
- Shyness and withdrawal when anxious
- Nervousness when meeting people
- Depression, including post-viral depression
- Nightmares
- Lack of concentration and poor memory
- Fear of a nervous breakdown.

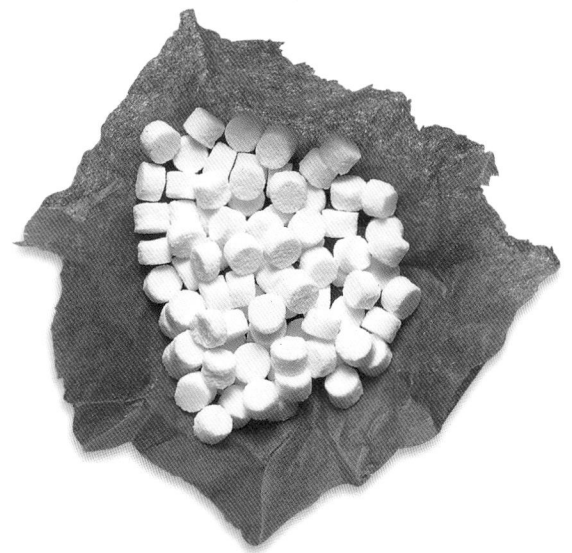

The Kali phos. remedy is prepared chemically from potassium carbonate, derived from potash and dilute phosphoric acid.

Physical aspects

- Weakness of limbs
- Neck and upper back pain
- Tension headaches
- Dizziness after rising from sitting or kneeling
- Chronic fatigue syndrome
- Discharges from colds and catarrh
- Productive coughs
- Diarrhoea
- Cystitis.

Modalities

- **Better:** for heat and movement.
- **Worse:** for worry.

Treatment Tips

Known as the 'great nerve soother', this is excellent in the treatment of all forms of exhaustion, particularly those brought on by stress.

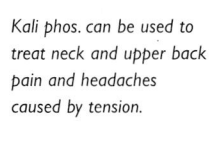

Kali phos. can be used to treat neck and upper back pain and headaches caused by tension.

Lachesis

Lachesis is derived from the venom of the bushmaster snake.

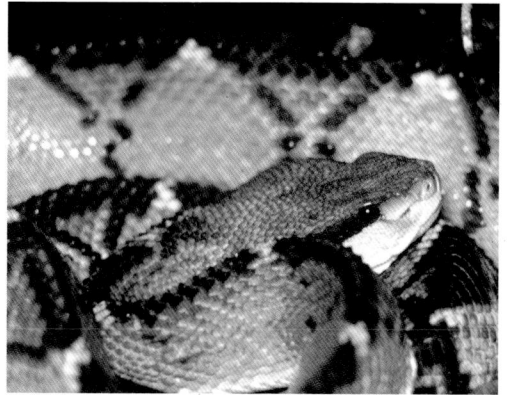

The fresh venom of the bushmaster snake can be dried and made into the remedy.

Treatment Use

Lachesis is useful when any of the following are indicated:

Mental and emotional aspects

● Hypersensitivity ● Talkative, rambling, self-absorbed nature ● Restlessness ● Fixed ideas and opinions, in particular about religion ● Fear of personal attack or burglary ● Suspicion of new people ● Jealousy and suspicion of loved ones ● No desire to mix with people ● Suppression of anger ● Nightmares ● Irritability ● Anger after the break-up of relationships ● Addictions, including alcohol, tobacco and drugs ● Premenstrual syndrome ● Post-menopausal depression ● Panic attacks.

Physical aspects

● Headaches, particularly on waking ● Puffy, bloated or swollen face ● Stomach-ache when craving stimulants ● Constrictive, sore throats ● Asthma ● Angina pain ● Palpitations and tightness or constriction of the chest ● Hot flushes ● Bloatedness ● Varicose veins ● Haemorrhoids ● Varicocele (varicose veins in the testes) ● Phlebitis and thrombosis ● Menopausal problems.

Modalities

● **Better:** in the open air; for eating and cool drinks.
● **Worse:** when trying to sleep; for touch; for tight clothing

Treatment Tips

Excellent for all circulatory problems. Also good for extreme stress when accompanied with pains and tightness in the chest.

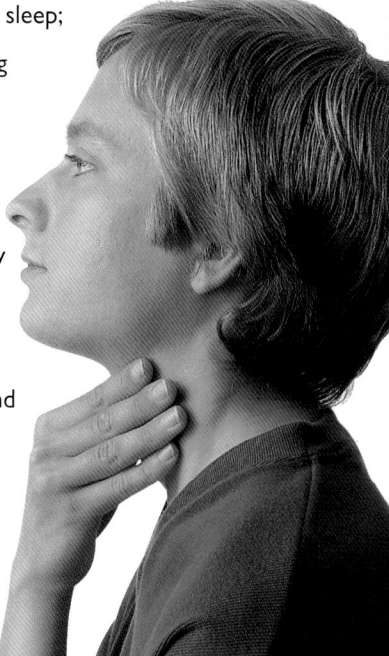

Swollen, sore throats are helped by Lachesis, which eases the pain and makes it easier to take in fluids that were previously difficult to swallow.

Ledum

Ledum is derived from the wild rosemary plant.

Treatment Use

Ledum is useful when any of the following are indicated:

Mental and emotional aspects

- Sleep disturbance with night sweats
- Impatience • Timidness.

Physical aspects

- Feelings of hotness and swelling triggered by stress • Wounds
- Stings with bruising and puffiness • Grazes and cuts • Bites
- It can prevent cuts, bites or stings from becoming infected • Injury to the eyes
- Arthritic and rheumatic pain affecting the ankles, knees or lower legs • Hot, burning sensations in the limbs • Gout.

Modalities

- **Better:** for cold compresses.
- **Worse:** at night; with heat.

The Ledum remedy can be used to help alleviate night sweats and sleeplessness.

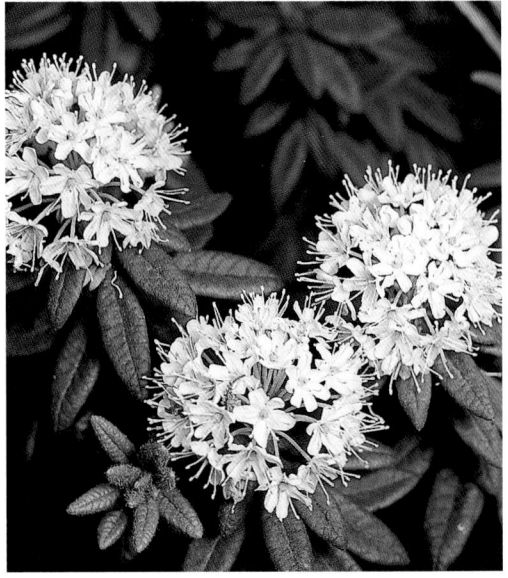

Fresh, flowering wild rosemary plants (Ledum palustre) are dried and powdered to make the remedy.

Treatment Tips

This is an ideal remedy for puncture wounds. It can prevent any infection caused through bites, stings and cuts.

This remedy is a useful addition to a homeopathic first-aid kit.

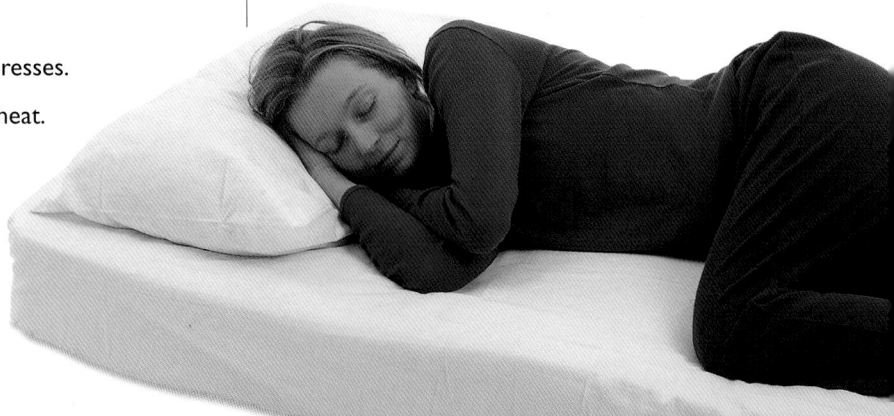

Lycopodium

Lycopodium is derived from the pollen dust of an evergreen herb.

Treatment Use

Lycopodium is useful when any of the following are indicated:

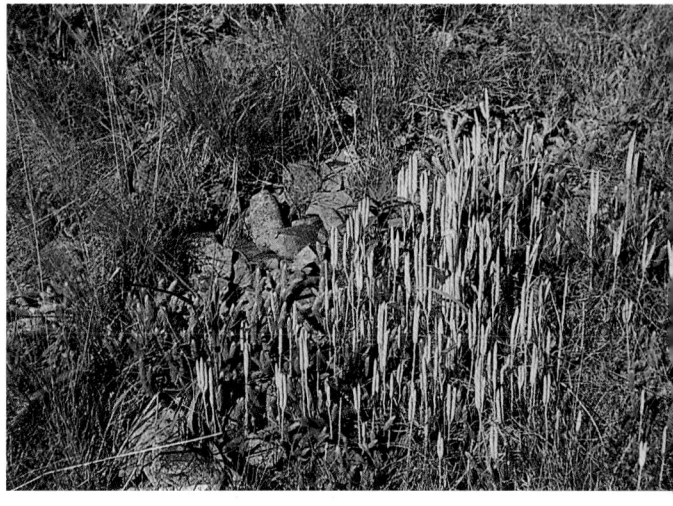

The flowering spikes of the lycopodium herb provide yellow pollen dust, which is shaken out of the plant and used for the remedy.

Mental and emotional aspects

● Lack of self-confidence ● Sexual fears ● Anxiety and fear of interviews and speeches ● Sensitivity ● Forgetfulness ● Irritation caused by minor matters ● Dislike of being contradicted ● Feelings of stress when meeting strangers ● Fear of ghosts, death and the dark ● Dislike of being alone ● Suppression of fears ● Agoraphobia ● Chronic fatigue syndrome ● Nervous breakdown ● Bulimia.

Physical aspects

● Digestive disorders including indigestion, irritable bowel syndrome, nausea, ulcers, hunger pains, feeling bloated after little food, flatulence, constipation ● Impotence ● Sore throats ● Dry cough ● Extreme tiredness followed by colds or influenza ● Bladder and kidney problems, including kidney stones ● Prostate problems ● Hair loss ● Restless legs at night ● Cold hands and feet ● Headaches over the eyes ● Shoulder pain ● Varicose veins ● Chronic eczema.

Modalities

● **Better:** for small meals and movement.
● **Worse:** for heat and stuffy environment.

Treatment Tips

The first remedy to use for digestive disorders.

The Lycopodium remedy helps cure digestive complaints, particularly indigestion.

Merc. Sol.

Merc. sol. is derived from the black oxide of mercury.

Treatment Use

Merc. sol. is useful when any of the following are indicated:

Mental and emotional aspects

- Slowness and sluggishness of thought
- Distrust of others • Fear of burglary and abuse • Poor memory and difficulty in recall
- Mental and emotional weakness and fatigue
- Chronic fatigue syndrome • Restlessness and anxiety • Deep insecurity
- Suspiciousness • Sensitivity to criticism
- Quick, sudden and aggressive temper
- Lack of willpower • Tendency to be arrogant • Emotional repression.

Physical aspects

- Stammering • Dribbling from the mouth

Liquid mercury is dissolved in dilute nitric acid, forming a greyish-black precipitate. This is used to make the remedy.

when sleeping • Tiredness in the limbs and feelings of weakness through the whole body • Body odour
- Cutting, burning pains • Gum and mouth problems • Mouth ulcers
- Bad taste in the mouth, in particular a metallic taste • Oral thrush • Sore throats
- Cold sores • Conjunctivitis with discharge
- Spasmodic coughs • Joint pain • Catarrh
- Scalp problems, eruptions and crustiness of the scalp • Bed sores.

Modalities

- **Better:** for rest in moderate temperatures.
- **Worse:** at night; for heat or changes in temperature.

Treatment Tips

An excellent remedy for problems with the mouth, especially mouth ulcers and gum problems.

Merc. sol. can be used to treat mouth and throat complaints, including gingivitis, halitosis and tonsillitis.

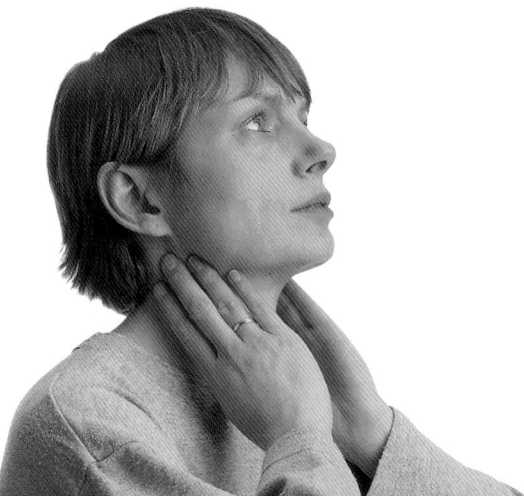

Natrum mur.

Natrum mur. is derived from a mineral rock salt called sodium chloride.

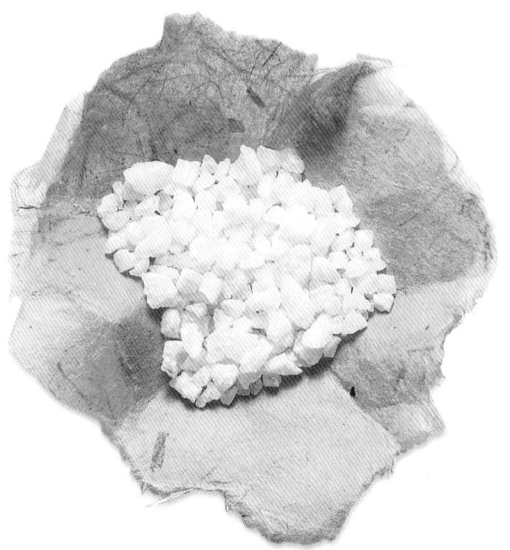

Rock salt is the source of this remedy. It is formed by the evaporation of salty water, which leaves a thick, salty crust behind.

Treatment Use

Natrum mur. is useful when any of the following are indicated:

Mental and emotional aspects

- Anxiety and depression caused by suppressed grief • Repressed fear
- Agoraphobia • Fear of thunderstorms
- Hypochondria • Agitation • Guilt
- Anorexia • Shock • Low self-worth
- Premenstrual syndrome • Quick changing of emotions without warning • Resentment
- Tendency to sulk or keep feelings locked up.

Physical aspects

- Sunstroke • Migraine • Eye strain
- Cold sores • Cracked and dry lips
- Mouth ulcers • Inflamed gums • Boils and warts • Anaemia • Constipation • Backache
- Irregular periods • Hair loss • Oily skin and hair • Coughs and colds • Palpitations.

Treatment Tips

A good remedy for people who brood on the past. Very good for treating emotional trauma such as anxiety or depression caused by loss, grief or separation.

The Natrum mur. remedy may help a fear of thunderstorms. Symptoms of anxiety may be made worse by thundery weather.

Modalities

- **Better:** for cool, fresh air.
- **Worse:** for heat and sunlight; on waking.

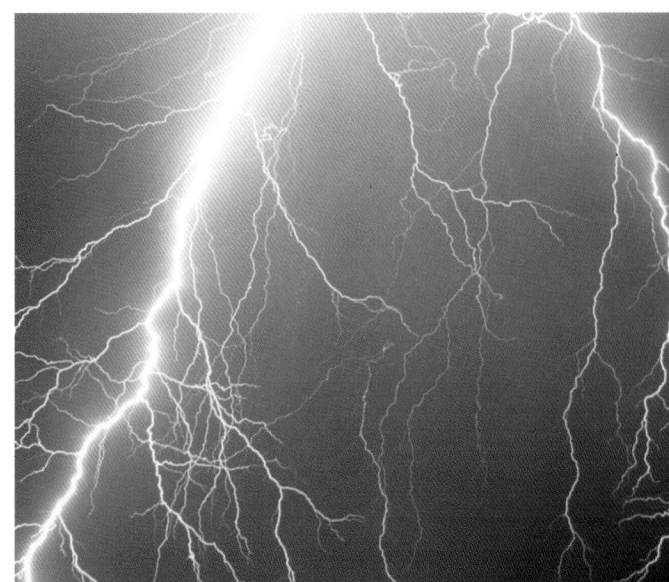

Nux vomica

Nux vomica is derived from the poison strychnine, which is extracted from the seeds of the *Strychnos nux vomica* tree.

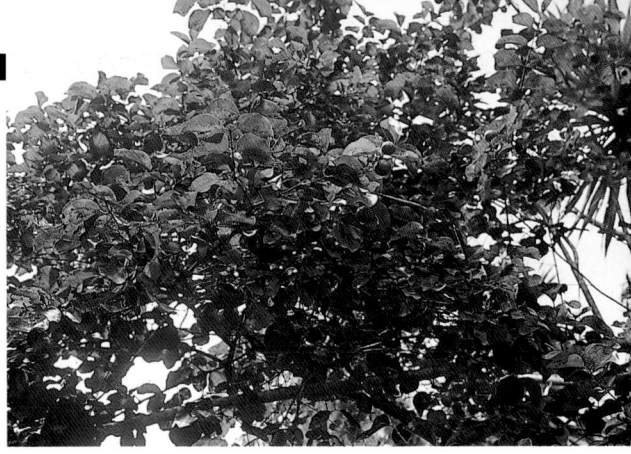

The leaves, bark and seeds of the the Strychnos nux vomica *tree all contain strychnine, but it is usually extracted from the dried seeds.*

Treatment Use

Nux vomica is useful when any of the following are indicated:

Mental and emotional aspects

● Tendency to over-indulge ● Cravings for stimulants such as alcohol, tobacco and rich foods ● Addictive nature ● Fear of failure ● Argumentative ● Critical ● Fear of spiders and beetles ● Dread of death ● Depression ● Insomnia ● Hyperactivity ● Frustration.

Physical aspects

● Digestive problems, such as indigestion and heartburn ● Food poisoning ● Vomiting ● Constipation ● Diarrhoea ● Stomach cramps ● Lower back pain ● Hiccups ● Headaches and migraines ● Hay fever ● Colds and influenza ● Blocked nose ● Heavy, aching muscles ● Fragility ● Morning sickness and cramp in pregnancy.

Modalities

● **Better:** for sleep.
● **Worse:** in the morning.

Treatment Tips

Excellent 'hangover' remedy. Also good for aiding digestion and promoting the appetite.

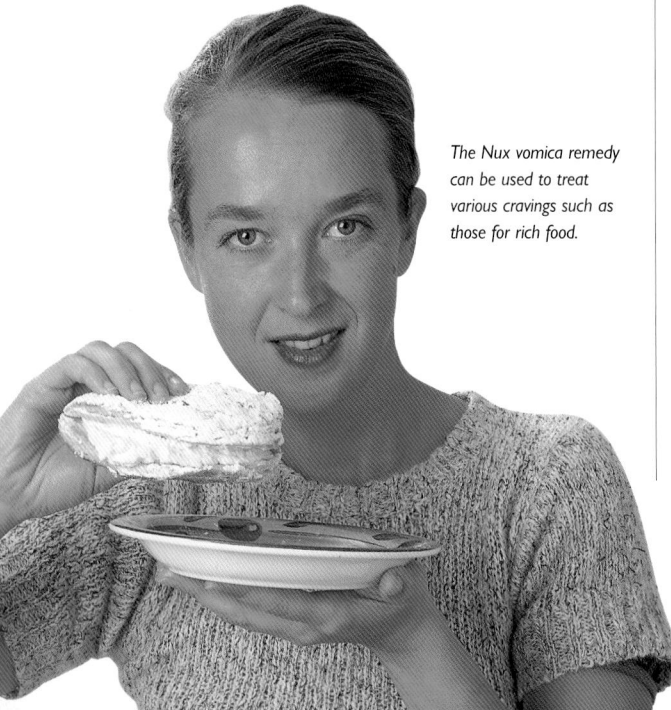

The Nux vomica remedy can be used to treat various cravings such as those for rich food.

This remedy is a useful addition to a homeopathic first-aid kit.

Phosphorus

Phosphorus is derived from a mineral found in phosphates and living matter. It is found in bones, teeth and bodily fluids.

Treatment Use

Phosphorus is useful when any of the following are indicated:

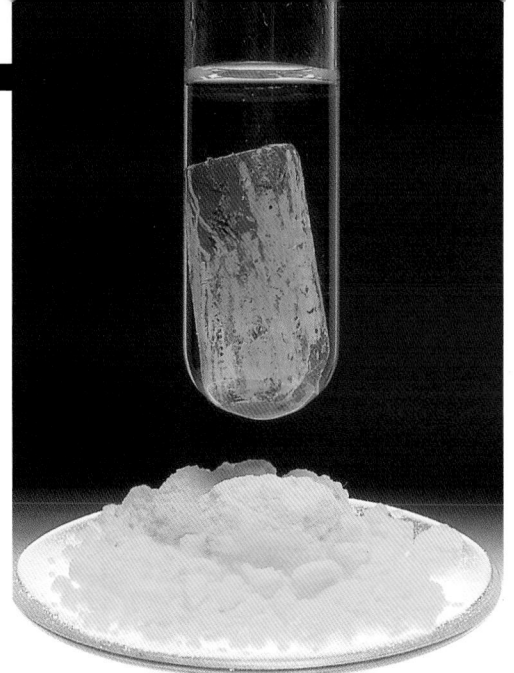

Phosphorus is a yellowish non-metallic mineral, derived from phosphates and living matter.

Mental and emotional aspects

- Hypersensitivity • Excessive imagination
- Easily angered • Fear of darkness and death
- Suppression of fear • Fixed ideas • Fatigue
- Craving for reassurance • Unnecessary worry about health • Nightmares and insomnia • Facial twitches • Shock
- Low spirits • Clairvoyant episodes
- Preference for company and fear of loneliness.

Physical aspects

- Unproductive, hard, dry cough with a tight, heavy chest • Low resistance to infections
- Sore throat with hoarseness • Pneumonia
- Bronchitis • Feels the cold • Asthma
- Bruising • Nose bleeds • Bleeding gums
- Heavy periods • Headaches • Vertigo
- Styes • Panic attacks • Exhaustion and fatigue • Food poisoning • Heartburn

- Back pain with a burning, hot sensation
- Dandruff • Weakness in the extremities.

Modalities

- **Better:** for warm, fresh air; touch and rubbing.
- **Worse:** for over-exertion; at night.

Treatment Tips

This is the ideal remedy for relieving ailments that are triggered by fear and anxiety as it helps to soothe the nervous system.

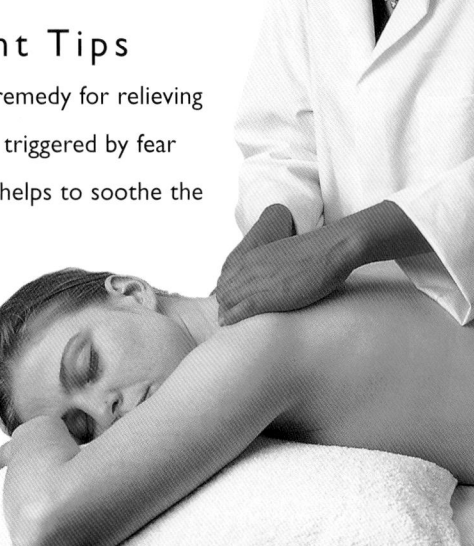

The symptoms helped by the Phosphorus remedy may be further alleviated by massage or rubbing.

Pulsatilla

Pulsatilla is derived from the pulsatilla plant, which is native to Scandinavia, Denmark, Germany and Russia. The fresh plant in flower is used.

Treatment Use

Pulsatilla is useful when any of the following are indicated:

Mental and emotional aspects

• Tendency to burst into tears without warning • Quiet temperament • Suppression of fear • Depression • Obsessive-compulsive behaviour • Fear of the opposite sex • Fear of the dark and ghosts • Very tearful when grieving • Bulimia.

Physical aspects

• Coughs and colds • Runny nose • Catarrh • Conjunctivitis • Digestive problems • Irritable bowel syndrome • All menstrual and menopausal problems, particularly if accompanied

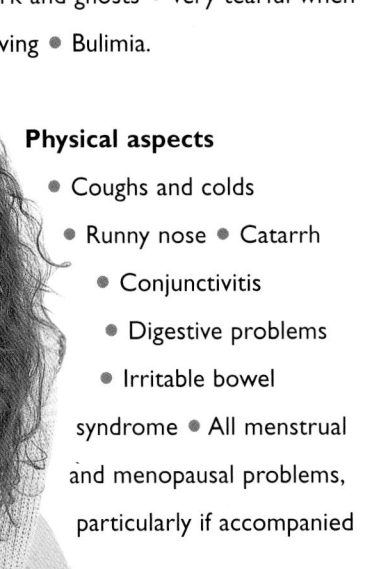

The Pulsatilla remedy is useful for depression and weepiness.

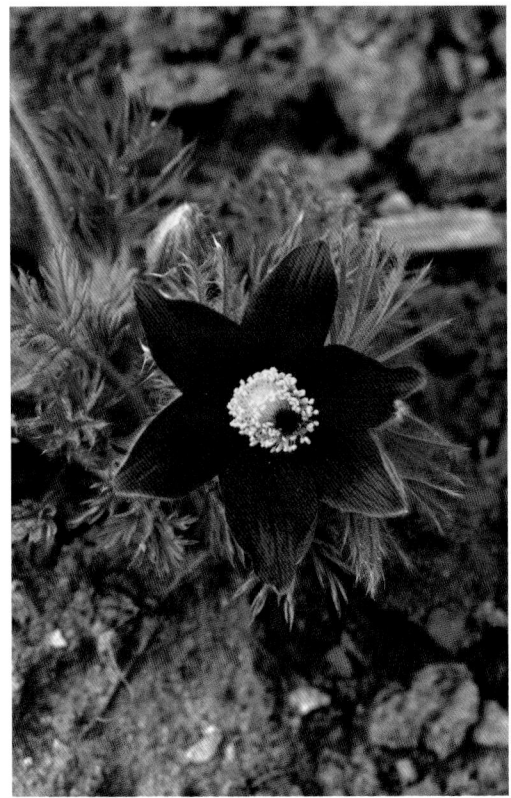

The flowers of the pulsatilla plant Pulsatilla nigricans *are crushed for their juices, which are used to make the remedy.*

by depression • Lower back pain • Headaches • Varicose veins • Arthritis • Styes • Incontinence • Skin problems.

Modalities

• **Better:** for crying and sympathy; cool, fresh air; gentle exercise.
• **Worse:** for heat; for rich or fatty foods.

Treatment Tips

This remedy works well on the mental state of the individual.

Rhus tox.

Rhus tox. is derived from the fresh leaves of the poison ivy plant.

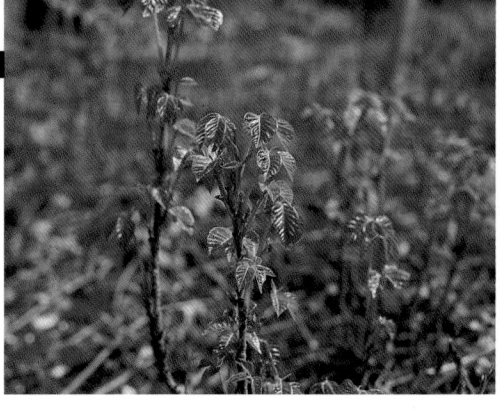

The leaves are collected from the poison ivy plant before it flowers and are pulped to make the remedy.

Treatment Use

Rhus tox. is useful when any of the following are indicated:

Mental and emotional aspects

- Irritability • Depression • Suicidal thoughts • Lack of joy in life • Anxiousness • Fear of being poisoned • Anxiety at night.

Physical aspects

- Skin problems, including eczema, dermatitis and blistering • Burning, itching, swollen skin • Cold sores • Nappy rash • Sciatica • Chicken pox • Shingles • Influenza • Sore, stinging eyes • Muscular aches and pains • Stiffness • Joint pain • Back pain • Arthritis and rheumatism • Sprains and strains • Jaw pain • Frozen shoulder • Neuralgia • Post-operative recovery • Repetitive strain injury.

Modalities

- **Better:** for movement; for a warm, dry atmosphere.
- **Worse:** for rest and stillness; for cold, damp weather.

Treatment Tips

This is an excellent remedy for muscular aches and pains. Eczema and other skin problems often respond to this remedy when others fail.

This remedy is a useful addition to a homeopathic first-aid kit.

The Rhus tox. remedy may help repetitive strain injury, which can be caused by spending long hours using a computer keyboard.

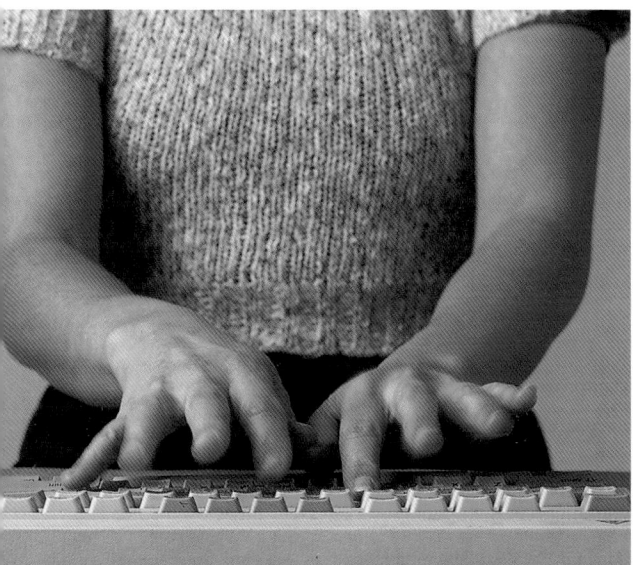

Ruta grav.

Ruta grav. is derived from the *Ruta graveolens* herb. The juice from the whole plant is used, before the plant flowers.

Treatment Use

Ruta grav. is useful when any of the following are indicated:

Mental and emotional aspects

- Low personal satisfaction
- Depression ● Critical of others and self ● Anxiety.

Physical aspects

- Aches and pains in bones and muscles ● Deep, aching pain
- Arthritis and rheumatism ● Lower back pain, where the pain feels deep and penetrating ● Repetitive strain injury
- Injuries to ligaments, tendons and cartilage
- Sciatic pain ● Chest and rib pain caused by coughing ● Eye strain and exhaustion from overwork ● Headaches, in particular from reading ● Constipation.

Modalities

- **Better:** for movement.
- **Worse:** for cold, damp weather; lying down.

Juice is extracted from the whole plant (Ruta graveolens) before it flowers.

Treatment Tips

This remedy acts upon the periosteum (the lining of the bone) and cartilage, so it is excellent for injuries to gliding joints such as the ankle and wrist. This remedy is also the first choice for repetitive strain injury – an inflammation of the tendon sheaths of the arm and wrist.

Ruta grav. can be used for deep aching pain and rheumatism. Damp weather can make the symptoms of such conditions worse.

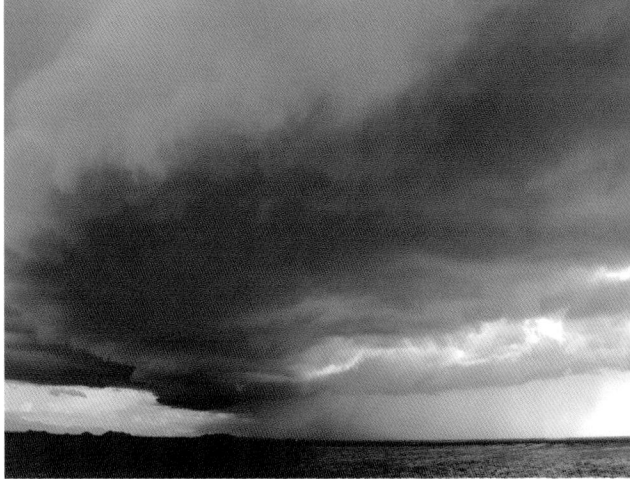

Sepia

Sepia is derived from the ink of the cuttlefish.

Treatment Use

Sepia is useful when any of the following are indicated:

Mental and emotional aspects

- Menopausal depression
- Exhaustion and slowness of thought • Feelings of weakness • Tendency to cry easily • Stress and anxiety • Feelings of being unable to cope • Fear of sickness and disease • Fixed ideas • Irritability • Grief, particularly on separation or relationship break-ups.

Physical aspects

- Chronic fatigue syndrome
- Menopausal problems, including hot flushes and night sweats • Ovarian, vaginal and

The Sepia remedy can be used to treat hot flushes during the menopause.

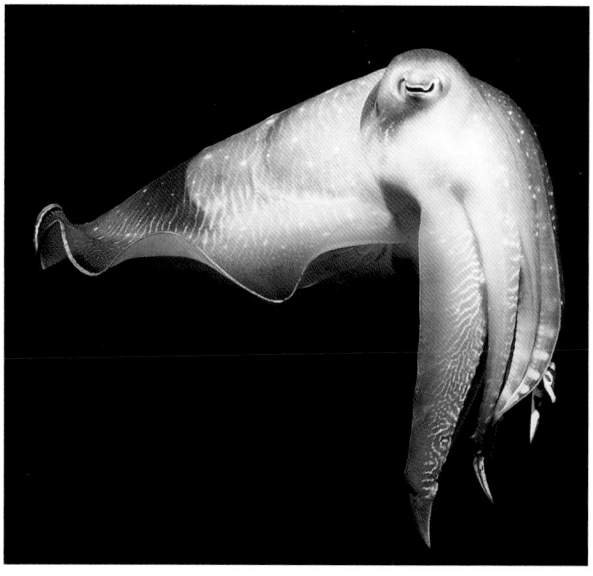

The cuttlefish squirts a dark ink for its protection. The pigments from the ink are used to make the remedy.

uterine complaints, including prolapse of the uterus • Heavy periods • Thrush • Backache • Flatulence and abdominal and stomach tenderness • Headaches and migraines • Constipation • Haemorrhoids and varicose veins • Hair loss • Tiredness • Dizziness • Sweaty feet.

Modalities

- **Better:** for sleep; warmth; gentle exercise.
- **Worse:** in the morning; for a sedentary lifestyle.

Treatment Tips

An excellent remedy for women, because it helps greatly with menopausal problems. It is also good for exhaustion.

S i l i c e a

Silicea is derived from the main part of most rocks and plant stems. It is also found in teeth, hair and bones. This remedy is mainly derived from quartz or flint.

Treatment Use

Silicea is useful when any of the following are indicated:

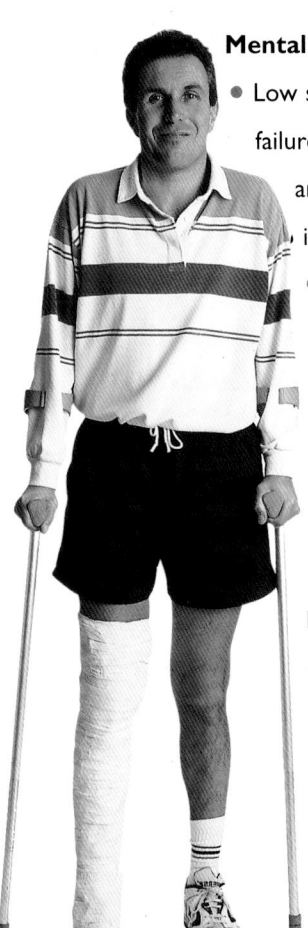

Rock crystal is a type of quartz. Traditionally, quartz or flint have been used to prepare the remedy.

Mental and emotional aspects

- Low self-confidence • Fear of failure • Lack of assertiveness and timidity • Anxiety about important events
- Exhaustion after periods of concentration
- Performance fear
- Obsessiveness about detail • Stubbornness
- Fear of commitment.

Physical aspects

- Weak immune system
- Weak nervous system
- Slowness of healing, particularly broken bones and fractures • Recurrent

The Silicea remedy can be used for helping fractured bones to heal.

coughs, colds and respiratory infections
- Ear infections • Sore, throbbing throat
- Swelling of glands • Catarrh • Chest infections, especially if a family history of tuberculosis • Boils • Headaches, especially if triggered by cold • Painful joints and bones
- Anorexia and under-nourishment in general
- Unhealthy skin, including acne • Slow bone growth in babies and children • Light-sensitive eyes • Poor sense of smell • Cracking at the corner of the mouth • Sensitive gums
- Constipation • Sweaty feet and head.

Modalities

- **Better:** for keeping warm.
- **Worse:** for cold damp weather; draughts.

Treatment Tips

A good remedy to use if an individual has low resistance to disease and is slow to recover from infection.

Staphysagria

Staphysagria is derived from the seed of the plant sometimes known as stavesacre or palmated larkspur. It was used by the Greeks and Romans as a remedy.

Treatment Use

Staphysagria is useful when any of the following are indicated:

Mental and emotional aspects

- Suppression of emotions, in particular anger
- Outbursts of temper • Fixated about an illness, symptom or emotional problem
- Likes to be alone • Sensitive to criticism and easily offended • Resentment and jealousy • Hypersensitivity • Sex addiction
- Workaholic • Over-indulgence in alcohol, tobacco or food.

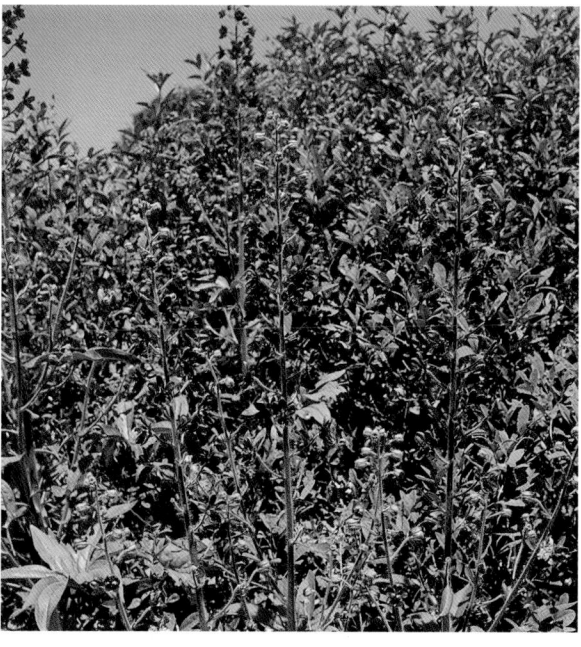

The seeds of the Delphinium staphysagria plant are used to make the remedy.

Physical aspects

- Post-operative trauma • Enlargement of prostate gland • Skin problems • Headaches
- Flatulence • Teething problems • Neuralgia
- Styes • Inflammation of the eyes

Modalities

- **Better:** for warmth.
- **Worse:** for suppressing emotions; touch.

Treatment Tips

It can be used to treat suppressed emotions and anger, and diseases stemming from these.

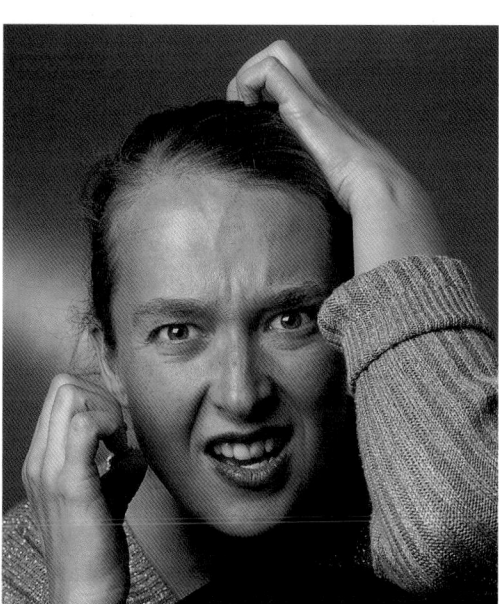

The remedy Staphysagria can be used to control suppressed rage.

Sulphur

Sulphur is derived from the mineral sulphur.

Treatment Use

Sulphur is useful when any of the following are indicated:

A powder called flowers of sulphur is extracted from the mineral sulphur and used to make the remedy.

Mental and emotional aspects

● Forgetfulness ● Inability to think clearly ● Lack of regard for others ● Laziness ● Irritability ● Self-centredness and selfishness ● Argumentative ● Aggressive tendencies ● Claustrophobia ● Fear of heights (vertigo) ● Fear of oppression ● Bulimia ● Insomnia ● Post-menopausal depression ● Alcoholism ● Addiction to smoking ● Lack of willpower ● Nightmares.

Physical aspects

● Burning, itching skin ● Eczema, dermatitis, psoriasis ● Thrush ● Nappy rash ● Catarrh ● Hot, sweaty burning feet ● Digestive disorders ● Constipation ● Diarrhoea ● Indigestion ● Loss of appetite ● Haemorrhoids ● Lower back pain ● Gout ● Headaches ● Conjunctivitis ● Red, sore and itchy eyes ● Offensive body odour ● Menopausal problems such as hot flushes and dizziness ● Hair loss ● Dry, itchy scalp ● Dry lips ● Sore throats ● Stiff knees and ankles.

Modalities

● **Better:** for warm, fresh air.
● **Worse:** early mornings and late nights; damp, cold weather; washing; prolonged sitting and standing.

Treatment Tips

Skin problems, particularly where the skin is red and itchy (such as eczema), respond well to this remedy. It is also a good general remedy for detoxification.

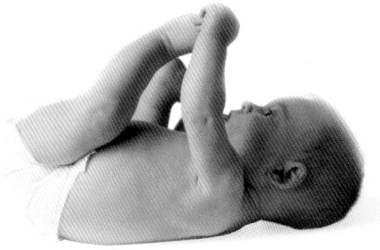

The remedy Sulphur can be used to treat skin conditions such as nappy rash.

Thuja

Thuja is derived from the leaves and twigs of the evergreen conifer tree, which is commonly known as the white cedar tree.

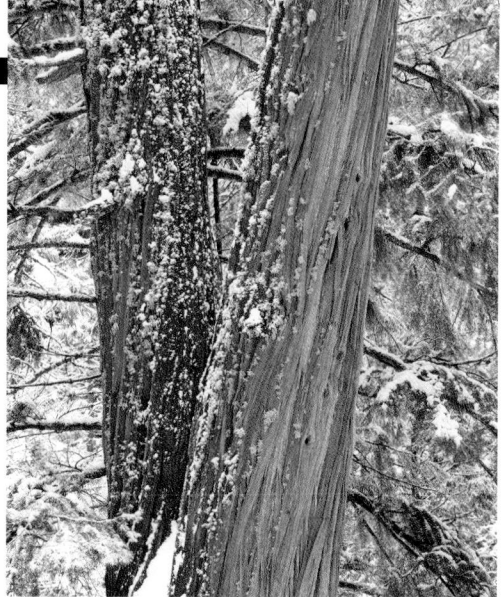

The leaves and twigs of the arborvitae conifer (Thuja occidentalis) are pounded to make the remedy.

Treatment Use

Thuja is useful when any of the following are indicated:

Mental and emotional aspects

● Anorexia ● Distorted ideas of body image ● Fear of strangers ● Facial twitches ● Fixed ideas ● Anxiety ● Cries easily ● Dyslexia ● Paranoia ● Interrupted sleep ● Lack of self-esteem ● Secretive ● Manipulative but weak.

Physical aspects

● Warts ● Verrucas ● Skin complaints ● Very oily skin ● Acne ● Perspiration with odour ● Headaches ● Polyps of the nose ● Styes ● Nail problems ● Haemorrhoids ● Loss of appetite ● Constantly cold ● Urethral and vaginal infections ● Menstrual problems including cramps.

Modalities

● **Better:** for movement.
● **Worse:** for cold and damp; at night.

Treatment Tips

Thuja is the first remedy of choice for dealing with warts and verrucas. In addition, it can be applied topically to provide back-up to the oral treatment.

In addition to its use in dealing with warts, verrucas and other skin complaints, Thuja remedy can be used to combat loss of appetite.

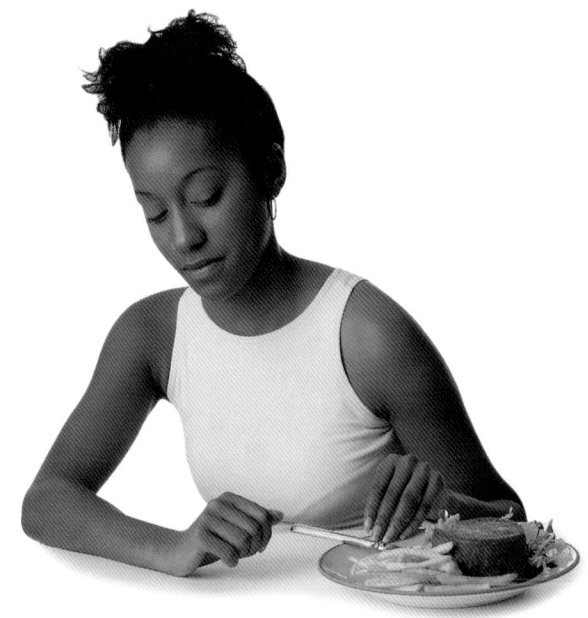

Zinc. Met.

Zinc. met. is derived from zinc.

Treatment Use

Zinc. met. is useful when any of the following are indicated:

Mental and emotional aspects

- Mental fatigue • Poor memory
- Restlessness • Depression • Alcoholism
- Irritability • Jumpiness • Constant fidgeting.

Physical aspects

- Exhaustion • Restless legs • Tiredness through lack of sleep • Weakness and exhaustion • Head feels heavy • Chilblains • Cramp • Varicose veins • Chronic fatigue syndrome • Bulimia • Sensitivity to noise • Anaemia.

Modalities

- **Better:** for bowel movement; emotional reassurance.
- **Worse:** after food.

Treatment Tips

A good remedy for lack of vitality or for treating exhaustion. It is also good for constant feelings of coldness.

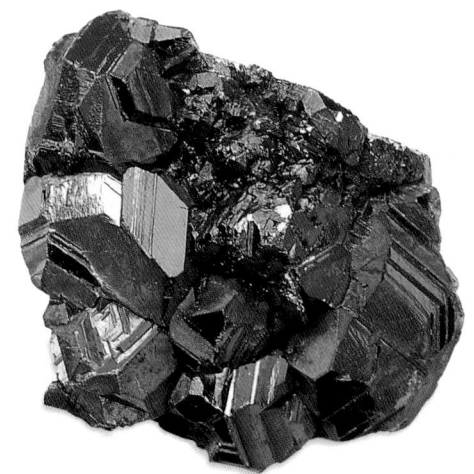

Zinc is a bluish metal; it is ground up to make the powder from which the remedy is made.

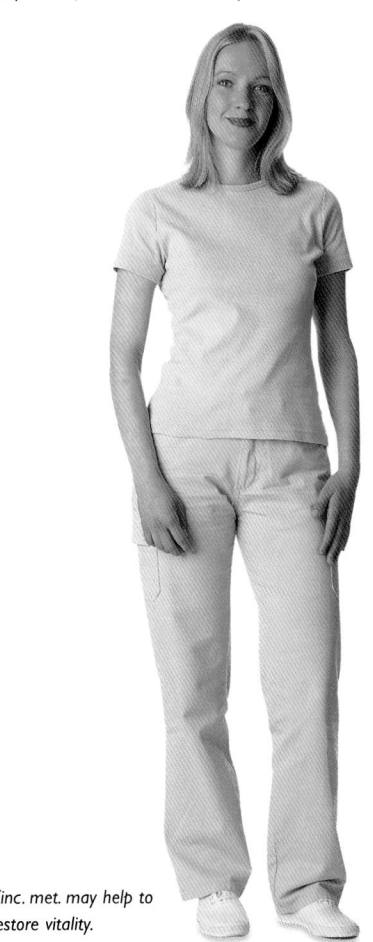

Zinc. met. may help to restore vitality.

Topical Applications

Some homeopathic remedies can be used in preparations that are applied directly to the skin. These are known as topical applications and are an ideal way to back up the oral remedies. They can also be used on their own or as a first-aid treatment. Topical treatments come in the forms listed below.

Forms of Topical Treatments

Creams: Easily absorbed.

Ointments: Greasier than creams in texture; best for larger areas.

Tinctures: Liquid remedies ready for dilution in water; best for cuts and grazes. Dilute according to instructions.

Massage balms: Remedies in vegetable oil base, ready for massage.

Sprays: Ready-mixed; useful for insect bites and stings (eg, pyrethrum spray).

The following remedies are the most widely available topical applications and are listed with the conditions they are usually used to treat.

Arnica: Bruising. Muscular aches and pains. Sprains and strains. After sport or exercise. Joint pain. Aching and stiff back. Tired, aching feet. First signs of repetitive strain injury. Frozen shoulder. Neck pain and stiffness. Sunburn (but do not apply to broken skin).

Calendula: Sensitive, dry, irritated, cracked and inflamed skin. Acne. Contact dermatitis. Eczema. Rashes. Cradle cap. Cold sores. Razor burn. Sunburn. Can be used on babies for minor irritations such as nappy rash and grazes. Good for cleaning cuts and wounds. Can be used as a facial moisturiser or aftershave balm.

Graphites: Eczema. Contact dermatitis. Psoriasis. Varicose eczema, or to help prevent it where skin is dry, thin and translucent. Extremely dry, itchy, sore skin. Sore skin in and around the nose accompanied by a cold. Cold sores. Use as a facial moisturiser to help clear eczema, dermatitis or allergic reaction to cosmetics.

Hamamelis: Sore, burning, itching skin. Varicose veins. Phlebitis. Haemorrhoids. Heavy, aching legs and feet, in particular after long periods of standing. *Always apply lightly around varicose sites. Do not use on broken skin.*

Hypericum: Cuts, sores, wounds, scrapes and grazes. Cold sores. Itchy, irritated and inflamed skin. Splinters. Nail irritations (nail-bed cuts or bitten, sore nails). Cracked, sore lips. Blisters. Sore, bleeding haemorrhoids.

Rhus tox.: Muscular aches and pains, in particular from physical over-exertion. Repetitive strain injury. Joint pain, including tennis elbow and knee injuries. Arthritis and rheumatism. Sciatica. Useful to use after Arnica, once the bruising has diminished. *Do not apply to broken skin.*

Ruta grav.: Stiffness and pain in tendons, ligaments, joints and muscles where there is a deep aching. Repetitive strain injury. Sciatica. Rib and chest pain brought on by coughs. Good for sports-related ankle and wrist pain. *Do not apply to broken skin.*

Thuja: Warts. Verrucas. Brittle, weak nails.

First-Aid and Travel Kit

 A homeopathic first-aid kit is a very useful item to have around the house, in the car or on holiday. Make sure it is readily available. You may wish to purchase a small remedy box in which to store your first-aid kit.

Several homeopathic pharmacies and suppliers provide a ready-made first-aid kit. Some of these consist of up to 18 remedies in small bottles or vials. It may not be necessary for you to have this many remedies. Look at the remedies listed in this section and decide which ones would be most useful. You may have already used some of the remedies or have worked out your constitutional type, and therefore know which ones work well for you.

KIT REMEDIES

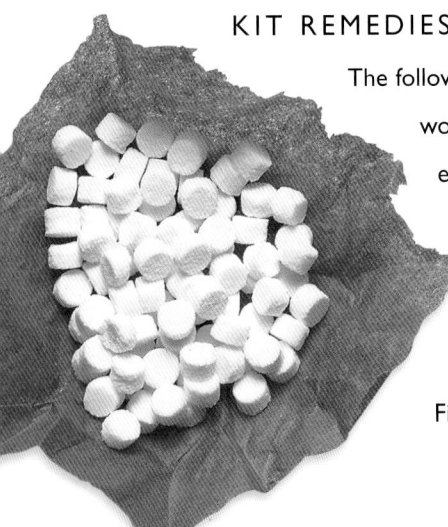

The following ten remedies would normally be enough to treat most first-aid situations.

Aconite

Panic. Fear. Pain. First signs of a cold or sore throat and fever. Inability to relax. Anxiety. To help induce sleep after a long journey. Any condition with a sudden onset.

Apis mel.

For bites and stings. Fluid retention and swelling. Swelling of legs and feet with travel.

Arnica

Shock. Injury. Bruising. Neck, back, shoulder and joint pain. Sprains and strains. Headaches. Jet lag. Topical application of Arnica cream or ointment can be used for bruising, sprains, strains and sunburn (but not on broken skin).

Cantharis

Chronic cystitis. Burning, stinging pain. Insect bites and stings. Sunburn.

Gelsemium

Sore throats. Coughs and colds. Influenza with shivering.

Graphites

Allergies. Reactions or break-outs of the skin due to change of climate or change of washing powders. Reactions to swimming pool chemicals. Eczema. Dermatitis. Topical application of Graphites cream can be used to soothe eczema, dermatitis or itchy, irritated skin.

Hypericum/Calendula mixture

Tincture for cleaning cuts and wounds. Ointment or cream for application on wounds, cuts and grazes or insect bites and stings.

Ledum

Puncture wounds. Splinters. Bites and stings.

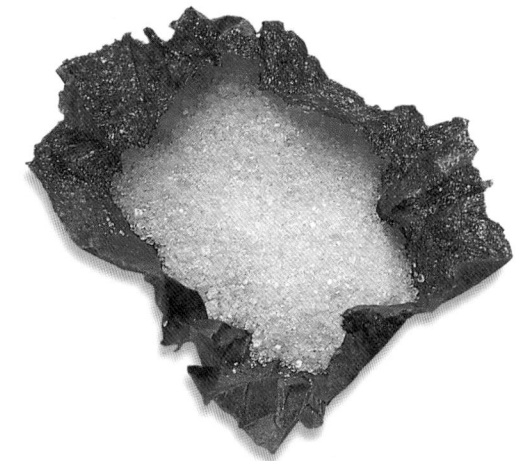

Nux vomica

Food poisoning. Travel sickness. Upset stomach. Jet lag. Hangover. Over-indulgence in rich foods.

Rhus tox.

Muscular aches and pains. Stiffness and over-exertion. Back and joint pain. Muscular aches and pain. Useful after skiing, trekking or activity holidays. The topical application of Rhus tox. can be used for muscular aches and pains, after sport or other exertion.

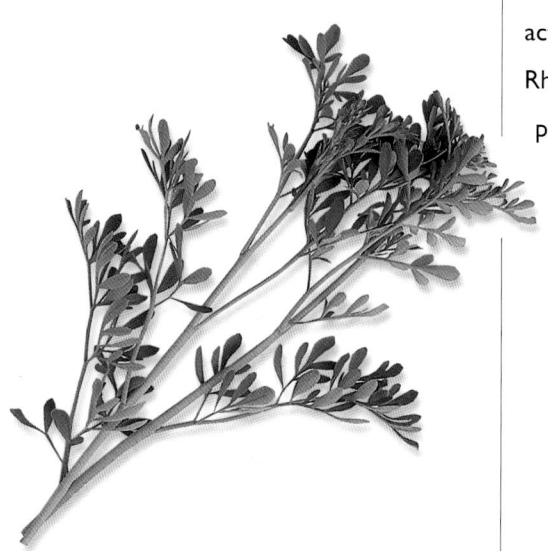

Useful Addresses and Websites

If you have trouble obtaining your remedy from a local pharmacist, chemist or health shop, then try the suppliers below. Most will supply ointments, creams and tinctures as well as the homeopathic tablets, boxes and carry cases.

Suppliers of Homeopathic Medicines

Ainsworths Pharmacy
36 New Cavendish Street
London W1M 7LH

British Institute of Homeopathy
Cygnet House
Market Square
Staines TW18 4RH

Helios Pharmacy
97 Camden Road
Kent TN1 2QR

The Homeopathic Supply Company
4 Nelson Road
Sherringham
Norfolk NR26 8BU

Nelson and Co. Ltd
73 Duke Street
London W1M 6BY

Olivers Wholefood Store
5 Station Approach
Kew, Richmond
Surrey TW9 3QB

Weleda (UK) Ltd
Heanor Road
Ilkeston
Derbyshire DE7 8DR

NHS Homeopathic Hospitals

Bristol Homeopathic Hospital
Cotham Hill
Cotham
Bristol BS6 6JU

Glasgow Homeopathic Hospital
1000 Great Western Road
Glasgow G12 OET

The Royal London Homeopathic Hospital
Great Ormond Street
London WC1N 3HR

Tunbridge Wells Homeopathic Hospital

Church Road

Tunbridge Wells

Kent TN1 1JU

Treatment with Author

The author of this section can be contacted by email: andrew@lmsltd.co.uk

This is an appointment and consultation service in London only. The author regrets that individual queries cannot be answered via this service.

See also: www.handsonreflexology.com

Homeopathic Organisations

The British Homeopathic Association

27a Devonshire Street

London W1N 1RJ

The Faculty of Homeopathy

The Royal London Homeopathic Hospital

Great Ormond Street

London WC1N 3HR

The Homeopathic Society

2 Powis Place

Great Ormond Street

London WC1N 3HT

Non-medically Qualified Homeopaths

Fellowship of British Institute of Homeopathy

Cygnet House

Market Square

Staines TW18 4RH

The Society of Homeopaths

2 Artizan Road

Northampton NN1 4HU

The United Kingdom Homeopathic

Medical Association

6 Livingstone Road

Gravesend

Kent DA12 5DZ

Please note that some homeopaths prefer not to have their address or telephone number listed on registers. Always check the qualifications of your homeopath. Personal recommendation is always the best way to find a good homeopath.

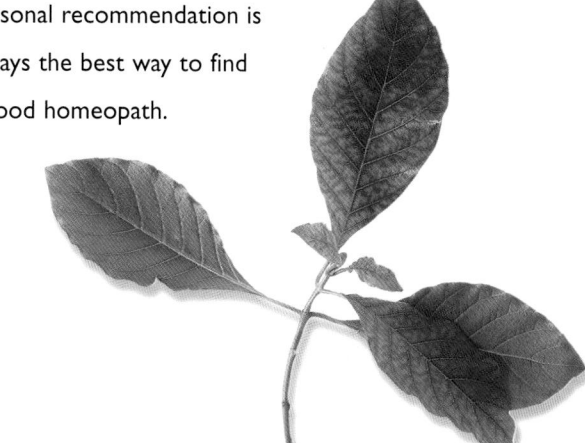

essential oils

Introduction

Humans love aromatic plants. When we pass a beautiful, scented flower our behaviour shows this very clearly. The fragrance is enough to stop us in our tracks, make us forget our train of thought and plunge our face into the petals to inhale the perfume. When we do, we forget the cares and troubles of the day for a moment, and the world seems to be a simpler place. Gardeners love to touch and smell the herbs and aromatic grasses that they grow themselves, sniffing the aromas that cling to the fingers, such as pungent rosemary or zesty peppermint, fresh lavender or tangy fennel. These mouthwatering scents make us relax and breathe deeply.

All these perfumes we are inhaling and enjoying so enthusiastically are essential oils, the natural fragrances of aromatic plants. These scents are manufactured by the plants

The pungent herb rosemary uplifts the senses and excites the tastebuds. It is easily grown in a pot outside.

themselves and held in their tissues, only to be released through touch or the heat of the sun. Of all the plants on the Earth, only about one per cent contain essential oils. Humans have enjoyed a special relationship with these species since antiquity, and we have used such plants for perfumes, incense and medicines.

Aromatherapy relies on essential oils to achieve gentle, nurturing effects on body and mind. The oils are used on the skin, in the bath and through inhalation to promote relaxation

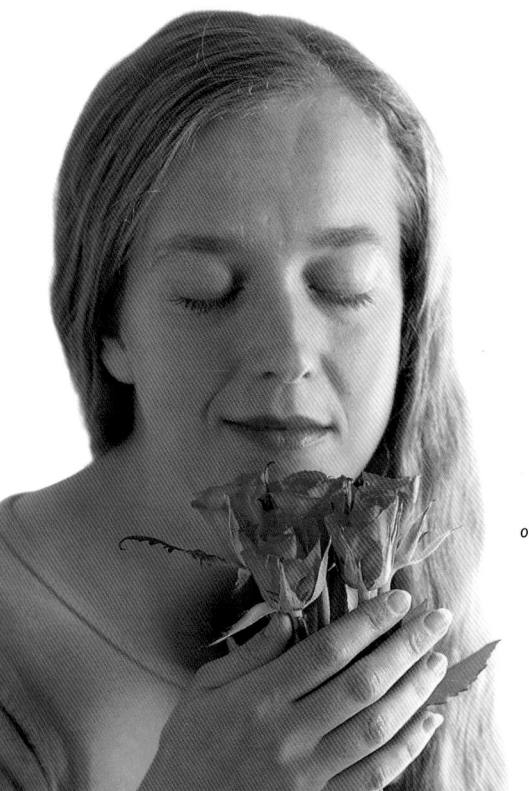

Flowers attract our sense of smell like a magnet. We are drawn to plants such as scented roses.

Relaxing in a bath with essential oils soothes the senses and can bring relief from aches and pains in the body.

and wellbeing. Essential oils and aromatherapy can make a very positive contribution to emotional and physical health, bringing a sense of inner peace and balance.

This section of the book takes you on an in-depth journey through the world of essential oils, where they come from and how they are obtained. It is an exploration of the particular plants that produce essential oils, revealing their unique role as a natural healing resource. The Essential Oils Index on pages 81–117 lists 36 common essential oils in detail, helping you get to know more about them and how to use them on yourself, friends and family. The methods are straightforward and easy to use in everyday situations. You will also find information about safety issues, buying and keeping the oils, and simple skincare routines.

You may well find that collecting essential oils, enjoying their aromas and learning about their different uses, becomes a fascinating pastime, something that develops from being a hobby into, quite simply, a way of life.

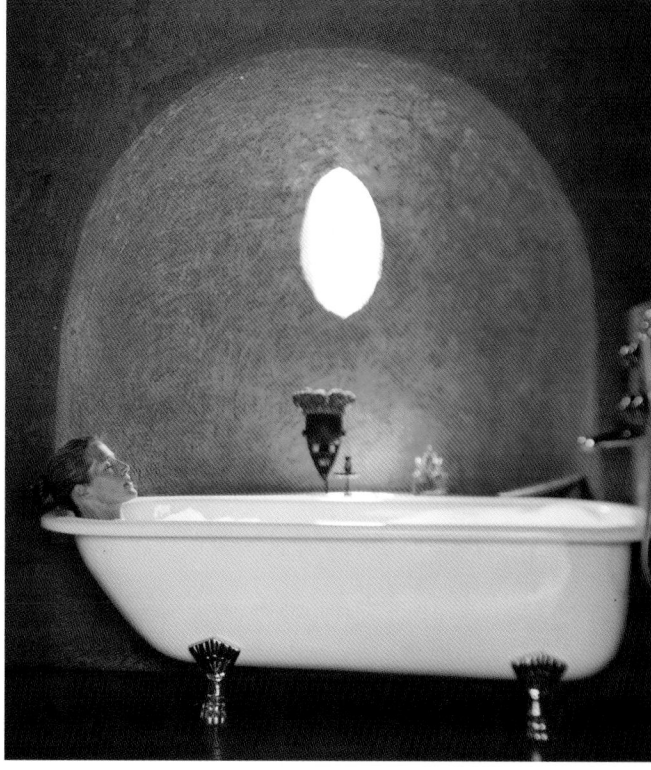

This section links the essential oils to the plants from which they are extracted. The botanical emphasis of this approach helps us to remember that all life on Earth is dependent on plants. As custodians of the planet we need to use these natural resources in a sustainable way if we are to continue to enjoy them.

Peppercorns yield a warming and stimulating essential oil that can ease painful joints and muscles.

Where Do Essential Oils Come From?

Essential oils are obtained from a small variety of aromatic plants. To understand essential oils, it helps to know something about how plants that provide essential oils function: through their roots, wood, leaves, flowers, fruits and berries. Essential oils may be found in any of these plant parts.

The Magic of Plants

Plants are the most astonishing interactive energy systems, able to respond to the most minute changes in environmental conditions at all times during their life span. They are in the business of survival, competition and reproduction, and over millions of years they have evolved precise mechanisms to achieve this, of which essential oils are one. Botanists are unsure why particular plants have evolved to contain essential oils. However, here are some suggestions.

Essential oils are found in a variety of plant parts. The roots, wood, leaves, flowers, fruits and berries can all yield up their precious perfumes.

other insects. This helps to protect delicate root tissue from damage and allows maximum water uptake.

Wood

Trees like sandalwood or cedarwood contain essential oils in the heartwood of their trunks

Essential oils in leaves may have a protective function. This is the ylang ylang plant – the beautiful blooms nestle within the large dark-green leaves and are protected from the elements.

Roots

Roots draw minerals and water into the plant tissue as well as giving stability to the growing plant. Aromatic roots such as turmeric or vetiver, which grow in hot tropical locations, are unsavoury to invading grubs, beetles and

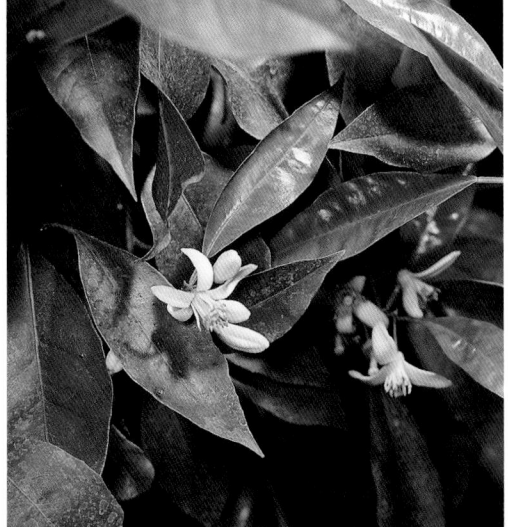

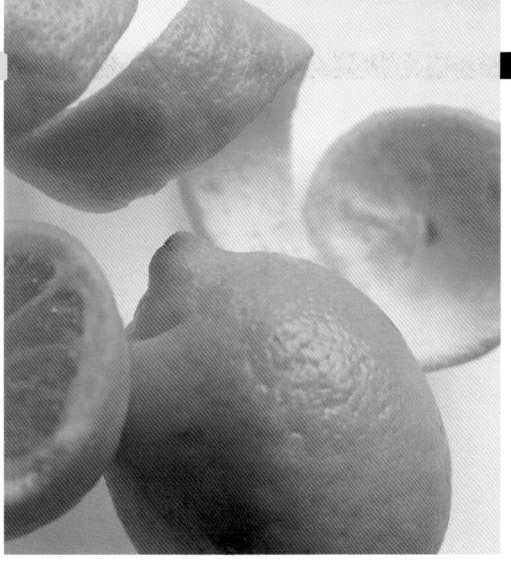

Essential oils that are found in the rind of fruits have a pungent and long-lasting aroma, making them popular scents.

and branches. There is some evidence that oils help to protect the inner structure of the wood from attack by beetles and other insects. Shrubs like frankincense and myrrh secrete resin, a sticky substance rich in essential oils, to protect themselves if their bark is cracked or damaged. The resin has been collected by humankind for thousands of years and burned as incense.

Leaves

In the leaves of any plant, the process of photosynthesis uses sunlight to convert carbon, hydrogen and oxygen to sugars. This process is vital for the growth of the plant, its eventual flowering and successful reproduction. Essential oils in the leaves may protect them from fungi or microbial attack, ensuring the maximum surface is available for the production of the plant's food.

Flowers

Some of the floral essential oils that are used in aromatherapy include subtle and exquisite fragrances such as lavender, rose, jasmine or orange blossom. The essential oils of other plants, such as frangipani, tuberose or mimosa, are very expensive to extract and are used in the formulation of some of the costliest perfumes. Flowers have only one purpose – to attract pollinating insects. The chemistry of attraction is a vital part of the insect–plant relationship. Some flowers have evolved aromas that mimic exactly the scent of specific insects. For example, the giant waterlily (*Victoria amazonica*) copies the pheremonal odour of a night-flying beetle, which has been pollinating the plant for centuries. Humans also have a long tradition of using the aroma of flowers to attract a mate – hence our love of perfumes.

Fruits and Seeds

Essential oils can be extracted from the rind of all citrus fruits. They are also found in the berries of bushes such as juniper. Fruits and berries are the end result of the flowering process. They tend to be aromatic in order to encourage animals or birds to eat them. The seeds are indigestible and are therefore excreted into the soil, giving the seed a better chance of germinating successfully.

How and Where are Essential Oils Obtained?

The production of essential oils involves a considerable investment of time, labour and skill. Plants are cultivated, harvested and processed to produce oils, which may then be shipped vast distances before reaching the consumer. Essential oils are a natural resource dependent on correct balances of soil composition, sun and rain to achieve good harvests year by year – just like any other natural crop.

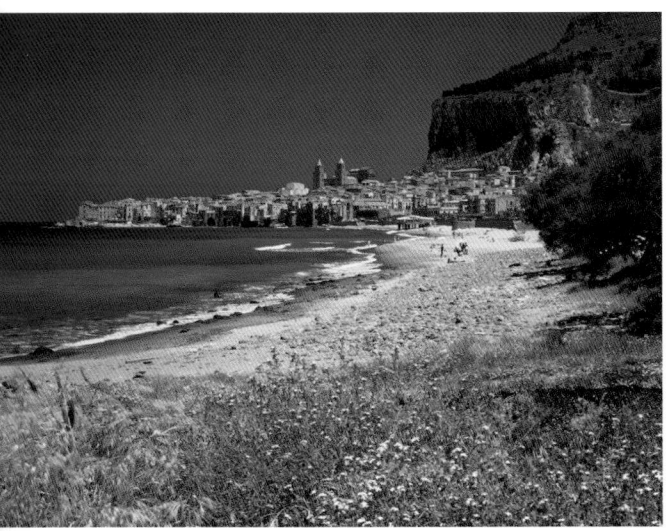

Many essential oils are found in distant locations worldwide. Mediterranean plants need sunlight to develop properly.

Geography

Essential oils are found in different plant groups all over the world. One of the most common is the botanical family *Labiatae,* which includes many Mediterranean plants such as rosemary, marjoram and lavender. Most of the oils used in aromatherapy come from plants grown in southern Europe and North Africa, as these need a lot of sunlight to produce their oils. The same geographical region is the home of many citrus fruits in the *Rutaceae* family, including succulent oranges, lemons and mandarins, whose peel is full of essential oil.

Further afield you find the trees, flowers and spices of India, for example, producer of jasmine, sandalwood, cardamom and patchouli oils. Indonesia produces some of the more unusual oils, such as vetiver, which has a smoky, earthy aroma. The best geranium oil comes from the island of Réunion in the Indian Ocean, while Australia is the biggest producer of tea tree oil.

Cardamom pods produce a warm, fragrant and spicy essential oil.

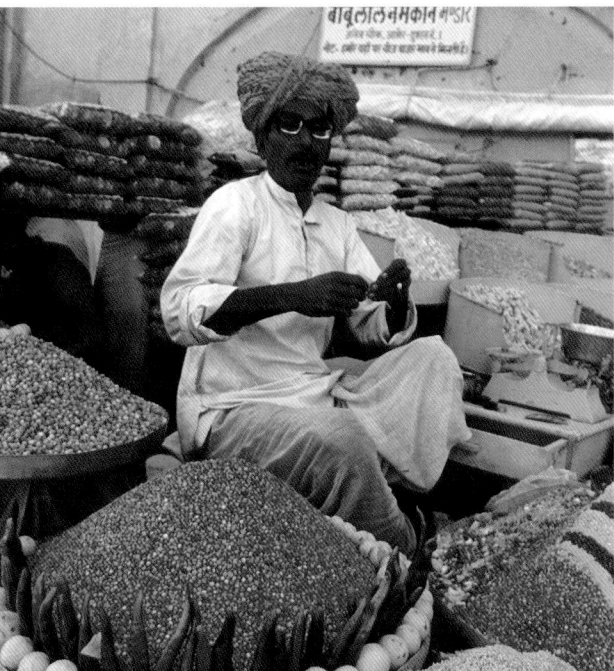

When buying an oil, check the Essential Oil Index (see pages 81–117) to see where it is produced and just how far it has travelled!

Cultivation

The cultivation of essential oils requires a lot of land to produce bulk supplies of plants. For example, it takes approximately half a tonne of lavender material to produce just one litre of essential oil. Successful lavender farms need many hectares of land.

Oils like vetiver are produced in developing countries where farmers use high levels of manual labour and traditional techniques. Very often the labour lies in the collection process where plants cannot be harvested

India is a huge producer of spices, aromatics and fragrances. Some of the more unusual oils come from this great continent.

mechanically. In Bulgaria, roses are picked off the bush by hand – roughly 50–100 rose blooms are used for one drop of essential oil.

More mechanised essential oil cultivation is found in Australia, where tea tree oil is produced on a large scale on plantations using modern machinery for harvesting.

Extraction Methods

Essential oils are held in sacs or special microscopic cells within the plant tissues themselves. To extract the oil, different techniques are used:

Steam distillation passes steam at high pressure through the plant material, releasing the globules of essential oil into the water vapour. The fragrant steam is cooled back to water, and the essential oil can then be skimmed off as it floats on the surface. This technique is used to extract most oils, including lavender and rosemary.
Expression involves pressing the oil directly out of citrus fruit peel.
Solvent extraction uses chemical solvents to dissolve aromatic compounds out of delicate plant tissues. The extract is refined to produce an 'absolute'. Jasmine oil is produced by solvent extraction.

What are Essential Oils Used For?

In the last ten years, more and more people have been using essential oils and aromatherapy has become very popular. However, it may surprise you to discover that essential oils have a long history of use, both in aromatherapy and in other areas.

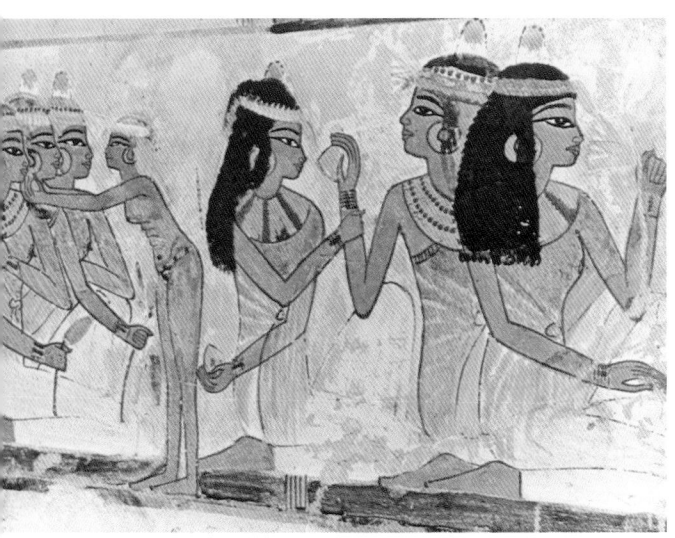

Ancient Egyptian men and women used aromatic fragrances to perfume the body and the hair.

was pressed into trays of fat, which were then heated in an oven or left out in the sun. The melted fat was strained and then allowed to set, and the solid, scented 'unguent' used as a fragrance on the skin and hair.

In the past, only the most wealthy could afford the rare and costly extracts that were available. Perfumes were a sign of wealth and status. At the beginning of the twentieth century, the development of synthetic aromatic chemicals meant that perfume formulae could be copied, which is what happens in the mass production of fragrances today. Natural essential oils and aromatic extracts continue to be used for the creation of new formulae for perfumes, which are then synthetically reproduced.

Perfumery

Essential oils have been the basic ingredients in perfume formulae since the invention of a form of distillation by Avicenna, an Arab perfumer, mystic and herbalist at the beginning of the last millennium. Even before that, essential oils were extracted by a method called enfleurage, in which aromatic plant material

Peppermint oil is used to flavour confectionery, including chocolates.

Food Flavouring

Many of the foodstuffs and drinks that we consume are flavoured with essential oils. Obvious examples include the use of peppermint and citrus oils in chocolate and other confectionery. However, many oils are used to give 'natural' flavours and fragrances to food products. They are used in preserved meats, alcoholic drinks, pickles and sauces. The amounts of essential oil used are very small and are carefully monitored to be at safe levels for internal consumption, because essential oils are extremely concentrated. In aromatherapy, essential oils are never swallowed. (See 'Essential Oil Safety Guidelines', pages 78–79.)

Pharmaceuticals

As well as being used in many foodstuffs, peppermint oil is used in pharmaceutical products such as toothpaste. Other essential oils that have pharmaceutical purposes include camphor and eucalyptus, which are used in commercial cough medicines, chest rubs and ointments for muscular aches and pains. Many of these products have been licensed since the early twentieth century.

Aromatherapy

Of all the tonnes of essential oils produced worldwide each year, only about five to ten per cent are used in aromatherapy. This is often a surprise to people, because they may be aware of essential oils only as the main ingredient in aromatherapy and not realise that they are so widely used elsewhere. In aromatherapy, it is very important that the oils used are totally natural and unadulterated with synthetics – trustworthy suppliers will buy directly from growers all around the world (for suppliers see page 125).

Essential oils such as that found in the citrus fruit orange are often used as food flavourings and preservatives.

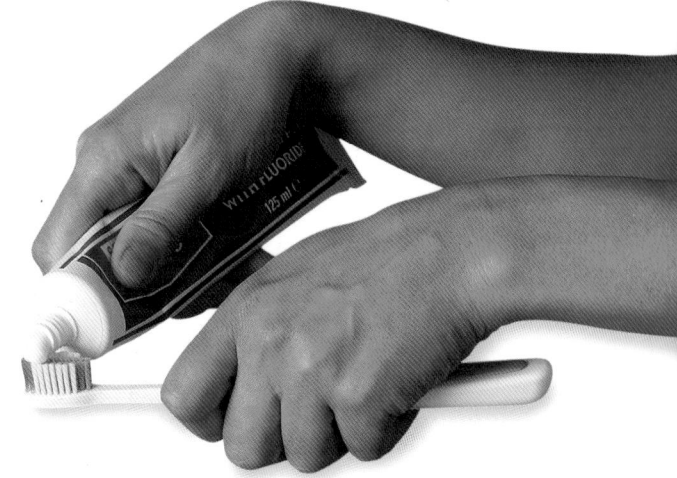

Essential oils such as peppermint or fennel are used to flavour different kinds of toothpaste the world over.

Essential Oil Safety Guidelines

Essential oils are completely natural. However, it is important to be aware that they are highly concentrated and need to be used safely and correctly. These guidelines will help you to check how to use essential oils in particular situations. It is advisable to consult your medical practitioner if you have any physical or psychological symptoms, as essential oils are not a replacement for professional medical treatment.

No to Oral Use

The most important safety guideline is simply this: do not take essential oils by mouth. They are highly concentrated substances and in large amounts they can do internal damage. If oils have been swallowed accidentally, seek medical help immediately.

Pregnancy Care

If you are pregnant, lactating or breastfeeding, it is especially important not to swallow any essential oils. Any oils you use on yourself for massage or in the bath should be in very weak dilutions. If you are making any of the blends in this book, you should use half the

Women who are pregnant or breastfeeding need to be very careful when using essential oils.

stated number of drops. You are best advised to use flower and fruit oils only, as these are very gentle. It is a good idea to consult a qualified aromatherapist for advice.

Skin Safety

Before being applied to the skin, essential oils should always be diluted in a carrier oil such as sweet almond or grapeseed because they are so concentrated. Provided that you do not have sensitive skin (a tendency to allergic reactions), you can use lavender or tea tree neat for first-aid purposes (two drops on a cotton bud applied to the affected area). If you are sensitive to nuts, it is best to avoid sweet almond oil and use grapeseed instead.

Phototoxic Oils

Essential oils from the citrus fruits – bergamot, grapefruit, orange, lemon, lime and mandarin – contain an ingredient that can cause skin

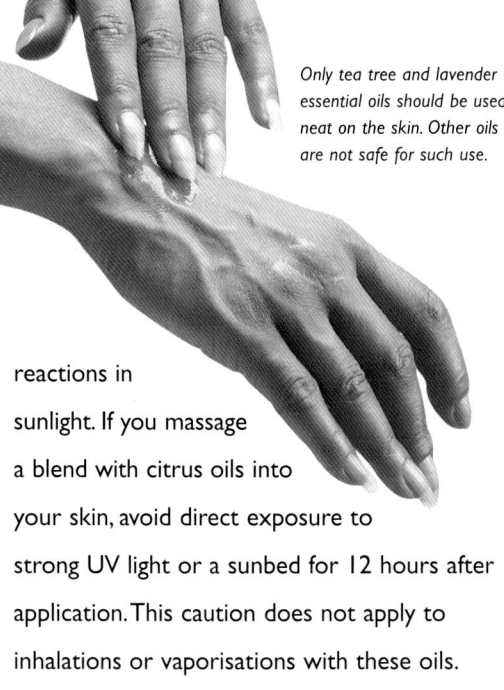

Only tea tree and lavender essential oils should be used neat on the skin. Other oils are not safe for such use.

reactions in sunlight. If you massage a blend with citrus oils into your skin, avoid direct exposure to strong UV light or a sunbed for 12 hours after application. This caution does not apply to inhalations or vaporisations with these oils.

High Blood Pressure

Rosemary essential oil is very stimulating and should be avoided if you have high blood pressure. Calming oils like lavender or ylang ylang are preferred for their soothing effects.

Epilepsy and Asthma

Again, rosemary essential oil has the potential to slightly increase the frequency of epileptic seizures, so it should be avoided by people who have epilepsy. Calming oils like sandalwood, neroli or orange are better suited for people with epilepsy. (Never attempt to apply oils during a seizure.) If you have asthma, it is advisable not to do inhalations with essential oils – use them for bathing, vaporisation and massage.

Babies and Children

Correct dosage of essential oils is especially crucial because of the delicate skin of small children. Follow these recommendations:

Babies up to 2 years: one drop of roman chamomile **or** rose otto **or** lavender in 20 ml sweet almond carrier oil for general skin care and baby massage.

Children 2–10 years: any blends made from this book should contain half the stated number of drops. If an odd number of drops is given, reduce this to just under half (e.g. reduce 3 drops to 1, or 5 to 2).

Children over the age of 10: can receive oils in the same dilutions as adults.

Elderly Skin

In cases where the skin is delicate and very transparent with visible veins, you should use half the stated number of drops in any blend you make from this book so that the skin is nourished by the oils more gently.

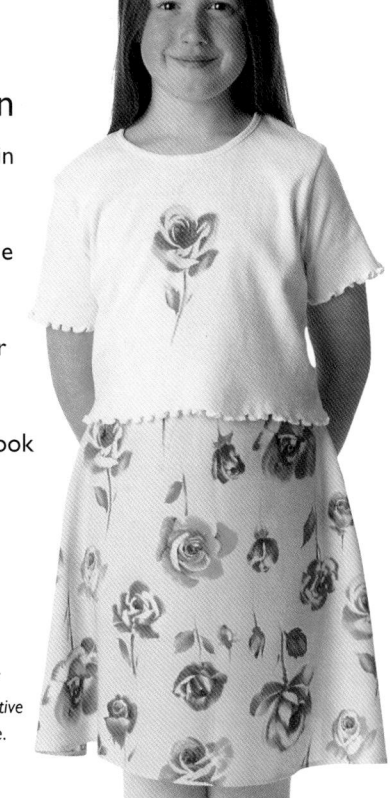

Blends for children (and the elderly) contain low amounts of essential oils. Young skin is sensitive while older skin is more delicate.

How Essential Oils are Used in Aromatherapy

Aromatherapy is what it says it is – the 'aroma' being the fragrances of essential oils, and the 'therapy' the way in which the fragrance is applied to relieve physical symptoms and promote mental wellbeing. There are several simple ways to use essential oils, including in baths, inhalation and massage.

Baths

For a 20-minute soak to relieve tension and stress, run the bath to a comfortable temperature. Sprinkle 4 drops maximum of one essential oil or 3 drops each of two essential oils as a combination onto the surface of the water. Agitate the water gently to disperse the oils before getting in. If you have dry or sensitive skin, you can dilute the essential oils in 20 ml full-cream milk or unfragranced bath oil before adding them to the water. A simple relaxing combination is 3 drops each of lavender and sandalwood.

Inhalation

This method helps to relieve colds, influenza or sinus problems. You need a large bowl just over half full of nearly boiling water. Sprinkle 2 drops each of eucalyptus and tea tree onto the surface, then cover your head with a towel and inhale the aromatic steam for 15–20 minutes. Remove your glasses or contact lenses so they don't steam up or irritate the eyes.

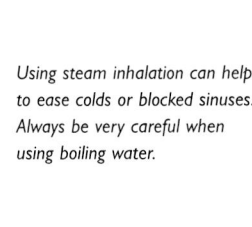

Using steam inhalation can help to ease colds or blocked sinuses. Always be very careful when using boiling water.

Vaporisation

Vaporisers gently heat up to evaporate the essential oil and disperse its fragrance into a room. You can buy a ceramic burner with tea light candles or one of the many electrical models available. You should follow the manufacturer's guidelines when using the oils though; generally 4 drops of one oil or 3 drops each of two as a combination will scent a room for up to two hours. You can use tea tree and lemon essential oils to remove

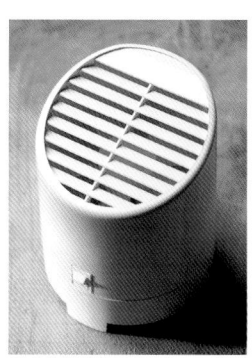

unpleasant odours, or choose a favourite aroma to create an environment that suits your mood.

An electrically powered fragrance diffuser can help ease breathing problems and is safe to be left on.

Massage

When using essential oils for massage, they first need to be diluted in a carrier oil. These are vegetable oils such as grapeseed, sweet almond or jojoba. Most of the massage blends in this book are based on a formula of using 10 drops of essential oils in 20 ml (4 teaspoons) carrier oil. The mixture should be stored in a clean glass bottle. Shake the mixture before use. This is a suitable dilution for massage on most skins and is enough to

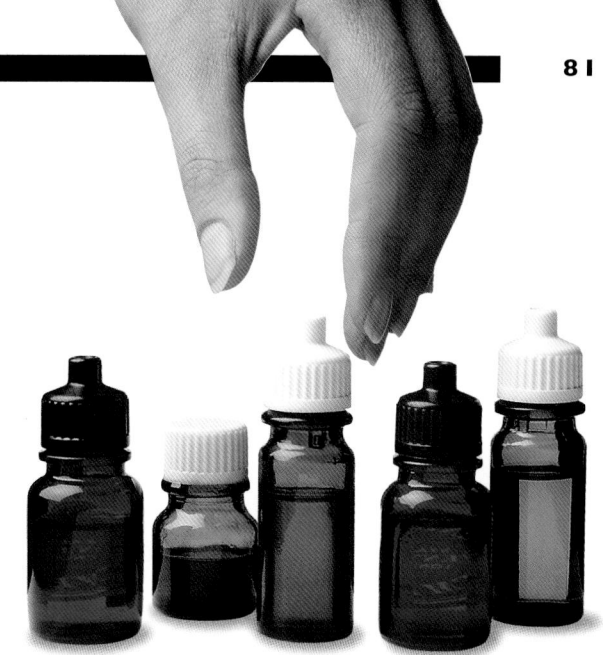

Drops of essential oil need to be counted very carefully when you are making up your blends. This is essential when treating children.

massage a full body, not including the face. Sensitive, very young or elderly skin requires only 5 drops in 20 ml. (See pages 120–121 for Special Massage Blends.) Your blends will last for a maximum of four weeks. If you want to make larger quantities, simply take 40 ml base oil and double the drops of essential oils in the blend formula.

Essential Oil Index

In this section, you will find 36 essential oils grouped according to the plant parts that produce them. Each essential oil file contains key information and blends to try out yourself to help ease physical conditions and rebalance mental and emotional states.

Root Oils

The energy of these oils is generally stabilising and grounding to the body. Originally they protect and strengthen the plants that produce them.

Ginger
Zingiber officinale

Plant profile: ginger is a key ingredient in the recipes of India and China. It is also used in Traditional Chinese Medicine for digestion and circulation problems. Ginger roots are dried before distillation, which means that the essential oil smells less pungent than the freshly chopped root.

Pungent ginger root yields a warming and spicy essential oil. It can improve energy levels.

Safety information: no issues.

Fragrance profile: a dry, musty aroma, which is sharper and spicier as it evaporates, leaving a lingering sweetness.

Main uses: eases indigestion; warms and soothes aches and pains in muscles; improves poor circulation; improves energy.

Suggested blends: for indigestion, add 2 drops peppermint, 3 drops ginger and 5 drops lemon to 20 ml of carrier oil and then massage into the abdomen gently.

Aches and pains can be eased by a taking a bath with 4 drops lavender and 2 drops ginger. Improve poor circulation by massaging a blend of 6 drops black pepper and 4 drops ginger in 20 ml carrier oil into the skin. You will notice the area becomes pink – this is an indication of improved circulation and is quite normal.

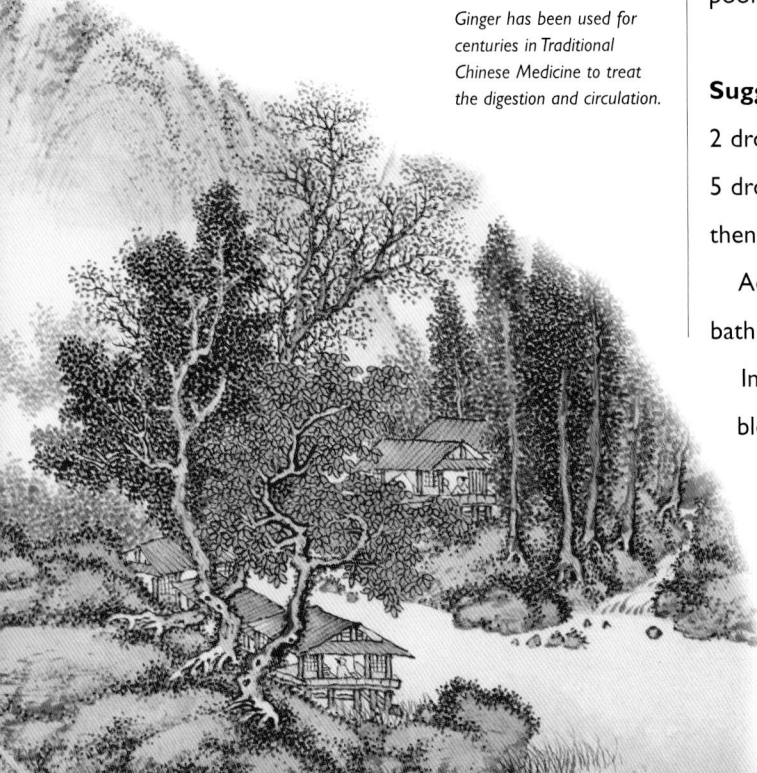

Ginger has been used for centuries in Traditional Chinese Medicine to treat the digestion and circulation.

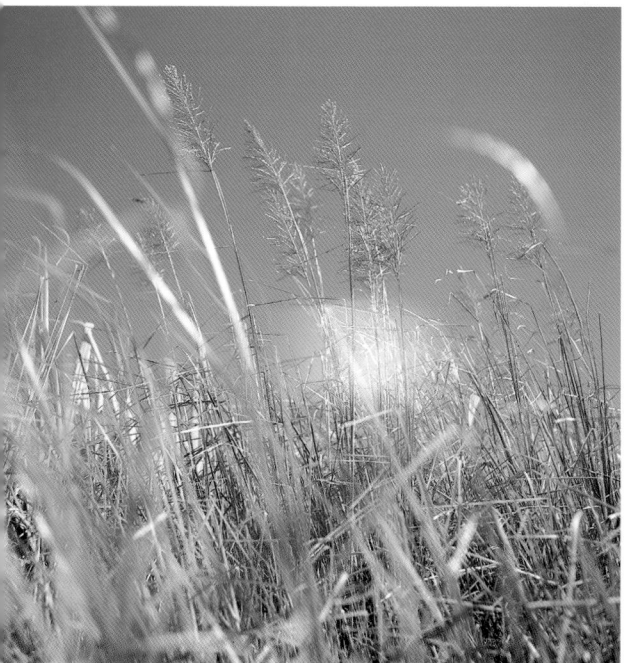

Vetiver

Vetiveria zizanoides

Plant profile: vetiver comes mainly from Indonesia, where it is known locally as *akar wangi*. It is a tough tropical grass that is economically important to growers. The upper leaves can be woven into mats and fibres, while the aromatic roots are harvested for distillation. Vetiver is also grown on the island of Réunion in the Indian Ocean.

Safety information: no issues.

Fragrance profile: a very unusual deep, earthy, smoky aroma, heavy and warm.

Vetiver is a very successful commercial crop in Indonesia as well as being a valuable essential oil.

Main uses: warms and relieves aches and pains, particularly backache; improves circulation; eases menstrual cramps; helps to ground and stabilise the emotions in cases of extreme stress.

Suggested blends: vetiver has a strong aroma, so no more than 2 drops are needed in a blend. For aches and pains and circulation, try 2 drops vetiver, 3 drops ginger and 5 drops lavender in 20 ml carrier oil for daily massage.

Menstrual cramps can be eased using a blend of 8 drops marjoram and 2 drops vetiver in 20 ml carrier oil, massaged over the lower abdomen twice daily.

Emotional insecurity can be calmed by taking a bath with 1 drop vetiver, 1 drop neroli and 3 drops lavender. You can also add these oils to 10 ml carrier oil and massage gently into the skin after your bath.

Massage an aching back with vetiver for relief from the pain. The warming scent is also very soothing to the mind and senses.

Angelica

Angelica archangelica

The whole of the angelica plant is aromatic. However, it is the root of the plant that is used in the distillation of the essential oil.

Plant profile: a herb that has been highly regarded in Western herbal tradition since medieval times; angelica is now cultivated for essential oil extraction in countries including Germany and Hungary. The whole plant is aromatic. It grows up to 2 metres in height and has dramatic spherical heads of tiny flowers. The pungent root has been used in herbal medicine for hundreds of years as a general cleanser and detoxifier.

Safety information: angelica essential oil is phototoxic. After any application to the skin, avoid direct exposure to strong sunlight or a sunbed for 12 hours. Angelica oil is best avoided in pregnancy.

Fragrance profile: sweet and aniseed-like, with a rich, warm and spicy note that is released as it evaporates.

Main uses: eases muscular aches, soothes arthritic joints and rheumatic pains; eases indigestion problems and wind and improves poor appetite; an overall energy tonic and revitaliser, especially in the springtime.

Suggested blends: for muscular aches and pains, add 2 drops angelica, 2 drops vetiver and 5 drops lavender to 20 ml carrier oil and apply using gentle massage.

Digestion problems can be eased by blending 3 drops peppermint, 4 drops ginger and 3 drops angelica in 20 ml carrier oil for massage over the abdomen.

A 'springtime blend' to help to energise and tone body and mind is 2 drops angelica, 3 drops juniper and 5 drops grapefruit in 20 ml carrier oil, to be massaged briskly into the skin after a bath or shower.

The angelica plant produces beautiful spherical flowerheads. These are made up of thousands of tiny flowers. Angelica is now specifically cultivated for essential oil extraction.

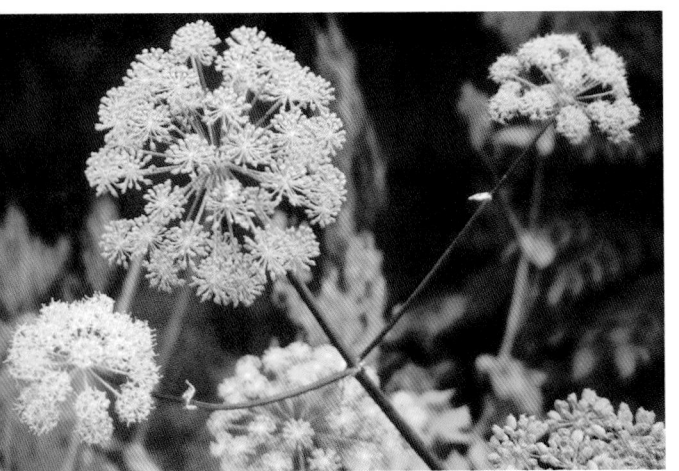

Turmeric

Curcuma longa/Curcuma domestica

Plant profile: turmeric is a plant that looks very like ginger, with tall shoots and abundant elegant leaves, and is a member of the same botanical family. The highly aromatic roots are bright yellow and are used to colour curries. The roots are cleaned and sun-dried before being ground as a spice or distilled for the oil. India, China and Indonesia are the main producers.

Safety information: no issues.

Fragrance profile: dry, musty and vegetable-like aroma; spicy and sweet as it evaporates.

Main uses: soothes and eases backache and muscular pains; improves circulation; tones and improves the digestion, easing stomach cramps and constipation. Very stabilising and grounding to overwrought emotions; warms and re-energises the body.

Suggested blends: for aches and pains, add 4 drops turmeric, 4 drops ginger and 2 drops vetiver to 20 ml carrier oil and massage the affected areas gently.

Yellow turmeric roots have many uses – they can be used as a cooking spice or an essential oil.

Cramps and indigestion can be eased by blending 4 drops turmeric, 2 drops lemongrass and 4 drops ginger in 20 ml carrier oil, and massaging the blend into the abdomen.

For emotional tension, add 1 drop turmeric, 2 drops neroli and 2 drops ginger to a warm bath and rest there for 20 minutes. This combination can also be added to 10 ml carrier oil and massaged into the skin afterwards.

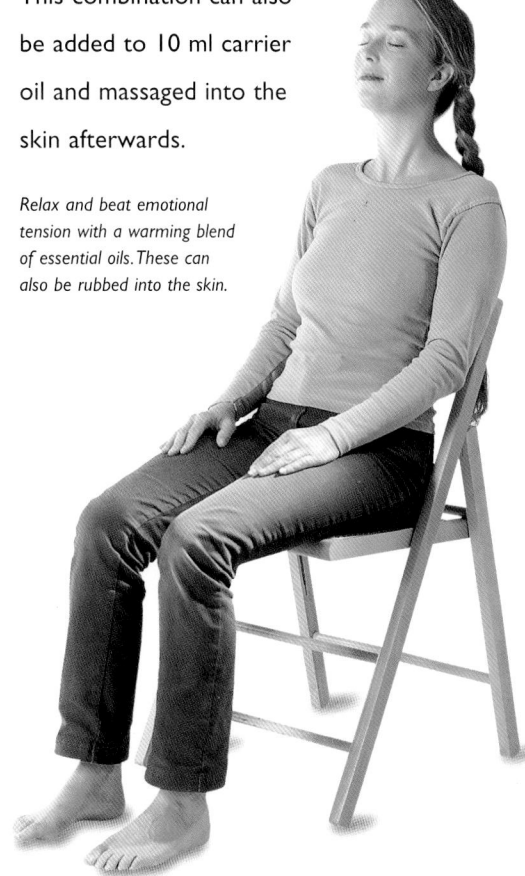

Relax and beat emotional tension with a warming blend of essential oils. These can also be rubbed into the skin.

Wood Oils

These oils are found in the aromatic heartwood in the centre of tree trunks and branches. They are at the centre of the growing, spreading height of the tree. The energy of these oils is more expansive, encouraging deep breathing.

Sandalwood

Santalum album

Plant profile: the best-quality sandalwood comes from the Mysore region of India near Bangalore. It takes approximately 30 years for the wood to mature to its full aromatic potential, so planting and harvesting is carefully rotated and controlled. The wood is used in the distillation of sandalwood oil. It is also powdered for making incense sticks and cosmetics, and can be carved into statues and boxes.

Safety information: no issues.

Fragrance profile: this beautiful oil should be thick and pale golden, with a subtle aroma at first, deepening to a rich, woody, spicy, sweet fragrance as it evaporates.

Main uses: eases tight chesty coughs, colds, sore throats; soothes dry chapped skin and improves the texture of all skin types; eases depression, anxiety and feelings of panic.

Suggested blends: for coughs, add 3 drops sandalwood, 3 drops cedarwood and 4 drops lemon to 20 ml carrier oil and massage gently over the chest area.

A rejuvenating skincare blend is 6 drops sandalwood, 2 drops patchouli and 2 drops rose in 20 ml jojoba oil, massaged into the face at night.

To ease anxiety or depression, add 3 drops sandalwood and 2 drops orange to a warm bath and rest for 20 minutes. Add the same oils to 10 ml carrier oil and massage into the skin afterwards.

Sandalwood brings a state of peace and calm to body and mind. It is also good for use on sensitive skins.

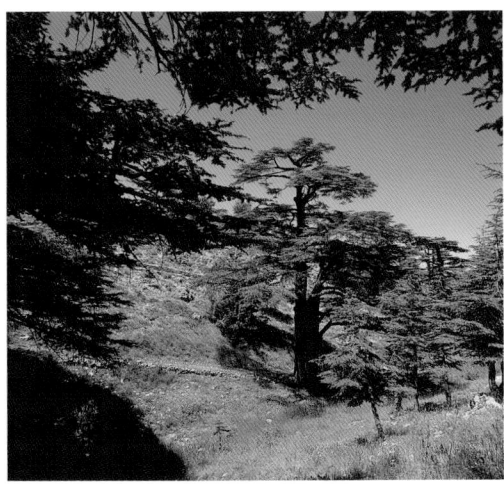

Atlas Cedarwood

Cedrus atlantica

Plant profile: these tall, majestic cedar trees come from the Atlas mountains in Morocco. They stand over 30 metres in height with a sweeping, tentlike appearance, and a wonderful aroma floats around them thanks to the essential oil in the red heartwood. Cedar was used extensively by the ancient Egyptians in the manufacture of furniture and ships because of the wood's resistance to insects – as well as its beauty.

Safety information: no issues.

Fragrance profile: sharp and fresh with a sweet, woody, soft undertone.

The ancient Egyptians used fragrant cedarwood to make beautiful and aromatic furniture.

Cedarwood trees are huge and majestic, and are wonderfully aromatic too. The oil comes from the red heartwood.

Main uses: eases bronchitis, chest infections, coughs; soothes cracked skin, eczema, acne and oily skin; assuages feelings of panic, calms and deepens the breath when under stress.

Suggested blends: for chest problems, add 3 drops cedarwood, 3 drops sandalwood and 4 drops lemon to 20 ml carrier oil and massage the chest. For cracked skin, try a blend of 3 drops cedarwood, 2 drops frankincense and 5 drops lavender in 20 ml carrier oil. For acne or oily skin, try 3 drops cedarwood, 2 drops tea tree and 5 drops lavender in 20 ml jojoba as a cleanser. For stress, vaporise 2 drops cedarwood and 3 drops lavender. Use these oils in 10 ml carrier oil to massage the neck and shoulders.

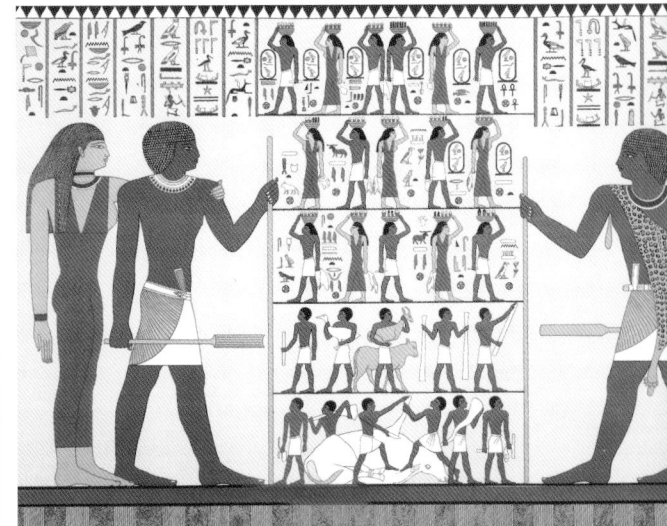

Resin Oils

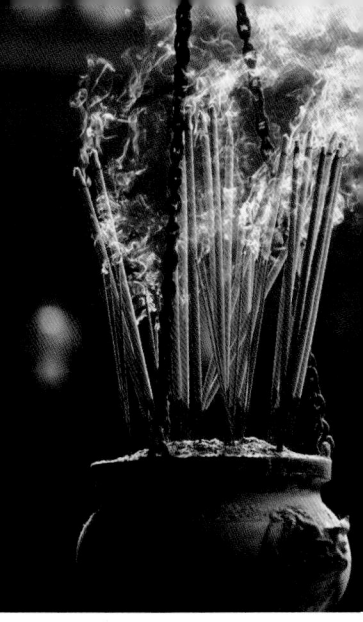

These sticky aromatic substances, the original incense ingredients, ooze out of the bark of certain trees and shrubs as a defence against injury. We too can use them to heal our skin.

Frankincense
Boswellia carterii var. thurifera

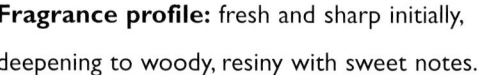

Frankincense is the original 'true incense' of antiquity and has been burned in places of religious worship for centuries.

Plant profile: frankincense is a robust desert shrub with delicate leaves and whitish papery bark. The name actually means 'true incense', and it has been burned in religious ceremonies since ancient times. The frankincense plantations of the pharaohs were seen as one of the most valuable commodities in Egypt and frankincense was used in the embalming process. Cuts were made in the bark to make the gum ooze out. It is still used for incense and distilled for the oil, mainly in Somalia and Oman.

Safety information: no issues.

Frankincense gum forms 'tears' or granules. This oozes out of the bark of the frankincense shrub when it is cut.

Fragrance profile: fresh and sharp initially, deepening to woody, resiny with sweet notes.

Main uses: disinfects and heals cuts, wounds, eczema and damaged skin; tones and rejuvenates all skin types, especially mature; eases chesty coughs or bronchitis; comforts anxiety and emotional stress.

Suggested blends: a good skin-healing blend is 4 drops frankincense, 2 drops lavender and 4 drops cedarwood in 20 ml carrier oil. Apply to the affected area twice daily. A tonic for mature skin is 4 drops frankincense, 3 drops neroli and 3 drops rose in 20 ml jojoba oil. For chesty coughs, try an inhalation of 3 drops frankincense and 3 drops cedarwood. To ease emotional stress and help you relax, vaporise 3 drops frankincense and 4 drops grapefruit.

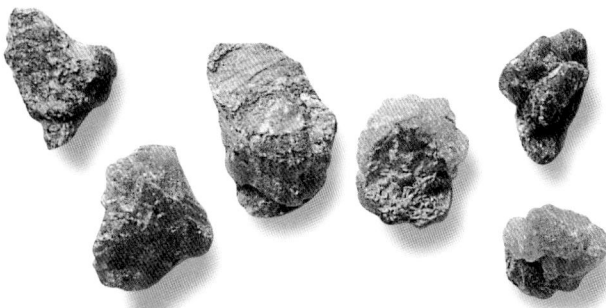

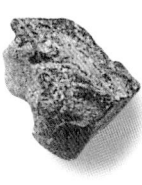

Myrrh

Commiphora myrrha

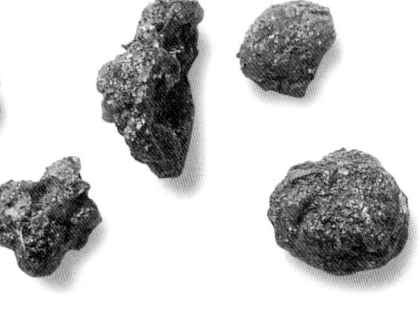

Plant profile: a thorny shrub, native to the arid climates of Somalia and Arabia, with papery bark and a reddish gum that oozes out when the bark is cracked or cut deliberately. Myrrh is soluble in water and has been used as a tonic for the teeth and gums since the time of Hippocrates (469–399 BCE), the father of Western medicine. Like frankincense, myrrh is prized for wound healing, and was used by the ancient Egyptians for embalming.

Safety information: myrrh is best avoided during pregnancy.

Fragrance profile: a dry, sharp and subtle aroma, which gradually deepens to reveal rich, sweet and spicy notes.

Main uses: heals and disinfects deep cuts, wounds, chapped and cracked skin, eczema; cleans and disinfects the mouth, easing sore gums and mouth ulcers; relieves bronchitis, chesty coughs; comforts and calms highly anxious emotional states.

Suggested blends: to help damaged skin, blend 3 drops myrrh, 4 drops tea tree and

Myrrh gum is reddish-orange in colour and was used in the embalming process in ancient Egypt.

3 drops frankincense in 20 ml carrier oil and apply 2–3 times daily. For problems in the mouth, add 2 drops myrrh to a glass of water, stir vigorously and use as a mouthwash (do not swallow). For chesty coughs, add 3 drops myrrh, 3 drops frankincense and 4 drops cedarwood to 20 ml carrier and massage the chest area especially at night. To de-stress, add 2 drops myrrh and 3 drops geranium to a bath – and relax.

Using myrrh as a mouthwash helps to keep teeth and gums healthy. Remember never to swallow any.

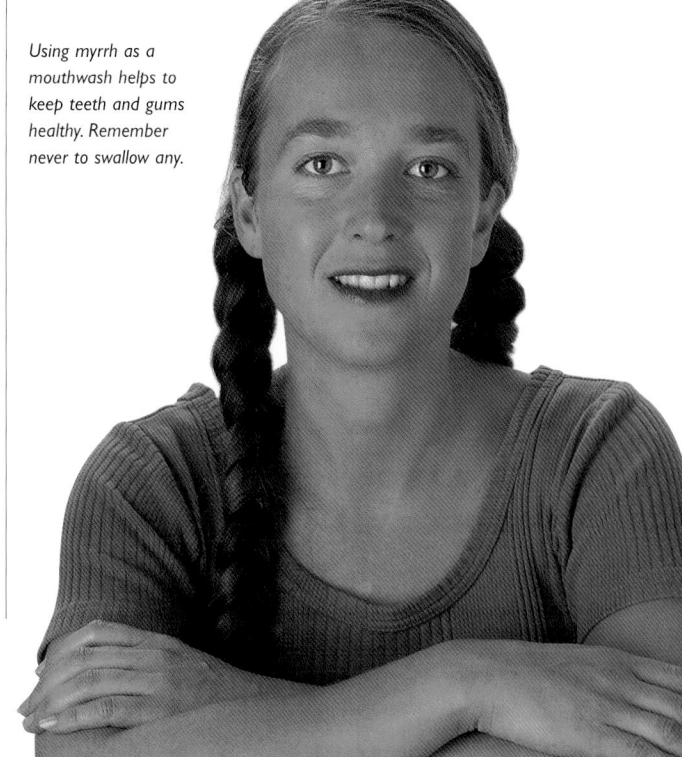

Leaf Oils

These oils are contained in the all-important leaves that manufacture the plant's food. They protect the leaf surface from damage by fungi and bacteria.

Marjoram
Origanum marjorana

French marjoram has a gentle woody aroma. The scent evaporates quite quickly.

Plant profile: this is the species otherwise known as 'French marjoram', and not Spanish marjoram, which is a type of thyme. French marjoram has been a favourite herb for cooking and has been widely used for centuries. It is low-growing, with small aromatic leaves and tiny white flowers that appear in summer. Originally from Mediterranean regions, it will grow well in more northerly climates if kept sheltered and in a sunny spot. The essential oil comes from France.

Safety information: no issues.

Fragrance profile: a warm, woody aroma that somewhat resembles camphor, gradually becoming sweet and soft.

Main uses: helps muscular aches and pains, stiffness and strains; eases menstrual cramps and mood swings; helps migraine, headaches and nervous tension.

Suggested blends: for muscular aches, add 4 drops marjoram, 4 drops ginger and 2 drops vetiver to 20 ml carrier oil for massage. Menstrual symptoms can be eased by massaging the abdomen with 4 drops marjoram, 4 drops lavender and 2 drops vetiver in 20 ml oil.

For headaches and nervous tension, add 4 drops marjoram, 2 drops peppermint and 4 drops lavender to 20 ml carrier oil and gently massage the forehead, neck and shoulders.

Using essential oils like marjoram can help headaches and menstrual problems.

Peppermint

Mentha piperita

Peppermint is a strongly scented herb and grows very easily and quickly in the garden.

Plant profile: peppermint is a tall vigorous mint with a very invasive habit – ask any gardener! It spreads rapidly through tough root systems, and will out-compete other more tender herbs in a plot unless it is contained in some way. The square, erect stems support deep-green aromatic leaves and, if left untrimmed the plant will produce tall heads of tiny white flowers. Peppermint essential oil comes mostly from the USA, where it is used to flavour toothpaste and chewing gum.

Safety information: if your skin is sensitive, use half the stated drops of peppermint in any blend due to the menthol content in the oil, which can act as an irritant.

Fragrance profile: pungent, fresh, zesty and minty aroma with sweeter notes later.

Main uses: eases stomach cramps, indigestion, constipation and nausea; helps muscular aches, stiffness, backache; eases headaches and migraine; clears the head and improves concentration.

Suggested blends:

indigestion symptoms can be helped by massaging the abdomen with 2 drops peppermint, 4 drops ginger and 4 drops cardamom in 20 ml carrier oil.

For aches and pains, massage daily with 2 drops peppermint, 4 drops rosemary and 4 drops black pepper in 20 ml carrier oil. To ease headaches, add 2 drops peppermint and 3 drops lavender to 10 ml carrier oil and massage onto the forehead and neck.

For clearing the mind, vaporise 2 drops peppermint and 3 drops lemon.

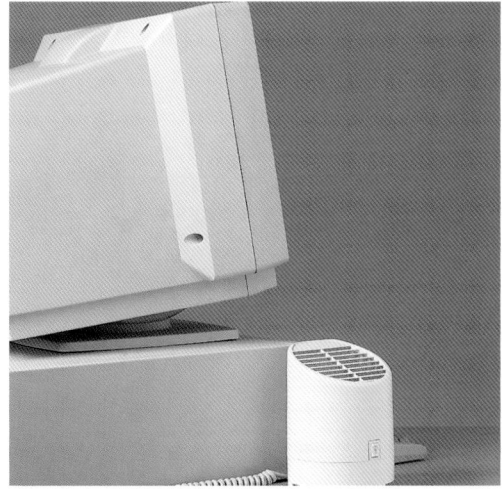

Vaporising peppermint essential oil in the office can clear your head and kick-start the mind.

Rosemary

Rosmarinus officinalis

Rosemary is an evergreen herb with a bracing aroma. It is used in cooking as well as aromatherapy.

Plant profile: the name 'rosemary' means 'rose of the sea', a reference to the original habitat of the plant on the dry, sandy coastline of the Mediterranean Sea. Even today, the best pungent oil comes from Spain or North Africa; the hotter and drier the climate, the better the aroma. Rosemary oil smells quite similar to eucalyptus because they have a fragrant ingredient in common: eucalyptol.

Safety information: rosemary is not advised for people with high blood pressure, as it is a stimulating oil. It should also be avoided by people who suffer from epilepsy.

Fragrance profile: strong, camphoraceous, fresh and herbal aroma with a definite eucalyptus tone.

Main uses: eases muscular aches and pains, backache, poor circulation; stimulates the scalp and eases dandruff; clears the breathing in colds, influenza or sinusitis; stimulates the mind and wakes up the brain.

Suggested blends: for aches and pains and for poor circulation, try using 4 drops rosemary, 2 drops lemongrass and 4 drops nutmeg in 20 ml carrier oil.

For a hair and scalp tonic, try adding 5 drops rosemary and 5 drops tea tree to 20 ml of unfragranced shampoo and then washing your hair as normal.

For easier breathing when suffering from colds or influenza, add 3 drops rosemary and 3 drops tea tree to a bowl of nearly boiling water and inhale the vapour for 20 minutes. To help stimulate the mind, vaporise 3 drops rosemary and 3 drops peppermint.

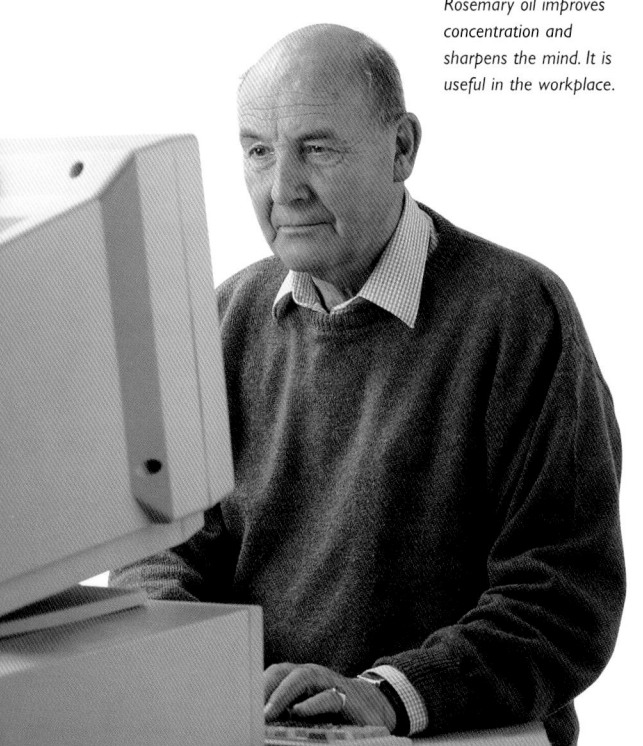

Rosemary oil improves concentration and sharpens the mind. It is useful in the workplace.

Cypress

Cupressus sempervivens

Plant profile: tall, evergreen cypress trees are an elegant feature of the landscape in Italy, France, Corsica, Sardinia, Spain and Portugal. The Latin name *sempervivens* means 'evergreen', a reference to the long life of the species. They are often planted near dwellings or near churches to signify eternal life. The oil comes from the young twigs and leaves, which are highly aromatic. Distillation takes place mostly in France or Spain.

Safety information: no issues.

Fragrance profile: earthy, smoky and green with camphoraceous and sweet notes.

Main uses: clears oily skin and blocked pores; improves lymphatic drainage and cellulite; eases spasmodic coughs and bronchitis; soothes fraught emotions.

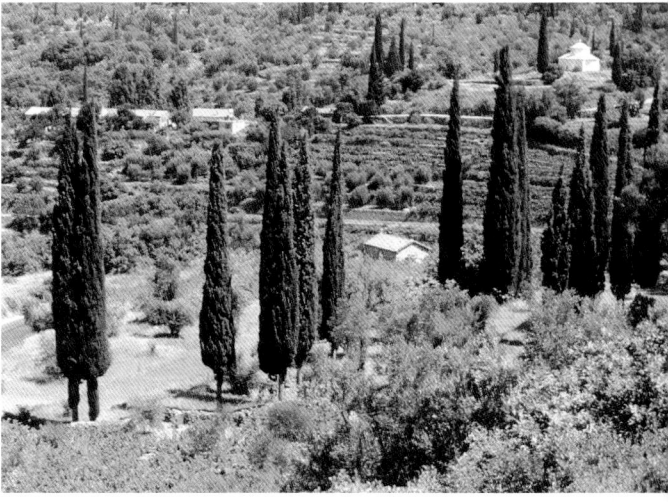

The tall dark shapes of cypress trees stand out clearly in a Mediterranean landscape.

Suggested blends: oily skin can be treated daily using 3 drops cypress, 3 drops tea tree and 4 drops grapefruit in 20 ml jojoba oil to cleanse and soothe the skin.

To counter cellulite, try using 4 drops cypress, 4 drops grapefruit and 2 drops juniper in 20 ml carrier oil for a vigorous daily massage on the affected areas.

To ease spasmodic coughs, do an inhalation with 3 drops cypress and 2 drops cedarwood twice daily; these oils can also be added to 10 ml carrier oil and massaged into the chest.

If your emotions are overstretched or you are suffering from stress, try taking a soothing bath with 3 drops cypress and 3 drops lavender and relax deeply.

Cypress essential oil is useful as a soothing skin treatment for an oily or blemished complexion.

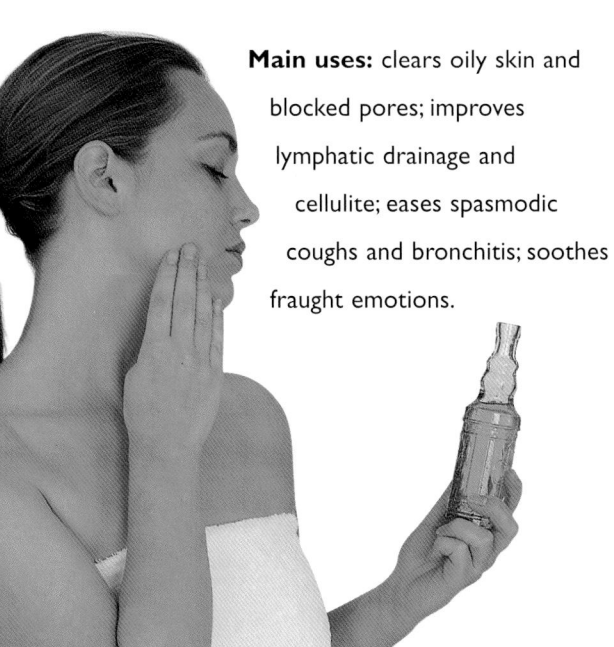

Petitgrain (orange leaf)

Citrus aurantium var. amara

Petitgrain is one of three oils taken from the bitter orange tree. Unlike most citrus oils, petitgrain is not phototoxic.

Plant profile: petitgrain is one of the essential oils produced by the bitter orange tree. The other oils are neroli (orange blossom) and bitter orange oil (expressed from the rind of the fruit). The leaves of the orange tree contain tiny sacs of essential oil, which are visible (like grains) to the naked eye when a leaf is held up to the sun – the French name of the oil means 'little grain'. The oil is an original ingredient of eau de cologne, popular since the eighteenth century. Most petitgrain oil comes from France or Paraguay.

Safety information: no issues. (Unlike orange, this oil is not phototoxic.)

Fragrance profile: a green, fresh, bittersweet aroma with a hint of citrus.

Main uses: tones, refreshes and balances oily and combination skins; eases stomach cramps, indigestion and wind; calms and soothes the mind, releasing tension and nervous exhaustion.

Suggested blends: for oily/combination skin, add 4 drops petitgrain, 2 drops patchouli and 4 drops lavender to 20 ml jojoba oil and use as a cleanser and skin-soother twice a day.

To ease stomach cramps, add 4 drops petitgrain, 2 drops peppermint and 4 drops roman chamomile to 20 ml carrier oil and massage the abdomen (half the dose of drops in 20 ml carrier can be used on children).

To relieve stress and calm the nerves, add 3 drops petitgrain and 3 drops sandalwood to a warm bath and relax.

Petitgrain is a fragrance note that can be found in many old-fashioned colognes.

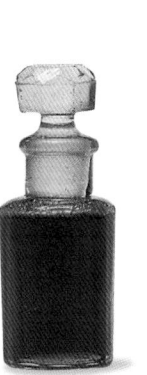
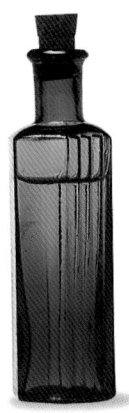
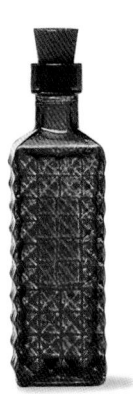
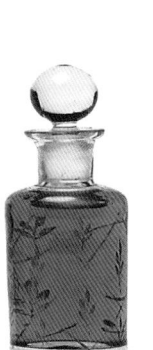
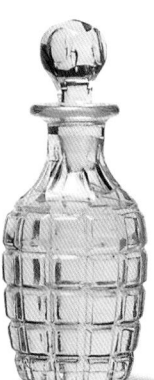
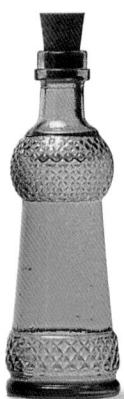

Patchouli

Pogostemon patchouli

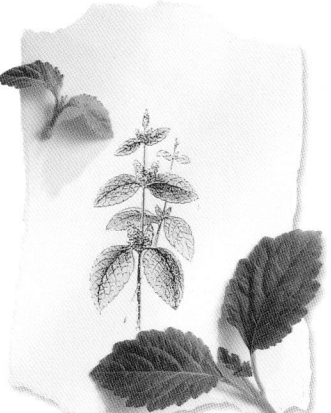

Patchouli leaves are soft, velvety and highly aromatic. The leaves are used in India to protect textiles from moths.

Plant profile: patchouli comes from India in the form of a thick, golden-brown essential oil with a very pronounced aroma. The leaves of the patchouli plant have a velvety texture thanks to thousands of tiny hairs on the surface. These contain microscopic sacs of essential oil, so that when you rub the leaf, the aroma is very strong on your fingers. Patchouli leaves are used to protect cloth from moths in India, and the oil is regarded as an insect repellent. It is also traditionally used in India as a skin conditioner and antiseptic.

Safety information: no issues.

Fragrance profile: a rich, velvety, musky aroma that develops spicy, earthy and sweet tones with time.

Main uses: helps to soothe cracked, chapped and dry skin and eczema; improves the complexion of mature and dry skins; increases sexual energy and helps to enhance sensuality.

Suggested blends: for dry, damaged or cracked skin, try creating a massage blend of 3 drops patchouli, 3 drops cedarwood and 4 drops roman chamomile in 20 ml jojoba oil and apply to the area as needed.

To improve the complexion, try adding 3 drops patchouli, 4 drops frankincense and 3 drops sandalwood to 20 ml carrier oil and massage gently into the face, especially at night (this blend is appropriate for men and women).

For a sensual massage blend, add 3 drops patchouli, 2 drops rose and 5 drops orange to 20 ml carrier oil.

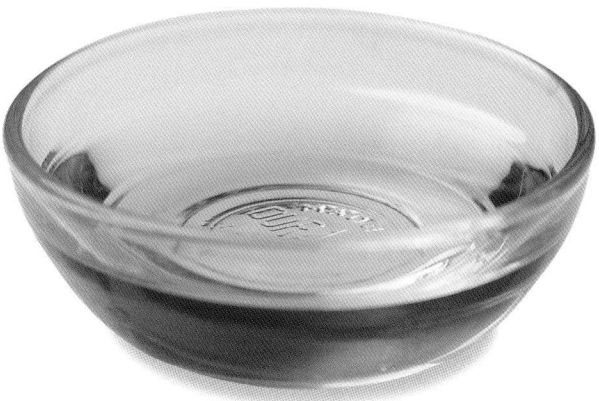

Patchouli makes a wonderful relaxing and sensual blend. The essential oil can increase and enhance sexual energy.

Eucalyptus
Eucalyptus globulus

Plant profile: there are more than 700 species of eucalyptus. In aromatherapy, several eucalyptus oils are used, of which *Eucalyptus globulus* is the most common. This evergreen tree from Australia can grow to a height of up to 90 metres when mature. The aromatic leaves are bluish-green on the upper surface and paler underneath. The leaves and the essential oil have been widely used as a household remedy in Australia from the days of the Aborigines in the treatment of fevers, respiratory conditions and skin infections.

Safety information: must not be swallowed – some cases of severe internal poisoning have occurred. Safe on the skin or as an inhalation.

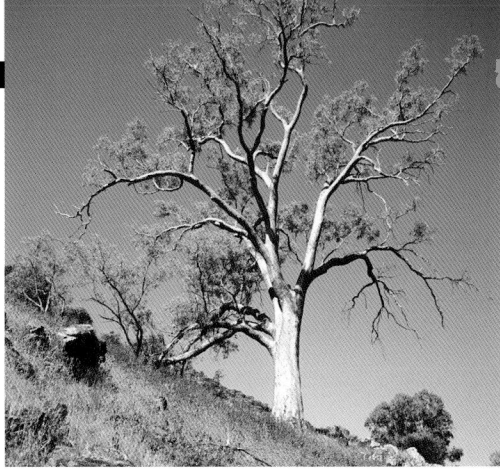

The eucalyptus tree is native to Australia and is an attractive evergreen with blue-green foliage.

Fragrance profile: extremely fresh and bracing, with woodier tones later.

Main uses: clears colds, blocked noses, sinusitis, chest infections; soothes burns, cuts, wounds and insect bites; eases muscular pains; improves circulation; improves concentration.

Suggested blends: for colds and chest problems, use 2 drops eucalyptus and 3 drops tea tree in an inhalation twice daily. Add the same combination of oils to 10 ml carrier oil and massage into the chest area.

For damaged skin, add 2 drops eucalyptus, 3 drops tea tree and 5 drops lavender to 20 ml carrier oil and apply twice daily.

For muscle pains, add 3 drops eucalyptus, 4 drops rosemary and 3 drops ginger to 20 ml carrier oil for massage.

To help improve levels of concentration, vaporise 3 drops eucalyptus and 3 drops rosemary.

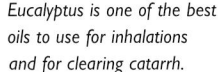

Eucalyptus is one of the best oils to use for inhalations and for clearing catarrh.

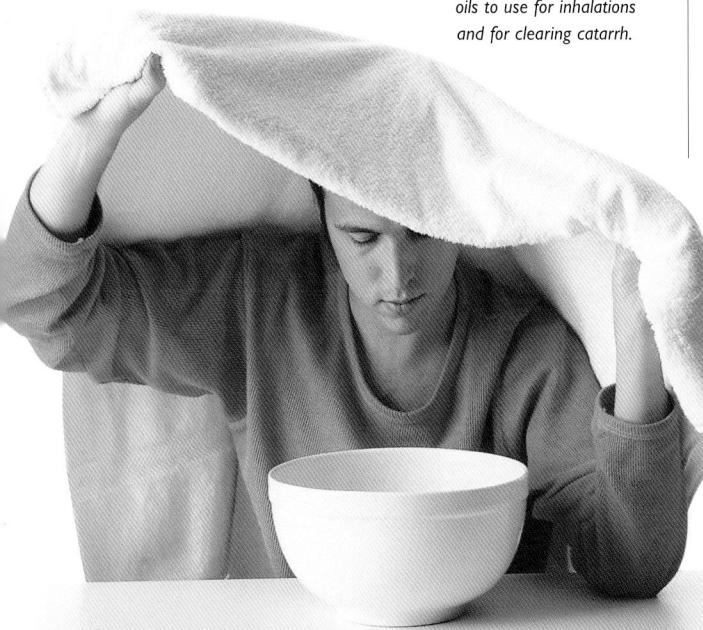

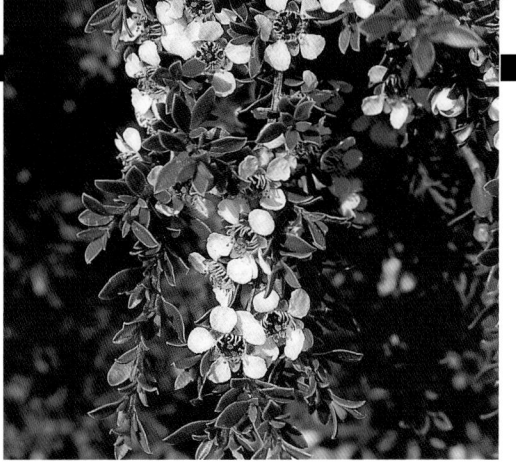

Tea tree essential oil is taken from the leaves of the tree and is very pungent and antiseptic.

Tea Tree
Melaleuca alternifolia

Plant profile: tea tree is native to Australia, where it has long been used by the aboriginal people as an antiseptic. The name 'tea tree' refers to the practice of drinking an infusion of the leaves as a healing herbal drink, first observed by the sailors on Captain Cook's ship in the eighteenth century. Production of the oil is now a huge commercial enterprise with a whole host of tea tree products available on the market, from toothpaste to foot powder. It is one of the most antiseptic plants ever discovered.

Tea tree can help to treat the symptoms of influenza. Inhale the oil from a tissue whenever necessary.

Safety information: safe to use neat on the skin (2 drops on a cotton wool pad applied directly to the affected area) except on individuals with sensitive or allergy-prone skin, for whom it must be diluted in carrier oil.

Fragrance profile: medicinal, green, camphoraceous aroma, pungent and strong.

Main uses: clears skin infection and acne; heals wounds and cuts; soothes insect bites; clears athlete's foot; helps influenza, colds, bronchitis; boosts general immunity.

Suggested blends: for skin infections, add 4 drops tea tree, 3 drops sandalwood and 3 drops lavender to 20 ml carrier oil and apply as necessary. To assist chest problems, use an inhalation of 3 drops tea tree and 3 drops lemon twice daily. To boost immunity, add 2 drops tea tree, 2 drops bergamot and 1 drop black pepper to a warm bath. Add this combination of oils to 10 ml carrier oil and massage the upper chest area. Do this daily during an episode of influenza.

Lemongrass
Cymbopogon citratus

Plant profile: lemongrass is an aromatic tropical grass from India. It is well known as a flavouring ingredient in Indian and Thai cooking. In India, the grass is used in traditional medicine to help reduce fevers and kill infections, and also as an insect repellent. The leaves are chopped just above ground level and, as with all grasses, new shoots are then produced very quickly.

Safety information: the oil is regarded as a potential irritant to already sensitive or allergic skin and is not advised for infants and young children. It should always be diluted in a carrier, even in bath blends.

Fragrance profile: a very strong, 'lemon sherbet' aroma that is zesty and sweet with a slightly heavy undertone.

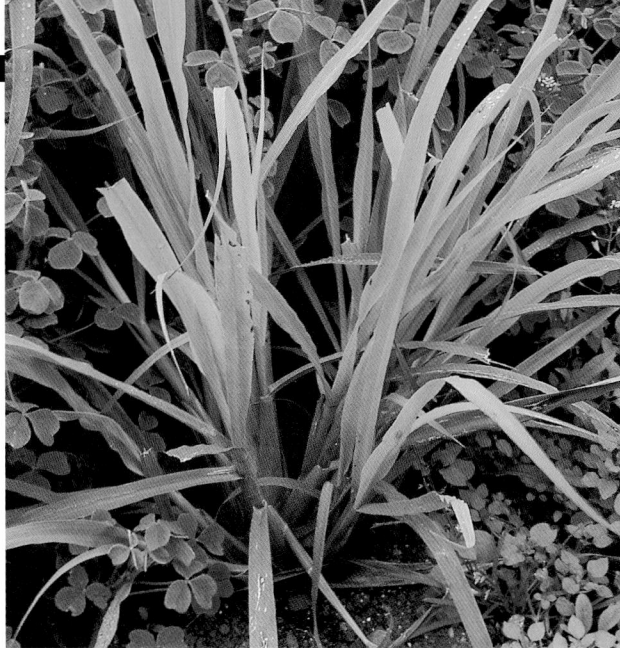

Lemongrass is a vigorous and aromatic tropical plant. It should always be diluted – even in blends for the bath.

Main uses: eases muscular aches, pains and stiffness; eases stomach cramps, indigestion and constipation; lifts depression or anxiety and improves the mood.

Suggested blends: for muscular aches, add 2 drops lemongrass, 3 drops rosemary and 5 drops cardamom to 20 ml carrier oil to massage the specific areas.

To ease stomach cramps or constipation, add 2 drops lemongrass, 4 drops coriander and 4 drops nutmeg to 20 ml carrier oil and massage the abdomen twice daily.

To improve mood and combat stress, add 2 drops lemongrass, 2 drops rose and 6 drops frankincense to 20 ml carrier oil.

Lemongrass is a key flavouring in most Thai dishes. Its zesty character can really lift a dish.

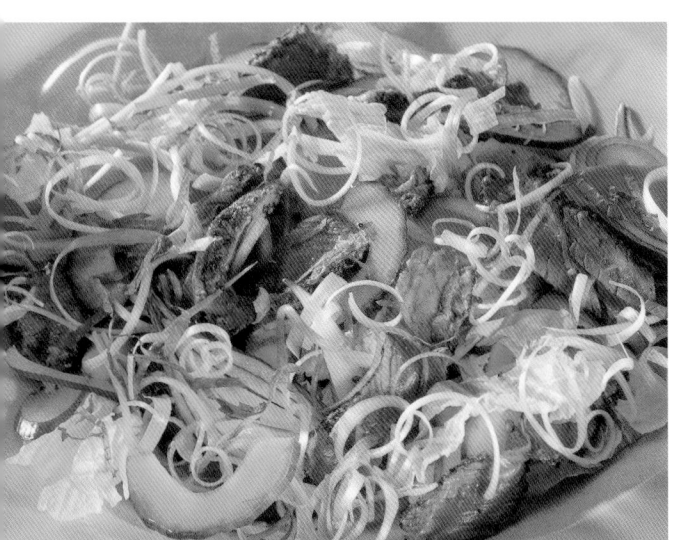

Palmarosa

Cymbopogon martini

Aromatic palmarosa is another grass grown in India. It has a similar fragrance to rose oil.

Plant profile: palmarosa is another aromatic grass from India, this time with a sweet smell and an altogether milder effect when used. In the past, it has often been used to adulterate or dilute pure rose oil, because the fragrance is somewhat similar and the grass is produced much more cheaply and in far larger quantities than rose. Palmarosa has a long-lasting aroma, which makes it a popular cosmetic ingredient in soaps, toiletries and perfumes.

Safety information: no issues.

Fragrance profile: a long-lasting, sweet and roselike aroma, which is soft and gentle with slightly lemony tones.

Main uses: soothes and calms irritated skin, acne, eczema, dermatitis; improves the facial complexion in all skin types, especially combination and mature; soothes cystitis and clears urinary tract infections; calms and de-stresses the nerves.

Suggested blends: for sensitive or irritated skin, add 3 drops palmarosa and 2 drops roman camomile to 20 ml carrier oil (note the low dilution) and apply as needed. To balance and rejuvenate the complexion, add 4 drops palmarosa, 3 drops frankincense and 3 drops sandalwood to 20 ml carrier oil and massage the face, especially at night. For cystitis or urinary problems, add 3 drops palmarosa and 3 drops sandalwood to a warm bath to soothe the area. To uplift your mood, add 3 drops palmarosa, 4 drops grapefruit and 3 drops orange to 20 ml carrier oil for an exotic and soft massage blend.

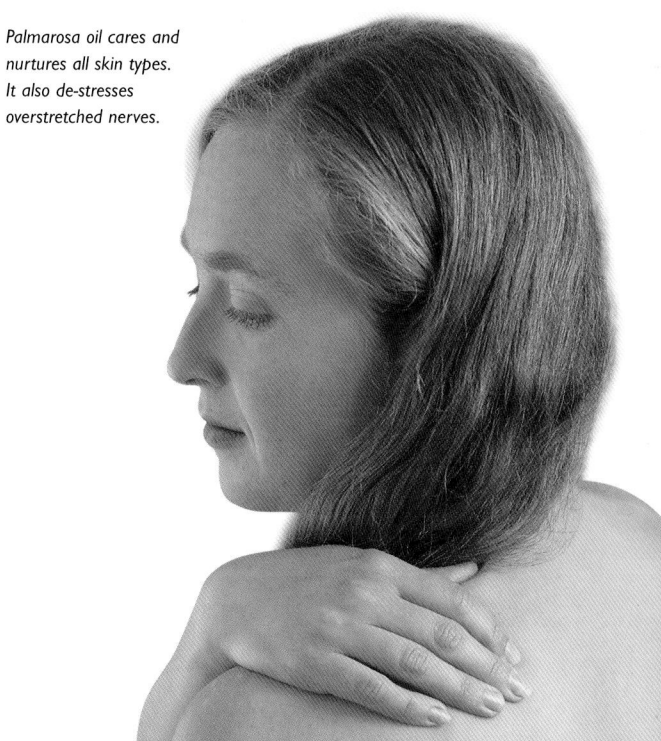

Palmarosa oil cares and nurtures all skin types. It also de-stresses overstretched nerves.

Flower Oils

These are some of the most exquisite fragrances you will encounter. Captured from the petals, they are the unique aromatic signal of that plant.

Lavender
Lavandula angustifolia

Plant profile: lavender oil is now widely produced in the UK, southern France, Tasmania, New Zealand and Bulgaria. Purple lavender fields make one of the most wonderful aromatic landscapes, filled with bees and butterflies busily enjoying the magnificent supply of pollen. Lavender oils vary in fragrance according to the altitude where they are produced – high altitude oils have sharper and fresher aromas, and low altitude ones are sweeter and softer.

Safety information: no issues. Lavender can be used neat (2 drops on a cotton wool pad applied directly to the affected area).

Fragrance profile: mainly soft, sweet and floral with camphoraceous and pungent notes.

Main uses: soothes cuts, burns, wounds, insect bites, sore skin; eases headaches, migraine and muscular aches and tension; soothes chesty spasmodic coughs; helps insomnia, nervous tension and anxiety; useful for both adults and children.

Suggested blends: for skin problems, add 4 drops lavender, 3 drops tea tree and 3 drops roman chamomile to 20 ml carrier oil and massage gently into the affected area.

Ease headaches by adding 3 drops lavender to 5 ml carrier oil and massaging the forehead and neck to provide relief.

To relieve coughs, an inhalation with 4 drops lavender and 3 drops cedarwood done twice daily can often be helpful.

To ease insomnia, vaporise 3 drops lavender and 3 drops orange to help you fall asleep.

Lavender fields are vibrantly purple and wonderfully aromatic. Bees and butterflies love visiting the plants that grow here.

Geranium

Pelargonium graveolens

The leaves of this geranium release a strong rosy aroma.

Plant profile:

this is a tropical geranium with velvety, frilly leaves. Rubbing the tiny surface hairs releases a strong, rosy aroma onto your fingers. The geranium grows as a shrub up to 1 metre in height and has pinkish flowers. The essential oil has a powerful floral aroma. The island of Réunion in the Indian Ocean produces the best-quality essential oil. Chinese and Egyptian geranium oils are also available but have a much heavier fragrance.

Geranium helps maintain a positive mood during the menstrual cycle.

Safety information:

no issues.

Fragrance profile:

rosy, sweet and strong, with a hint of lemon and fresh green notes.

Main uses: soothes cracked and inflamed skin, eczema, dermatitis, acne and congested or oily skin; eases premenstrual symptoms such as lack of energy, bloatedness and fluid retention; soothes mood swings and helps to balance hormonally related emotional upsets.

Suggested blends: for skin problems, add 3 drops geranium, 3 drops sandalwood and 4 drops lavender to 20 ml carrier oil and apply to the area as needed.

To ease premenstrual symptoms, try adding 2 drops geranium and 3 drops petitgrain to a warm bath. You can also use the same combination of oils in 10 ml carrier oil for an uplifting massage afterwards.

To help balance mood swings, add 3 drops geranium, 3 drops lemon and 4 drops orange to 20 ml carrier oil and massage into your skin. This will give you a floral and citrus uplift.

Ylang Ylang

Cananga odorata

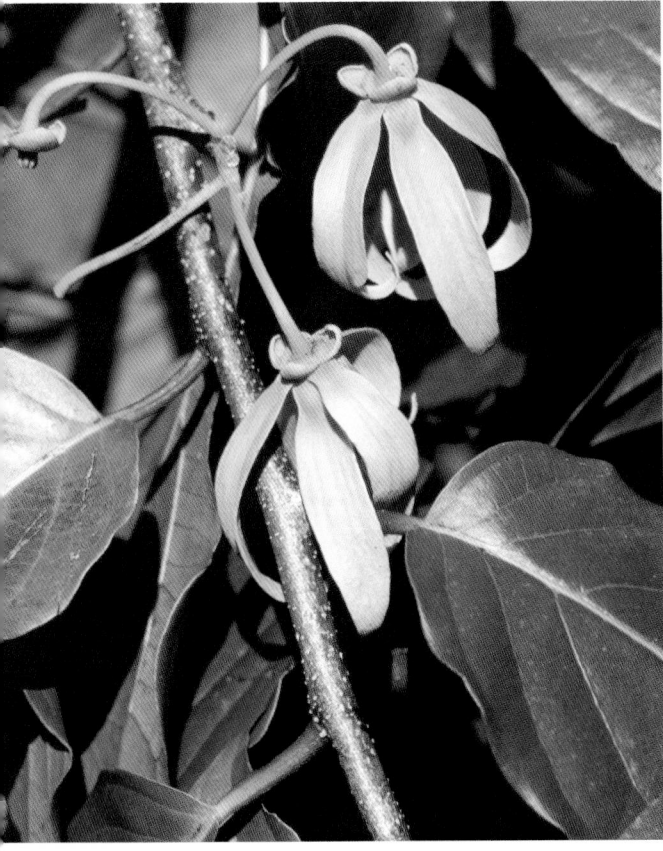

Ylang ylang flowers are beautiful exotic blooms, which yield large amounts of deeply scented essential oil.

Plant profile: all the way from Madagascar, a magical island off the coast of East Africa, comes the 'flower of flowers' – ylang ylang. Beautiful, lush, golden-yellow flowers with velvety petals produce a wonderful oil with a strong resemblance to jasmine. There is such a high content of fragrance in the flowers that the essential oil can be drawn off three times during the process of distillation, giving rise to three grades of essential oil. The first collection of oil is known as the 'perfume' grade and is the best quality.

Safety information: no major issues. Some individuals find the strong floral aroma brings on a headache.

Fragrance profile: sharp and sweet, becoming deeply floral, jasmine-like, heady and soft with time.

Main uses: tones oily and combination skins; reduces panic attacks and stress-related anxiety symptoms; soothes and calms emotional stress and overstretched nerves.

Suggested blends: to tone oily skin, add 2 drops ylang ylang, 3 drops sandalwood and 5 drops frankincense to 20 ml jojoba oil and use as a cleanser and skin-soother twice daily.

For panic and anxiety attacks, add 2 drops ylang ylang and 3 drops lavender to a warm bath, and add the same combination of oils to 10 ml carrier oil for a relaxing neck and shoulder massage afterwards.

To soothe the nerves and ease anxiety, add 2 drops ylang ylang, 2 drops patchouli and 5 drops orange to 20 ml carrier oil and massage your body gently.

Rose

Rosa damascena

Plant profile: costly and labour-intensive to produce, rose is one of the most beautiful of all essential oils. The little damask rose from Kazanlik in Bulgaria produces the finest quality rose oil, although Turkish, Moroccan and Russian rose oils are also excellent. Rose 'otto' is simply distilled rose oil – between 50 and 100 blooms are needed per drop. An 'absolute' of rose, chemically extracted, is also available at a slightly lower cost. Look out for pure rose oil already diluted in jojoba as a more affordable and still effective way to use this oil.

Safety information: no issues.

Fragrance profile: honey-sweet, slightly lemony and soft, with richness and depth.

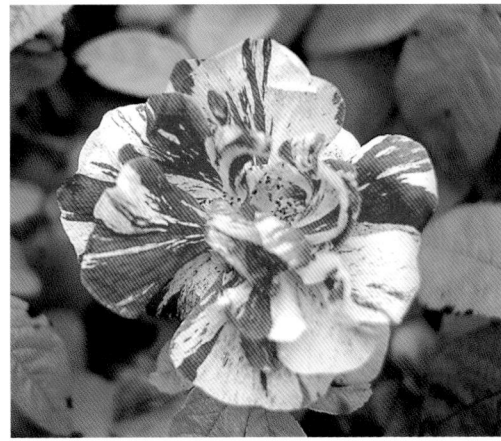

The damask rose has a uniquely glorious aroma. It is one of the most costly oils to produce but is worth every drop.

Main uses: tones and rejuvenates all skin types, especially dry, sensitive and mature; eases premenstrual and menopausal symptoms; helps release feelings of grief and separation, restoring the heart.

Suggested blends: to tone the skin, add 2 drops rose, 4 drops frankincense and 4 drops sandalwood to 20 ml jojoba oil (halve the number of drops for sensitive skin).

To help relieve premenstrual or menopausal symptoms, add 4 drops rose, 3 drops neroli and 3 drops mandarin to 20 ml carrier oil and massage into the body.

To ease grief, add 2 drops rose and 3 drops orange to a bath. Use the same combination in 10 ml carrier oil for a massage afterwards.

Pure rose oil trickled into a bath releases an amazing fragrance, which can relieve stress almost instantly.

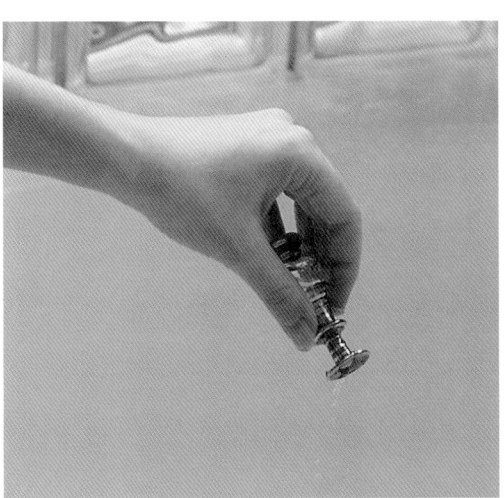

Roman Chamomile

Anthemis nobilis

Plant profile: the name 'chamomile' is originally from the Greek *kamaimelon,* which means 'ground apple'. This derives from the fact that the chamomile plant is low-growing and smells strongly of apples. In its non-flowering variety, this species of chamomile is often used to make a fragrant lawn. The flowers, however, are required for distillation.

The oil has a pale blue colour due to the presence of a substance known as 'azulene', which has anti-inflammatory properties. The oil is now cultivated successfully in the UK.

Safety information: no issues.

Fragrance profile: fruity (apple-like), sweet, fresh and soft.

Main uses: soothes cuts, burns, sore, dry skin, nappy rash; eases menstrual cramps, premenstrual low energy and tension; soothes headaches, migraine; helps insomnia, nervous exhaustion, tension, restlessness and stress-related problems.

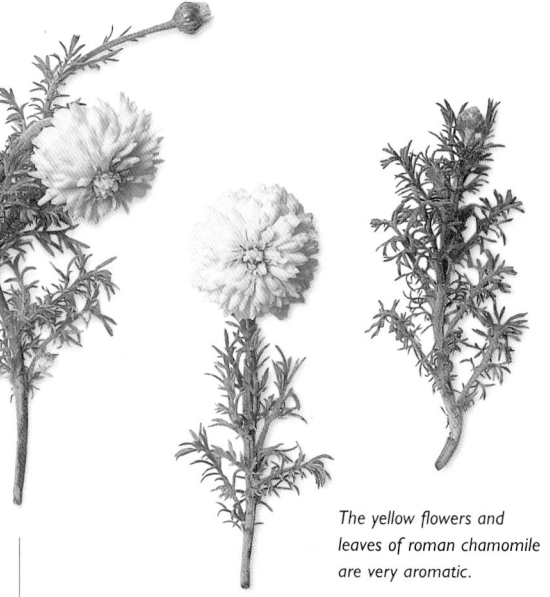

The yellow flowers and leaves of roman chamomile are very aromatic.

Suggested blends: for skin problems, add 3 drops roman chamomile, 4 drops lavender and 3 drops palmarosa to 20 ml carrier oil and apply as necessary; for baby nappy rash, use 1 drop only of chamomile in 20 ml carrier oil for an extremely gentle application.

To ease menstrual symptoms, add 3 drops roman chamomile and 2 drops marjoram to a warm bath, then add this combination of oils to 10 ml carrier oil and massage the lower abdomen.

For insomnia and restlessness, try vaporising 3 drops roman chamomile and 3 drops lavender in the bedroom before turning in for the night.

Babies and younger children respond well to the fragrance of roman chamomile essential oil.

Neroli (orange blossom)

Citrus aurantium var. amara

Plant profile: the essential oil from orange blossom is named after princess Neroli, an Italian noblewoman of the Renaissance period who perfumed her gloves with Neroli flowers. The oil has an enchanting aroma, and is costly and labour-intensive to produce, as the fragrant white flowers of the bitter orange tree have to be picked by hand. Neroli essential oil is mostly distilled in France and Morocco. Look out for pure neroli diluted in jojoba from quality essential oil ranges, as this is a more affordable way of trying this fragrance.

Safety information: no issues.

Fragrance profile: creamy-sweet, citrusy, rich and soft with green undertones.

Main uses: tones and rejuvenates the complexion, especially dry, mature or undernourished skins; helps scar tissue, wounds, cuts; eases nervous indigestion and irritable bowel symptoms; helps calm panic, shock and sudden emotional upsets.

Suggested blends: for skincare, add 3 drops neroli, 4 drops frankincense and 3 drops

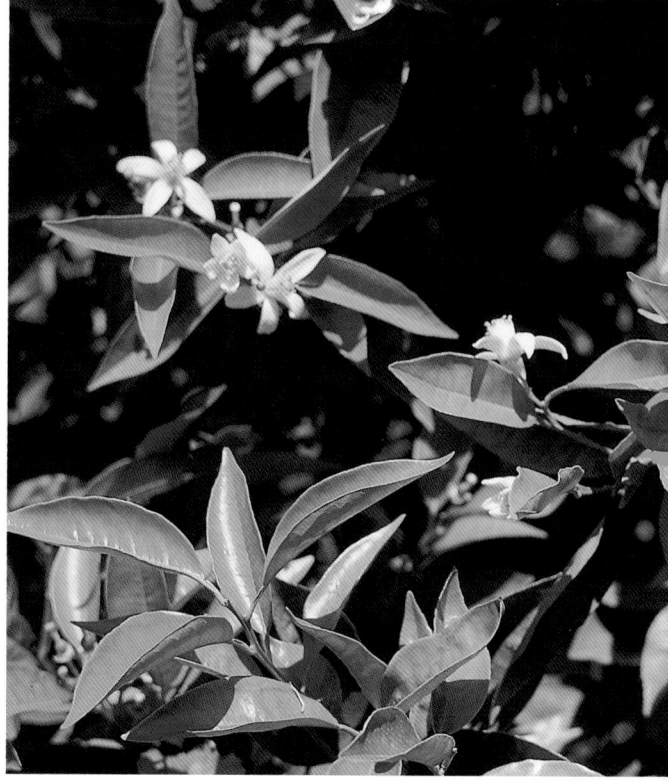

Each orange blossom has to be picked by hand, making neroli – along with rose – one of the more expensive essential oils.

patchouli to 20 ml jojoba for a nourishing facial massage oil.

To heal damaged skin, add 3 drops neroli, 4 drops lavender and 4 drops myrrh to 20 ml carrier oil and apply to the area twice daily.

For nervous indigestion, add 4 drops neroli, 3 drops peppermint and 3 drops ginger to 20 ml carrier oil for gentle abdominal massage whenever necessary.

To help shock and panic, simply place 2 drops neroli on a tissue and inhale the fragrance until calm is restored.

Berry and Seed Oils

These are aromatic packages of pungent fragrance, often designed to attract animals and birds. They ingest the seeds and then eventually release them into the earth, helping plant reproduction.

Nutmeg
Myristica fragrans

Aromatic nutmegs have a spicy, cheering fragrance. They can be used in cakes and biscuits to give a distinctive flavour.

Plant profile: the nutmeg tree grows in Indonesia and Sri Lanka. The fruits are covered with a layer called mace, which is removed before processing. The highly aromatic nutmegs are steam-distilled to give a fragrant essential oil. In Western herbal tradition, nutmegs were prized for their digestive tonic and muscle-warming properties. In medieval times they were so valuable they were kept locked away.

Safety information: a strong oil, so should be used in moderation.

Fragrance profile: warm, sharp, spicy and sweet with a distinctive softness later.

Main uses: eases muscular aches and pains, arthritic pain and cold extremities; soothes and calms indigestion, stomach cramps, nausea; helps to re-energise the body after illness, speeding convalescence, uplifting the spirits and restoring the circulation.

Suggested blends: for aches and pains, add 2 drops nutmeg, 4 drops cardamom and 4 drops grapefruit to 20 ml carrier oil and massage into the affected area. To soothe the digestion, add 2 drops nutmeg, 4 drops peppermint and 4 drops ginger to 20 ml carrier oil for abdominal massage. As a restoring tonic, add 1 drop nutmeg, 2 drops black pepper and 2 drops orange to a warm bath and relax in the water. Add the same oils to 10 ml carrier oil and massage into the skin afterwards.

Blends made using nutmeg can ease muscular cramps.

Black Pepper

Piper nigrum

Plant profile: this plant is a trailing vinelike climber with lovely, heart-shaped, dark green leaves and clusters of white flowers that become the berries – or peppercorns. These turn from red to black as they mature (white pepper has had the outer layer removed). Black peppercorns are steam-distilled to yield the essential oil. The tropical plant is native to India, and the oil is produced there as well as in Indonesia and Malaysia.

Safety information: no issues.

Fragrance profile: warm, musty, sharp and spicy, with heavier sweet notes later.

Main uses: warms and stimulates blood circulation; helps to ease aches and pains; soothes indigestion, stomach cramps and constipation; strengthens the immune system, especially against influenza.

Suggested blends: to help stimulate poor or sluggish circulation, add 4 drops black pepper, 2 drops lemongrass and 4 drops cardamom to 20 ml carrier oil and massage into the affected area as needed.

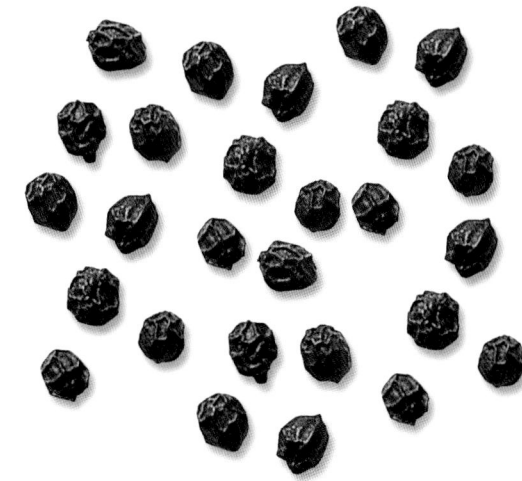

Black peppercorns yield a warm and pungent oil, which has a very spicy aroma. Black pepper essential oil can boost the immune system and ease indigestion.

To help ease indigestion or constipation, add 3 drops black pepper, 3 drops peppermint and 4 drops neroli to 20 ml carrier oil and massage the abdomen twice daily.

As a tonic for the immune system, add 1 drop black pepper, 2 drops tea tree and 2 drops bergamot to a warm evening bath and soak for at least 20 minutes. Add the same oils to 20 ml carrier oil and massage the chest area afterwards.

Poor circulation can be helped by vigorously massaging the area in question with the pepper blend.

Cardamom

Elettaria cardamomum

Essential oils like cardamom improve the mood and warm the affected areas. Cardamom is a good energy tonic too.

Plant profile: a member of the same plant family as ginger, cardamom produces aromatic flowers that turn into little seed pods filled with tiny black seeds. The pods are traditionally chewed in India to sweeten the breath after eating spicy food, and the wonderful aroma of cardamom is also used to flavour Indian ice cream and confectionery. Cardamom is commonly used in Eastern medicinal traditions as a lung tonic and immunity-boosting plant remedy.

Safety information: no issues.

Fragrance profile: warm, fruity, sweet and spicy with a mouthwatering pungent freshness.

Main uses: soothes and opens the chest, helping breathing and congestion; warms and soothes stomach cramps and indigestion; uplifts the mind and gives a positive feeling when energy is low.

Suggested blends: to improve breathing, add 3 drops cardamom and 2 drops cedarwood to a bowl of nearly boiling water and inhale the vapour, repeating twice daily; add the same oils to 10 ml carrier oil and massage the chest area afterwards.

To help ease digestion problems, massage the abdomen twice daily with 3 drops cardamom, 3 drops coriander and 4 drops orange in 20 ml carrier oil.

As a tonic to raise low spirits, add 3 drops cardamom and 2 drops mandarin to a warm bath and relax in the water. Add the same oils to 10 ml carrier oil and massage into the skin afterwards.

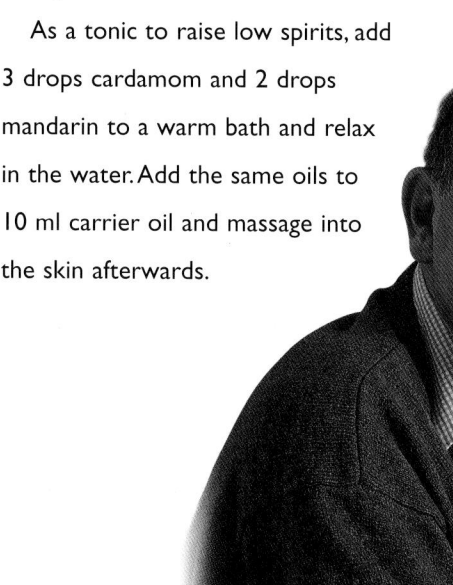

May Chang

Litsea cubeba

May chang has berries that smell like lemon sherbert! It is not a suitable oil for babies and young children.

Plant profile: a tree from China with delicate leaves and little whitish-yellow flowers that become highly lemon-scented tiny fruits. The oil from the berries of the may chang tree is used a great deal in China as a mood enhancer and as a tonic to the heart; it calms and regulates the heart rhythm when used in massage. It is similar to lemongrass, but has a much lighter and sweeter fragrance.

Fresh lemony scents, such as may chang, have a cheering effect on the body and mind and can help ease mood swings.

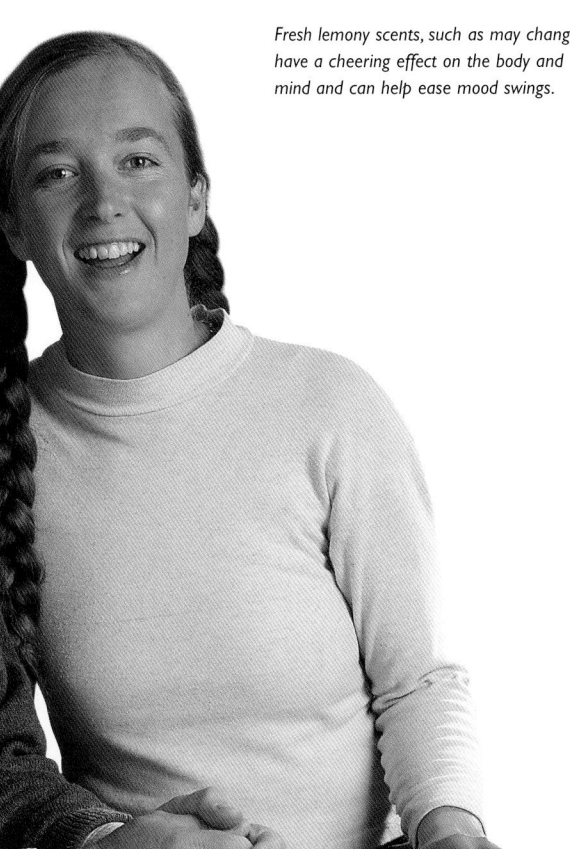

Safety information: avoid using this oil on sensitive or damaged skin. It is not suitable for babies or children. Always dilute this oil, even if you are using it in the bath.

Fragrance profile: soft, sweet and fruity with a strong 'lemon sherbet' aroma that is zesty and mouthwatering.

Main uses: eases muscular aches and pains, strains and backache; eases panic or stress attacks; uplifts depression and anxiety, mood swings and tearfulness.

Suggested blends: for aches and pains, add 2 drops may chang, 4 drops juniper and 4 drops lavender and massage affected areas.

Panic and stress attacks can be eased by simply placing 2 drops may chang on a tissue and inhaling the aroma for a few minutes. Add 2 drops may chang and 3 drops neroli to a warm bath and relax in the water to recover.

Uplift moods and ease depression by massaging the body with a blend of 2 drops may chang, 2 drops rose and 6 drops frankincense in 20 ml carrier oil.

Juniper

Juniperus communis

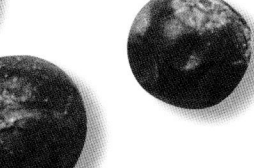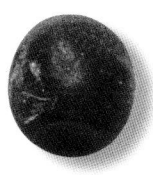

Blue-black juniper berries are sharp and pungently scented. They take up to two years to turn black.

Plant profile: juniper is a vigorous shrub with dark green spiky leaves. The essential oil comes mainly from Germany, where the plant grows well, and also from parts of Croatia. The berries on the juniper bush take up to two years to turn black and produce the best-quality oil. Juniper is also used in making gin, and in northern European cooking it is used to give pungent flavour to root vegetables. In herbal medicine, juniper is considered to be a strong diuretic and internal cleanser.

Safety information: this is best avoided during pregnancy, and also by people with any serious kidney complaints.

Fragrance profile: pungent, peppery and camphoraceous, with sweeter, softer notes developing later.

Main uses: helps to clear lymphatic congestion and detoxify the system; opens the chest and eases breathing in respiratory complaints; freshens the mind and helps improve concentration.

Suggested blends: to help detoxify, add 2 drops juniper, 2 drops angelica and 6 drops grapefruit to 20 ml carrier oil for a vigorous daily massage to affected areas of the body.

To help respiratory complaints, add 2 drops juniper and 3 drops eucalyptus to a bowl of nearly boiling water and inhale the vapours. Do this twice daily.

To help concentration, vaporise 3 drops juniper and 3 drops lemon in a room; this also helps to clear the atmosphere and neutralise any stale or unpleasant odours.

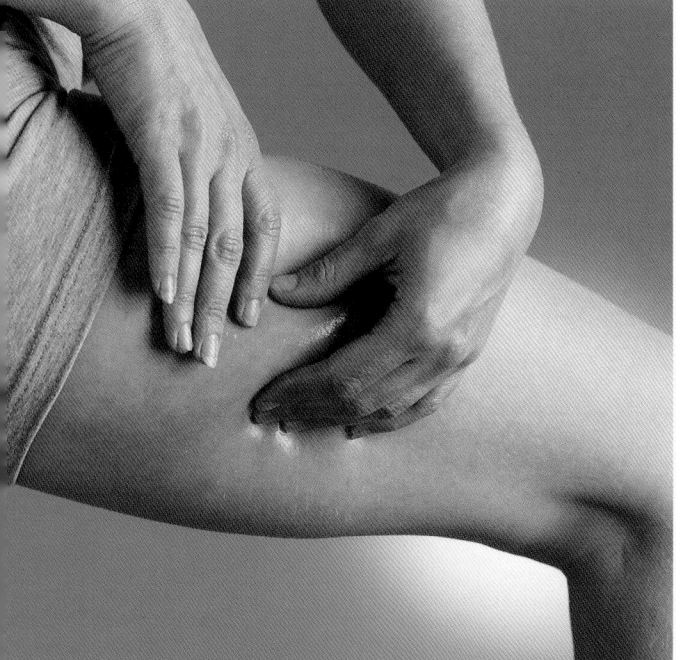

Massage blends with juniper can help improve areas of poor circulation in the legs. A vigorous daily massage is recommended.

Coriander Seed

Coriandrum sativum

Plant profile: the coriander plant is a highly aromatic herb with deliciously flavoured dark green leaves. It is easy to grow in the garden and makes a pungent addition to salad greens and a wonderful garnish for Indian dishes. The coriander plant produces umbels – umbrella-like stalks topped with little white flowers that eventually turn to brownish-coloured aromatic seeds. These are distilled to produce the essential oil in Eastern European countries, including Russia and Croatia.

Safety information: no issues.

Fragrance profile: woody, spicy and sweet with a slight hint of musk.

Main uses: warms and soothes muscular stiffness and aching joints; helps build immunity, especially in the case of influenza; eases mental exhaustion and overstretched nerves.

Coriander is a herb widely used in cooking and herbalism. It has attractive heads of white flowers.

Coriander seeds are a pungent spice and are used frequently in Indian cuisine. The leaves are also used as a delicious garnish.

Suggested blends: to warm muscles, add 3 drops coriander, 3 drops black pepper and 4 drops ginger to 20 ml carrier oil and massage twice daily. To help boost the immune system, add 2 drops coriander and 3 drops lemon to a bath; add the same oils to 10 ml carrier oil afterwards and massage into the chest area.

To ease exhaustion, add 2 drops coriander, 1 drop neroli and 2 drops lavender to a bath; the same oils can be added to 10 ml carrier oil afterwards for a massage. This routine can also help improve the quality of sleep.

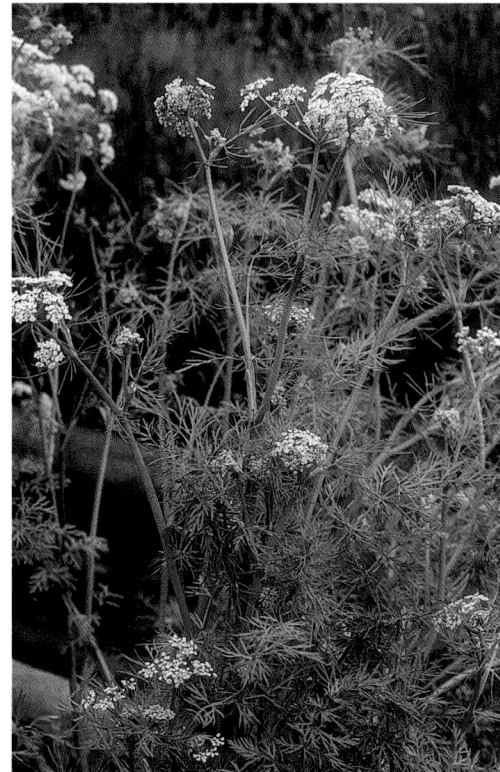

Fruit Oils

These oils are packed into tiny fragrant globules in the rind of citrus fruit. Fresh and zesty, they are mouthwatering aromas, loved by adults and children.

Orange (sweet)
Citrus sinensis

Plant profile: most orange essential oil that is commercially available is from the sweet orange tree, which originated in China. The essential oil is expressed, or crushed out of the rind of the fruit. The bitter orange tree (*Citrus aurantium*) produces petitgrain and neroli essential oils.

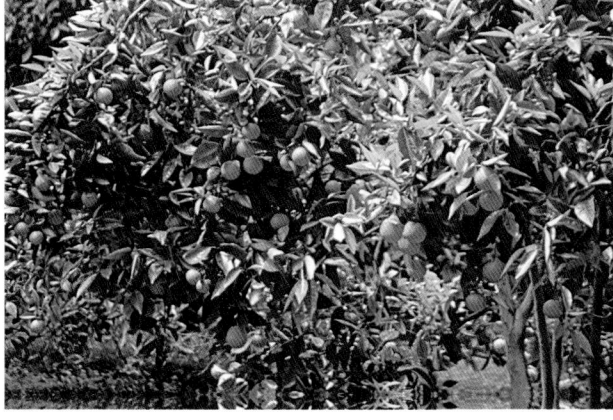

Orange trees are covered with delicious-smelling leaves, flowers and fruits. Orange essential oil is popular with young and old alike.

Safety information: very mildly phototoxic; avoid exposure to strong sunlight or a sunbed for 12 hours after skin application.

Fragrance profile: sweet, warm, fresh and citrusy.

Main uses: soothes stomach cramps and indigestion (especially in children); rejuvenates congested and

Children particularly love the sweet soft aroma of orange essential oil. It is a popular Christmas smell!

slack skin; uplifts depression, mood swings, anxiety and emotional stress.

Suggested blends: for stomach problems, add 4 drops orange, 2 drops peppermint and 4 drops ginger to 20 ml carrier oil and massage the abdomen 2–3 times daily (halve the number of drops in 20 ml for children).

To rejuvenate tired skin, add 4 drops orange, 4 drops frankincense and 2 drops cypress to 20 ml jojoba.

To ease anxiety, add 2 drops orange, 1 drop rose and 2 drops sandalwood to a bath; use this blend in 10 ml carrier oil for massage.

Lemon

Citrus limonum

Lemon rind is packed full of fresh and zesty essential oil. It is a good oil to assist concentration and sharpen the mind.

Plant profile: the finest essential oil of lemon is considered to come from trees grown in Sicily, although the fruit is also cultivated in California, Florida and Israel. The evergreen tree is thorny and has shiny, dark green, aromatic leaves that produce an essential oil called *petitgrain citronnier*. The fragrant flowers turn into the fruit, which when ripe are a warm golden yellow. Essential oil of lemon is expressed, or squeezed out of the peel of the fruit.

Safety information: mildly phototoxic; avoid any exposure to strong sunlight or a sunbed for at least 12 hours after application of the oil to the skin.

Fragrance profile: green, citrusy and fresh, zesty and bright; softer and more sherbety tones develop with time.

Main uses: helps build immunity against colds, influenza and other viral infections; detoxifies the system and assists lymphatic drainage; freshens the mind and helps to improve concentration.

Lemon trees grow all over the Mediterranean, and particularly in Sicily. They are a wonderful sight in the summer.

Suggested blends: to help boost the immune system, vaporise 3 drops lemon and 2 drops tea tree in a room to disinfect the air; add the same oils to 10 ml carrier oil to massage the chest area twice daily.

To help detoxify the body, add 4 drops lemon, 2 drops angelica and 4 drops juniper to 20 ml carrier oil and massage the legs and other affected areas twice daily.

To assist concentration and improve alertness, add 3 drops lemon and 3 drops rosemary to a vaporiser; this is especially helpful when studying.

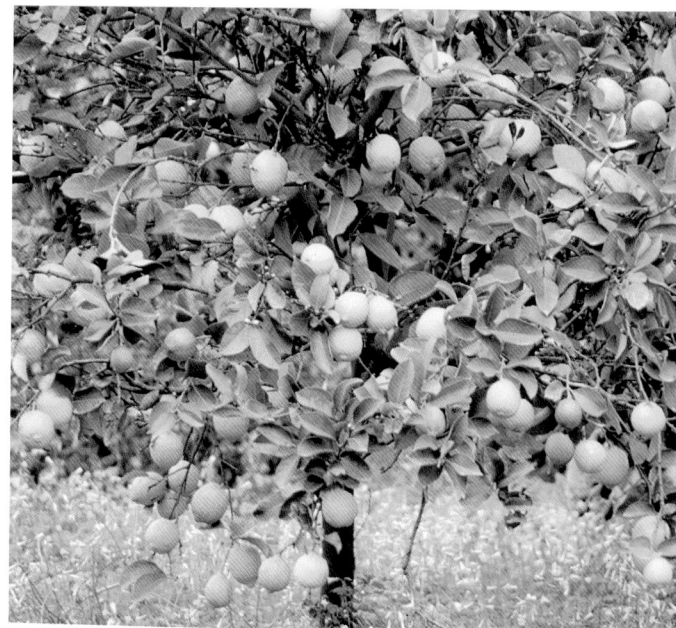

Mandarin

Citrus reticulata

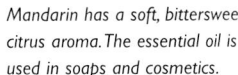

Mandarin has a soft, bittersweet citrus aroma. The essential oil is used in soaps and cosmetics.

Plant profile: this small citrus tree is evergreen and its fruit has an immediate association with Christmas. The fruit and the expressed oil are produced mainly in Brazil, Spain and Italy. Because it is so mild and pleasant, mandarin is used as a flavouring in many confectionery items, liqueurs and soft drinks, as well as in soaps, toiletries and perfumes. It is a favourite with children.

Safety information: very mildly phototoxic; avoid exposure to strong sunlight or a sunbed for 12 hours after application to the skin.

Fragrance profile: fresh, pungent and sweet with a bright citrus zest; softer and more floral tones developing with time.

Main uses: clears congested and oily skin; soothes stomach cramps and nervous indigestion (especially in children); eases insomnia, restless sleep and troubled dreams.

Suggested blends: for oily skin, add 4 drops mandarin, 3 drops cypress and 3 drops juniper to 20 ml jojoba oil and use as a cleanser and skin-soother for evening treatment.

To ease digestion problems, add 4 drops mandarin, 2 drops roman chamomile and 4 drops lavender to 20 ml carrier oil and gently massage the abdomen twice daily (halve the number of drops in 20 ml for children).

To help induce restful sleep, add 3 drops mandarin and 3 drops lavender to a vaporiser.

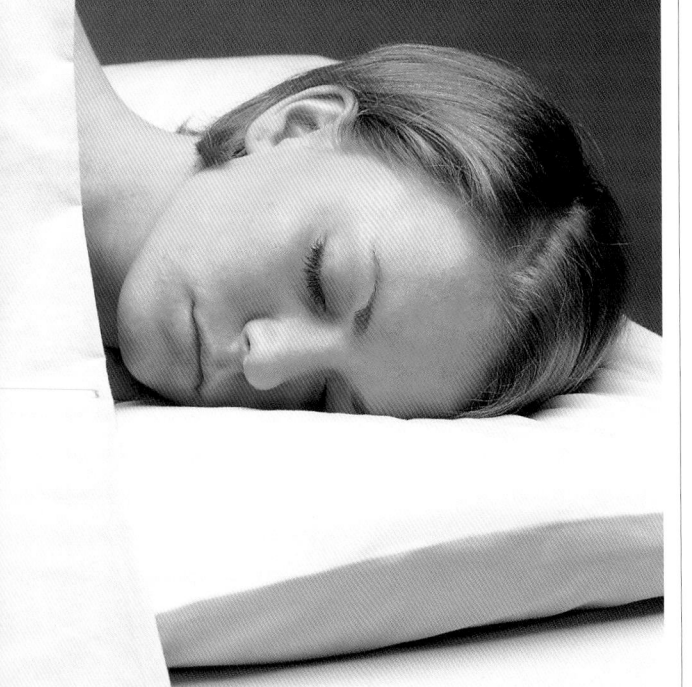

Vaporising mandarin essential oil at night helps to improve sleep and ease any lingering anxiety.

Grapefruit

Citrus x paradisi

The large golden grapefruit produces a different aroma to its other citrus relatives.

Plant profile: grapefruit is a hybrid which may have been derived from an old variety of fruit called the shaddock. It is now cultivated extensively in Florida in its familiar golden and pink-fleshed varieties. The essential oil is expressed from the peel, and grapefruit has an aroma quite different from its citrus relatives, thanks to the presence of sharp bitter constituents that give it freshness and zest.

Safety information: mildly phototoxic; avoid exposure to strong sunlight or a sunbed for 12 hours after application to the skin.

Fragrance profile: green, bittersweet, zesty and fresh, with a soft, powdery afternote.

Main uses: helps clear toxins and improve areas of cellulite; eases the chest and breathing in colds and influenza; eases anxiety, depression and stress, helps to relieve insomnia and disturbed dreams.

Suggested blends: for detoxification purposes, first use a skin brush on dry skin to boost the circulation, then add 4 drops grapefruit, 3 drops lemon and 3 drops juniper to 20 ml carrier oil for an evening massage of the affected areas. To help relieve chest infections, add 3 drops grapefruit and 2 drops cedarwood to a bowl of nearly boiling water and inhale the vapour for 20 minutes; add the same drops to 10 ml carrier oil afterwards and massage the chest.

To ease insomnia and anxiety, add 2 drops grapefruit and 3 drops sandalwood to a warm evening bath and relax in the water; add the same drops to 10 ml carrier oil and massage the skin afterwards.

Massaging the chest with grapefruit essential oil can ease congestion and help breathing problems.

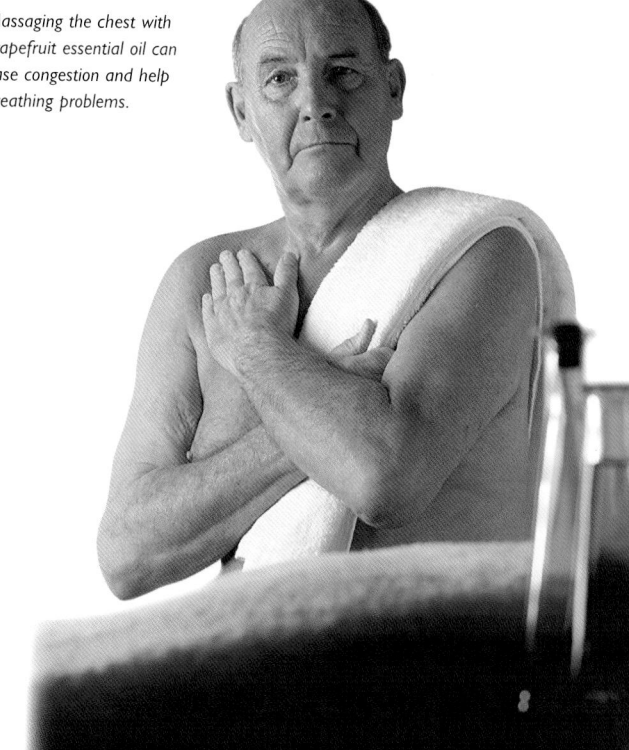

Bergamot

Citrus bergamia

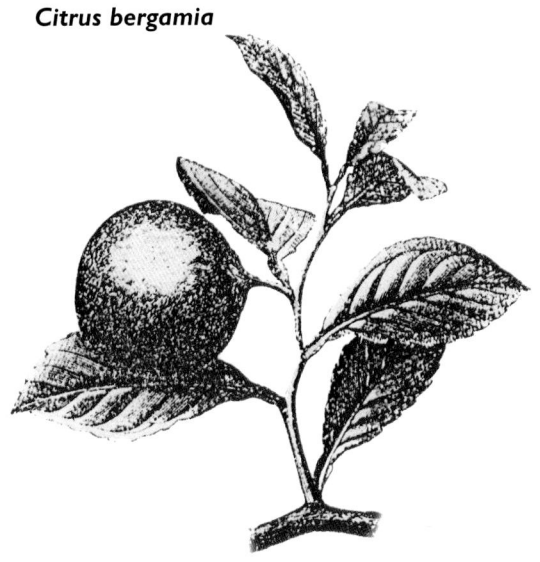

Bergamot is a small and very bitter orange. It is grown in Italy, where it has been used in traditional remedies for many years.

Plant profile: bergamot is a small bitter orange grown in the Lombardy region of Italy near the town of Bergamo. The fruit has long been used in the traditional medicine of the area as a remedy for fevers and low immunity. The essential oil from the peel is best known as the flavouring of Earl Grey tea, giving the drink a fresh, citrusy flavour.

Safety information: bergamot is strongly phototoxic; avoid exposing the skin to strong sunlight or sunbeds for at least 12 hours after application. FCF (furano-coumarin free) bergamot oil is available with the phototoxic constituent removed, but the aroma of the oils is much reduced.

Fragrance profile: fresh, bright, citrusy and sweet, developing softer, rounder and warmer tones later.

Main uses: boosts immunity, helps to combat colds, influenza and respiratory complaints; eases the symptoms of vaginal thrush; soothes anxiety, depression, helps to lift low spirits and combat stress.

Suggested blends: to help boost the immune system, add 2 drops bergamot, 2 drops tea tree and 1 drop black pepper to an evening bath and relax in the water; then add the same drops of essential oil to 10 ml carrier oil and massage the chest area.

For thrush, add 2 drops bergamot and 3 drops sandalwood to a warm bath to soothe the area.

To ease stress and anxiety, vaporise 3 drops bergamot and 3 drops frankincense to create a warm and uplifting aroma.

Bergamot and tea tree oils help to improve general immunity.

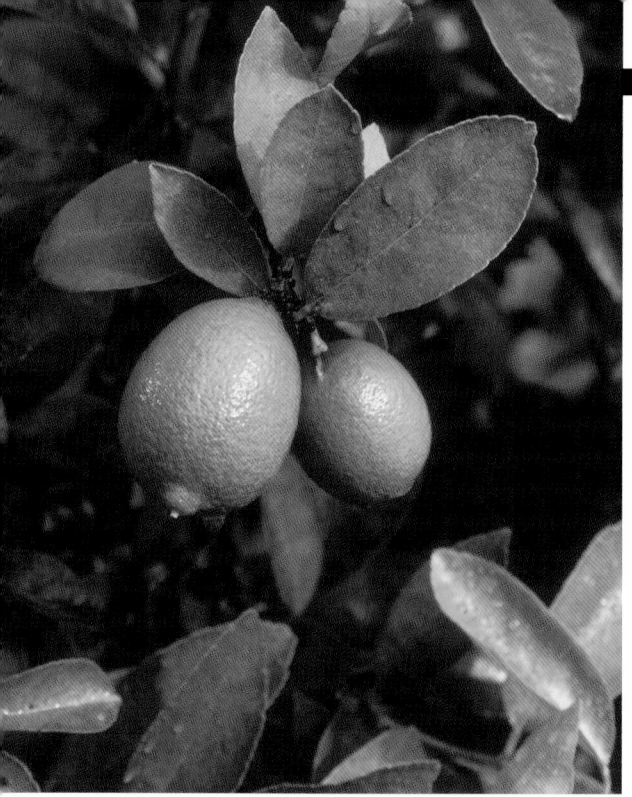

Fresh green limes are popular in Caribbean cooking. They are also an excellent source of vitamin C.

Lime

Citrus aurantifolia

Plant profile: an evergreen citrus tree, this is thorny with smooth aromatic leaves and small white flowers which turn into the fruits. Limes are about half the size of lemons and are a rich green in colour. Limes are an excellent source of vitamin C and are widely used in cookery recipes from the West Indies. The oil is expressed from the peel. The main centres of production are Florida, Cuba and Central America.

Safety information: lime is moderately phototoxic; you should avoid exposing the skin to strong sunlight or a sunbed for at least 12 hours after application.

Fragrance profile: bitter, green and fresh with a powerful zest and sharp fruity notes.

Main uses: helps detoxify and improve areas of cellulite; eases chest infections, respiratory complaints and catarrh; clears the head and improves concentration.

Suggested blends: to help detoxify, first use a skin brush to stimulate the circulation, then add 2 drops lime, 3 drops juniper and 5 drops cypress to 20 ml carrier oil and massage affected areas, as an evening treatment.

To relieve respiratory complaints, add 3 drops lime and 3 drops eucalyptus to a large bowl of nearly boiling water and inhale the vapours, twice daily for 20 minutes.

To clear the head, increase alertness and improve the atmosphere in stuffy rooms, vaporise 3 drops lime and 3 drops peppermint.

Vaporise a mixture of peppermint and lime essential oils to help improve concentration.

Simple Essential Oil Skincare

Essential oils can be used as the basis of a simple and effective skincare routine. They are particularly effective when used at night, because lying horizontally promotes an excellent supply of blood to your face, allowing maximum absorption of essential oils through the skin. Use the chart below to identify your skin type and choose the blends that will be most suitable for you.

Skin types

Normal – smooth and supple, clear in appearance, fine-textured
Dry – dull-textured, dehydrated, tends to tighten up in wind or warm temperatures
Mature – evident expression lines and slackness around eyes end mouth, less elasticity
Oily – shiny, with large obvious pores, tendency to blemishes
Combination – a greasy patch over forehead, nose and chin; dry cheek areas
Sensitive – often very pale, sensitive to sunlight and cosmetics, allergic tendency

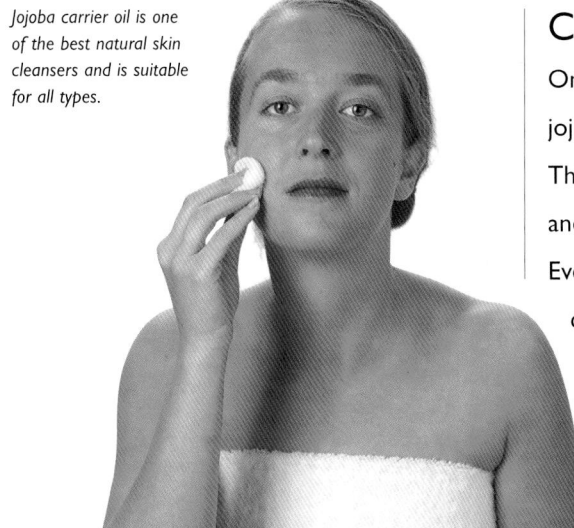

Jojoba carrier oil is one of the best natural skin cleansers and is suitable for all types.

Cleanse

One of the best all-round skin cleansers is jojoba oil, a liquid wax from the jojoba bean. This wax is very similar to the skin's own oils, and literally dissolves dirt out of the pores. Even greasy skin can benefit, and jojoba conditions all skin types beautifully. A small amount of blend on a cotton wool pad goes a long way. Try using the cleansing blend before you get in your bath, so the steam from the bath can further open the pores before you use your toner.

Choose one of the following blends and add to 20 ml jojoba oil:

Normal/dry/mature skin: 2 drops frankincense, 4 drops sandalwood, 4 drops orange.

Oily/combination skin: 2 drops juniper, 3 drops cypress, 5 drops lemon.

Sensitive skin (half the proportions): 2 drops roman chamomile, 3 drops lavender.

These blends should be used within 4 weeks. They can be kept at room temperature or for longer in the fridge.

Tone

Good chemists, drug stores and essential oil suppliers sell floral waters, the by-products of the distillation process, which make very good toners. Use a small amount on a cotton wool pad to freshen the skin before the moisturising treatment. The following flower waters are recommended:

Normal/dry/mature skin: pure rose water or pure neroli water.

Floral waters from the distillation process make very gentle skin toners. Good chemists will stock them.

Oily/combination skin: pure lavender water.

Sensitive skin: pure chamomile water or pure rose water. Floral waters will last up to six months if kept in the fridge.

Moisturise

Night time facial treatment oils have a shelf life of about four weeks and can be made up either in sweet almond oil, recommended for dry or mature skins, or jojoba, for all skin types.

Add to 20 ml of your chosen carrier oil:

Normal/dry/mature skin: 2 drops rose, 3 drops neroli, 5 drops frankincense.

Oily/combination skin: 3 drops geranium, 3 drops cypress, 4 drops lemon.

Sensitive skin (half proportions): 3 drops roman chamomile, 2 drops rose.

Massage a small amount into your face for 10 minutes, using upward strokes on your cheeks and tiny circles around your eye sockets and over your forehead. Be careful not to wipe the blend into your eyes.

Special Massage Blends

Here are some special massage blends for you to try, for physical, mood-related and seasonal reasons. They are all designed to be made up in 20 ml carrier oil, such as sweet almond, jojoba or grapeseed, a lighter and less greasy base oil. They all have a four-week shelf life. Massage relevant areas gently, using relaxing sweeping movements. Sometimes you may wish to work on yourself, but it can be soothing to let someone else – a close friend or partner – massage you.

Physical Tonics

Here are four blends for hard-working areas of the body which are constantly under strain.

Super muscle tone: for sports massage to energise and strengthen the muscles – 4 drops rosemary, 2 drops lemongrass and 4 drops ginger.

Barefoot bliss: a massage blend to help cool and soothe tired and aching feet after a long day – 3 drops peppermint, 3 drops black pepper and 4 drops lavender.

Chest relief: a wonderful blend for chest massage to ease respiratory problems –

Massage blends firmly into the limbs for the best effect.

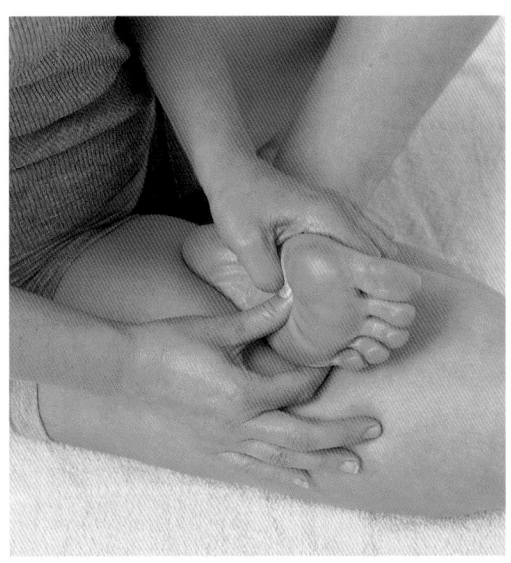

A foot massage warms and relaxes tired feet. It feels even better if someone else does it for you!

3 drops cedarwood, 3 drops frankincense and 4 drops lemon.

Neck and shoulder rescue: ask a friend or your partner to massage this blend into your aching muscles – 2 drops vetiver, 3 drops ginger and 5 drops lavender.

Mood Mixtures

Here are some ideas for more subtle blends with rich aromas. You will find them useful for lifting the spirits and easing emotional stresses and strains.

Beat the blues: 3 drops orange, 4 drops grapefruit and 3 drops sandalwood makes a wonderful relaxing, uplifting and de-stressing blend for massage.

PMT reviver: at that low time in your monthly cycle, try a blend of 4 drops palmarosa, 2 drops patchouli and 4 drops bergamot for an evening massage blend.

On cloud nine: when you need to escape without a care in the world, try 4 drops grapefruit, 2 drops neroli and 4 drops cardamom for a dreamy aroma.

Tropical retreat: create an exotic mood with 2 drops ylang ylang, 4 drops mandarin and 4 drops sandalwood – this is a fruity, rich and floral feast for the senses.

Seasonal Treats

As your energies vary, you may find that you need different massage blends to pick you up at different times of the year. Massage is particularly effective after a bath, as the skin absorbs the blend better. Spending time being massaged also helps improve your sleep – when you rest like this, your whole body can restore itself and your mind can be at peace.

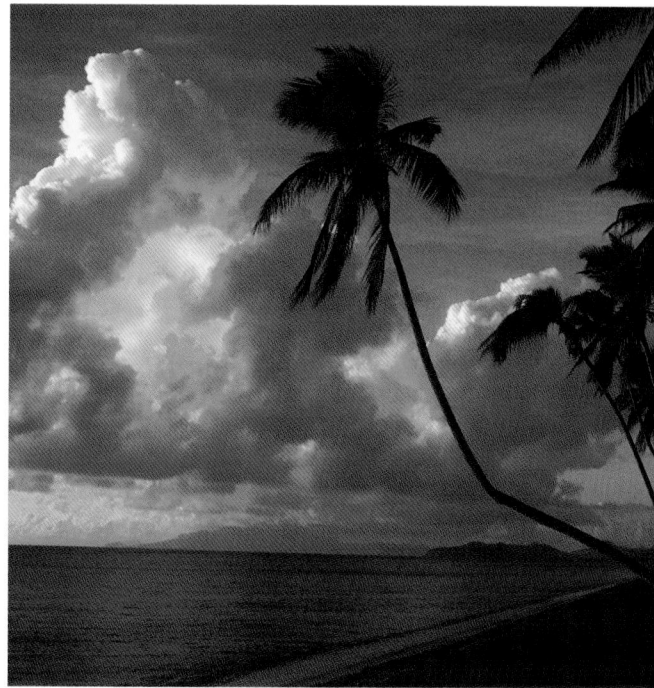

Inhale the aromas of the oils in the blends and float off into your own haven of tranquillity – a tropical beach, for example.

Springtime freshener: to help to revitalise and energise you after the long drag of wintertime – 4 drops lemon, 3 drops juniper and 3 drops peppermint.

Summer skin food: use the following blend in 20 ml jojoba oil to nourish the skin deeply – 3 drops sandalwood, 2 drops patchouli and 5 drops frankincense.

Autumn spiritual reviver: to uplift you as the nights draw in – 4 drops mandarin, 3 drops may chang and 3 drops coriander.

Winter energiser: for aches, stiffness and low vitality – 2 drops vetiver, 3 drops lemongrass and 5 drops nutmeg.

Essential Oils in Everyday Life

Essential oils are a wonderful and natural way to keep your environment fresh and to raise your energy levels. They are very portable and can easily be adapted to suit different locations and needs. Here are some ideas for using oils simply and effectively.

Home

In your home, essential oils help to personalise your living space.

Kitchen

This is one of the most frequently used and also most potentially accident-prone areas. Always keep lavender and tea tree to hand – you can use either oil neat for cuts, burns, scalds and other mishaps (put 2 drops on a cotton wool pad). A kitchen spray to remove stale odours and freshen work surfaces at the end of a day can be made in a pump-action spray bottle filled with 100 ml water, 10 drops peppermint and 15 drops lemon. Shake the bottle and spray mist into the air, or spray surfaces and wipe them down.

A pump-action spray bottle helps to spread essential oils over a much wider area.

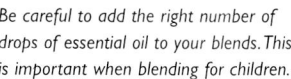

Be careful to add the right number of drops of essential oil to your blends. This is important when blending for children.

Dining room

A vaporiser adds atmosphere to a dinner party. For example, a Christmas gathering can be fragranced with 3 drops mandarin and 3 drops nutmeg, or a summer party with 3 drops may chang and 3 drops orange. One dose of essential oils in a vaporiser will last up to 2 hours.

Living room

Again, a vaporiser can clear the atmosphere, neutralise pet odours and freshen the air. A combination like 3 drops tea tree and 3 drops lemon helps if someone has a cold or influenza. After a party the night before, 3 drops peppermint and 3 drops rosemary is very uplifting and refreshing.

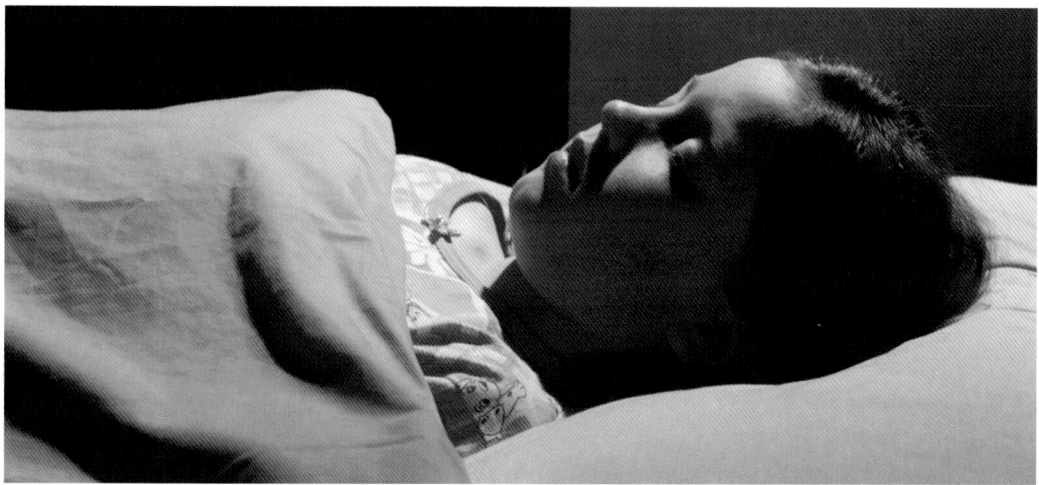

Child's bedroom

An electrical vaporiser is recommended for safety reasons. Essential oils can really help sleep. Add 3 drops lavender and 3 drops orange for a soothing aroma; or 3 drops lavender and 3 drops eucalyptus if there are chest problems. Try to start the vaporiser at least 10 minutes before your child goes to bed – this spreads the fragrance into the room as they fall asleep.

Travel

Essential oils can help you on the move.

Car

Vaporisers are available that plug into the cigarette lighter socket, or you can put oils on a tissue. On long journeys, 3 drops peppermint and 3 drops rosemary will help you stay alert.

Using essential oils while you are on the move will enable you to have a more restful journey.

Vaporising oils in a bedroom will improve the quality of sleep and scent the room delightfully as well.

Trains and planes

Carry one or two essential oils with you and add a few drops onto a tissue to inhale. Lavender will help you relax, peppermint and rosemary will wake you up, and lemon or tea tree will help ease sinus congestion.

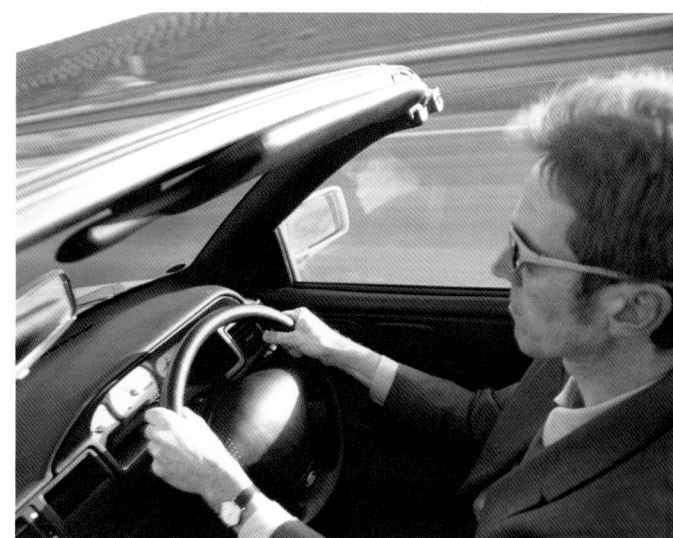

Buying and Storing Essential Oils

Here are some simple guidelines to follow to help you get the best out of your essential oil collection.

Buying Oils

There are many essential oil suppliers now selling to the public, and there is, unfortunately, a huge variation in the quality and therapeutic effectiveness of the oils available. True essential oils are not just a manufactured product, they are produced year by year and harvests can be affected by many environmental changes. Cheap essential oils are much more likely to be synthetic copies than the genuine article. Check that your supplier sources oils directly from growers.

You need to buy your oils in dark glass bottles to protect them from UV light. Oils should also have a drop dispenser in the neck of the bottle to release one drop at a time to help you calculate your blends. This is also an important safety feature: open-necked bottles

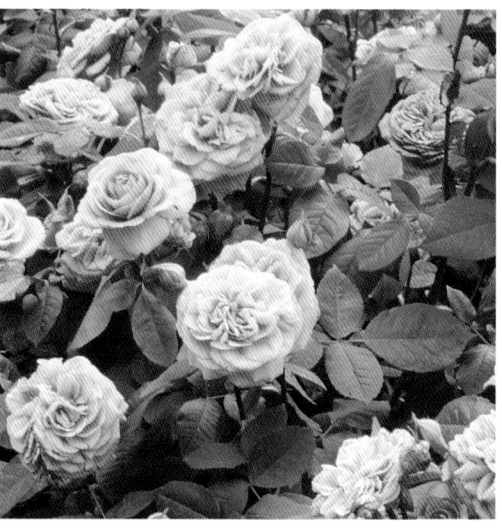

Many plants are expensive to harvest and these oils can be costly to buy. However, their divine scent makes it all worthwhile!

are a risk to children, who may swallow the contents. In any case, keep all essential oils well out of children's reach.

Storing Oils

Essential oils degrade with time. Their constituents oxidise and become unstable, smelling rancid. The cooler and more tightly closed they are kept, the longer the shelf life. How long you keep your oils depends on the storage temperature: in the fridge, most oils last up to two years, citrus oils one year.

Dark glass bottles with integrated stoppers or drop dispensers are vital if you are planning to use a lot of essential oils.

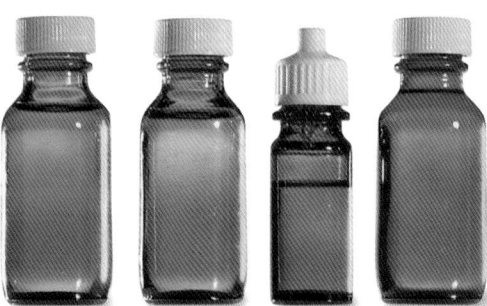

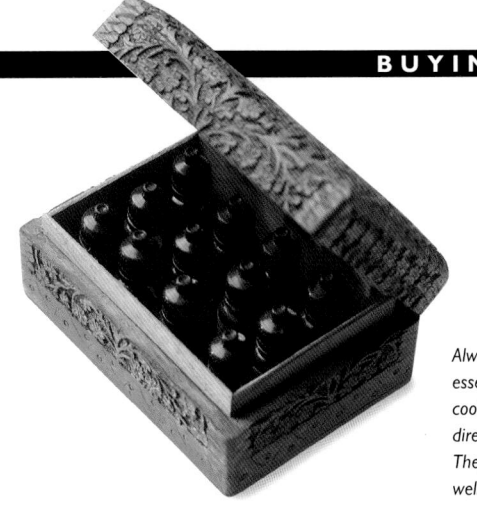

Always keep essential oils cool and out of direct sunlight. They also keep well in the fridge.

At room temperature, most oils last up to one year, citrus oils six months. The shelf life is calculated from the first day you open a new bottle. Write a date on the label or place a sticker on the bottle to remind you of the use-by date. If you are keeping oils in the fridge, you are advised to put them in an airtight box first to stop the fragrances spreading to your milk and dairy products! Out of the fridge, keep the oils tightly closed, in the dark and in a cool place. Do not use essential oils once they have gone past their shelf life, because they are then more likely to cause skin reactions.

Keeping essential oils in the fridge extends their shelf life. Make sure that the bottles are airtight at all times.

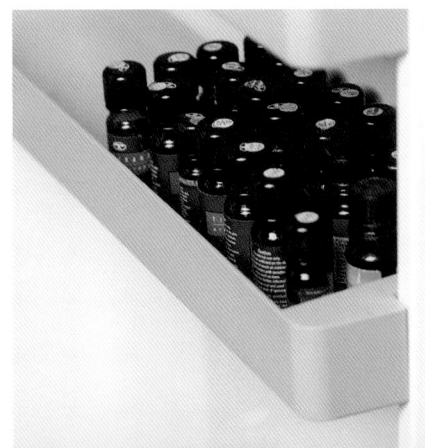

Recommended Suppliers

The following suppliers do mail order and sell high-quality ranges of essential oils.

Aromatherapy Products Ltd (suppliers of the Tisserand range, selling to 30 countries) Newtown Road, Hove, East Sussex BN3 7BA, UK
Tel: +44 (0)1273 325666;
Fax: +44 (0)1273 208444
Call them for your nearest stockist or mail order enquiries.

Essentially Oils Ltd
8–10 Mount Farm, Junction Road, Chipping Norton, Oxfordshire OX7 6NP, UK
Tel: +44 (0)1608 659544;
Fax: +44 (0)1608 659566
www.essentiallyoils.com
email: sales@essentiallyoils.com
Mail order enquiries welcome.

In the USA you are recommended to contact **National Association for Holistic Aromatherapy (NAHA)** for details of suppliers: 2000 2nd Avenue, Suite 206, Seattle WA 98121, USA
Tel: +001 (206) 2560741
www.naha.org

Glossary

Camphoraceous note

a medicinal and sharp aroma, such as marjoram.

Carrier oil

a vegetable oil used to dilute essential oils.

Cellulite

waterlogged fatty tissue deposits, particularly on thighs.

Citrus note

fresh and fruity aroma like citrus fruit.

Constituent

a fragrance ingredient of an essential oil (most oils contain up to 150).

Detoxifying

assists in the removal of toxins from the system.

Distillation

extraction of essential oils through steam followed by condensation.

Drop dispenser

a mechanism in the neck of a bottle to dispense one drop of oil.

Expression

pressing essential oils out of citrus fruit peel.

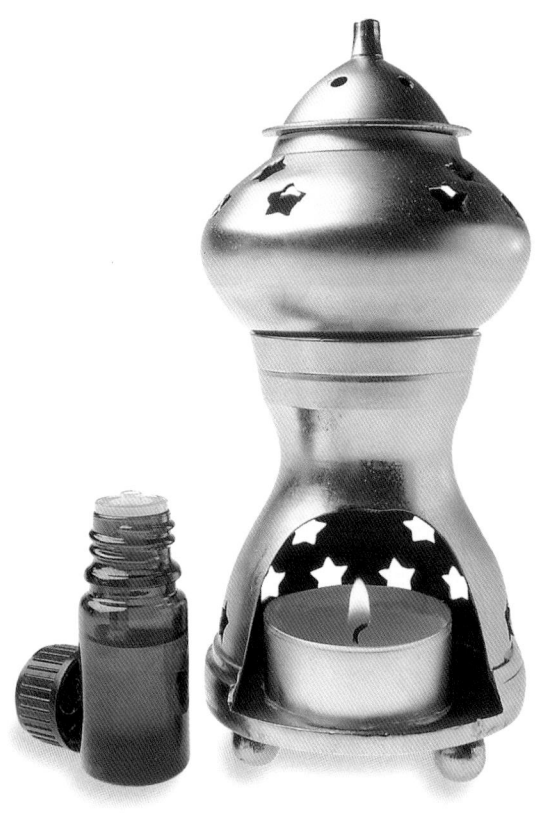

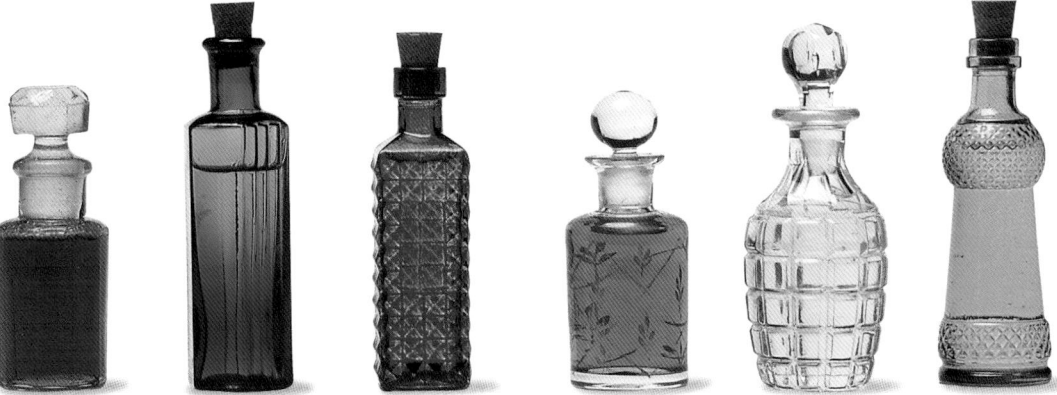

Floral note

a sweet flowery fragrance, such as rose.

Floral water

the by-product of distillation, delicately fragranced, very mild on the skin.

Inhalation

breathing in essential oils to clear the chest.

Photosynthesis

plant process of sugar production using sunlight.

Phototoxic

causing skin reactions in sunlight.

Pungent note

a warm and sometimes spicy aroma.

Sensitive skin

delicate, allergy-prone skin with a tendency to rashes.

Shelf life

length of time an essential oil can be kept before it degrades.

Solvent extraction

fragrance extraction using chemical solvents.

Synthetic fragrance

an aroma created by artificial chemicals.

Vaporiser

a unit designed to spread the fragrance of essential oils into a room.

Useful Addresses and Websites

United Kingdom

Aromatherapy and Allied Practitioners' Association (AAPA)
8 George Street, Croydon, Surrey,
CRO 1PA, UK
Tel: 020 8680 7761
www.aromatherapyuk.net
e-mail: aromatherapyuk@aol.com

International Federation of Aromatherapists (IFA)
182 Chiswick High Road, London W4 1PP, UK
Tel: 020 8742 2605
www.int-fed-aromatherapy.co.uk

International Society for Professional Aromatherapists (ISPA)
ISPA House, 82 Ashby Road, Hinckley,
Leicestershire LE10 1SN, UK
Tel: 01455 637987
www.the-ispa.org

National Institute of Medical Herbalists
56 Longbrook Street, Exeter, Devon
EX4 6AH, UK
Tel: 01392 426022

Register of Qualified Aromatherapists (RQA)
PO BOX 3431, Danbury, Chelmsford, Essex
CM3 4UA, UK
Tel: 01245 227957
e-mail: admin@R-Q-A.demon.co.uk

School of Herbal Medicine
Bucksteep Manor, Bodle Street Green, Nr
Hailsham, East Sussex BN27 4RJ, UK
Tel: 01323 834800

N.B. In 2002, the IFA, ISPA and RQA are intending to amalgamate as one body called the International Federation of Professional Aromatherapists (IFPA).

USA

American Alliance of Aromatherapy

PO BOX 750428, Petaluma, CA 94975, USA

Tel: +001 (707) 778-6762

California School of Herbal Studies

PO BOX 39, Forestville, CA 95436, USA

www.cshs.com

Herb Research Foundation

1007 Pearl Street, Suite 200, Boulder,

Colorado, CO 80302, USA

www.herbs.org

National Association for Holistic Aromatherapy (NAHA)

4509 Interlake Ave N, 233, Seattle WA

98103–6773, USA

Tel: +001 (206) 547-2164

www.naha.org

Australia

Australian College of Natural Medicine Inc.

609-611 Camberwell Road, Camberwell,

Victoria 3124, Australia

Tel. +0061 03 9859 9288

e-mail: acum@vicnet.net.au

International Federation of Aromatherapists

PO Box 786, Templestowe, Victoria 3106,

Australia

Tel. +0061 1902 240 125

www.ifa.org.au

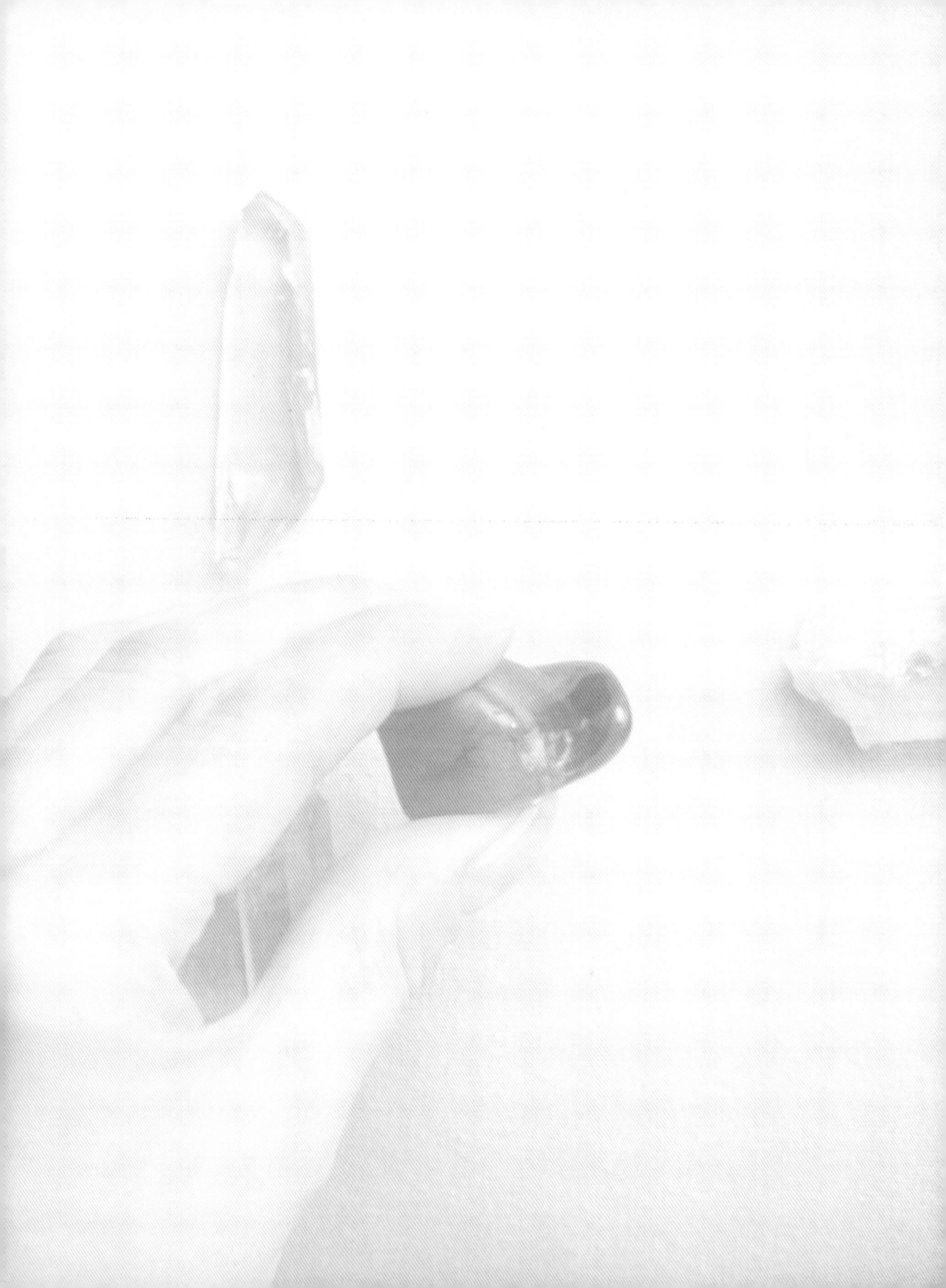

crystals

Introduction

The amazing world of crystals and jewels never ceases to fascinate us. Even in our everyday language we talk about a brilliant idea being 'a gem', or about things being 'as clear as crystal'. Ask anyone what is the most valuable thing they can think of and many will answer 'diamonds' – didn't Marilyn Monroe claim they were 'a girl's best friend'?

An engagement ring containing a diamond or other gems is given as a symbol of something rare and precious that will last for ever. At the heart of our deep and long-lasting regard for these valuable and beautiful glittering gifts of the Earth is the idea that they are eternally special.

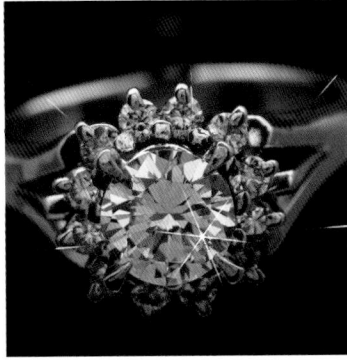

Engagement rings containing diamonds are a symbol of eternal and enduring love.

Fortunately, as well as precious stones, there are crystals like quartz, amethyst, moonstone or garnet, which are also beautiful and much more affordable, either as jewellery, stones for a collection or for healing purposes. This section will explore all of these aspects, especially the use of stones as tools for balancing the energies of body, mind and spirit. This is a practice with deep historical roots; many stones have ancient associations with different physical or mental conditions. In India to this very day, gems are ground to a powder and mixed with water, then drunk for their healing properties, just as they were hundreds of years ago. In the Crystal Index, found later in this section on pages 147–179, we shall link 32 minerals and stones to their different colours and learn their geological

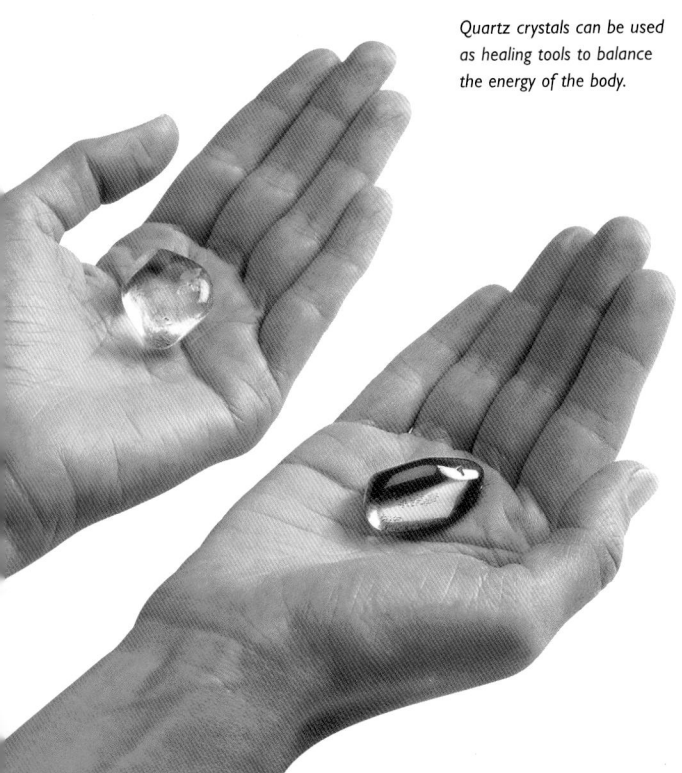

Quartz crystals can be used as healing tools to balance the energy of the body.

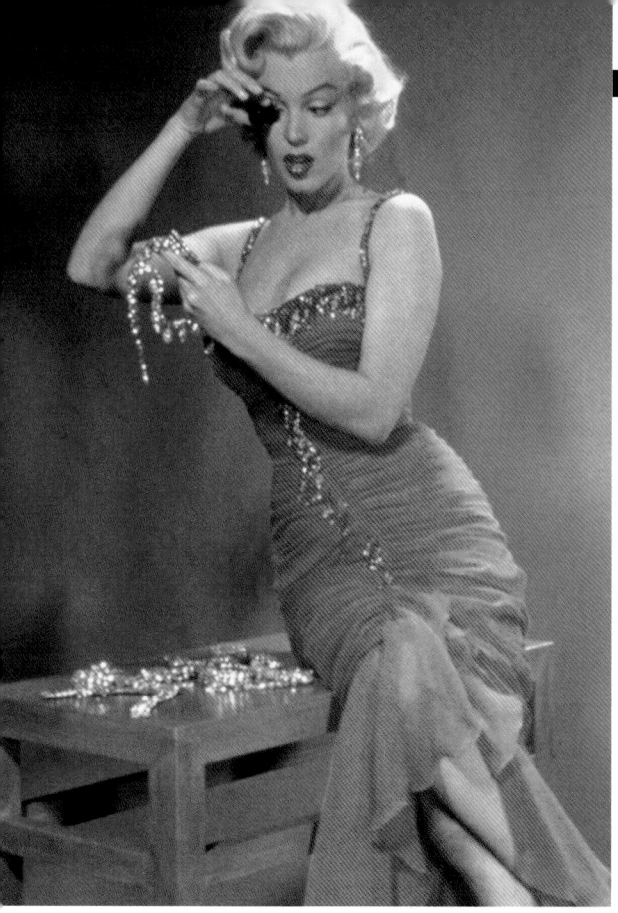

The brilliant lustre of diamonds endeared them to Marilyn Monroe's character Lorelei Lee in Gentlemen Prefer Blondes.

characteristics, as well as their history and healing uses.

Crystals can be used to beautify and clear the energies of your environment, as tools for meditation and contemplation, and of course can also be worn on your person. Perhaps the wearing of jewellery will take on a different meaning when you discover some of the fascinating geological and historical facts about the stones. You may find that you have already instinctively brought crystals into your environment and

the information given on particular stones will help you to realise why.

Bringing crystals into your personal space is a way of creating a connection with the Earth, since all crystals are born and grow within our planet's structure. If you use them with care and respect, crystals will share with you the positive energy of their light, colour and beauty. Whether you simply collect or wear them or use them to enhance your energy, crystals are a source of wonder. Enjoy this crystal journey through the worlds of geology, history, legend and healing.

The vibrant purple hues of an amethyst crystal have a soothing effect on the mind.

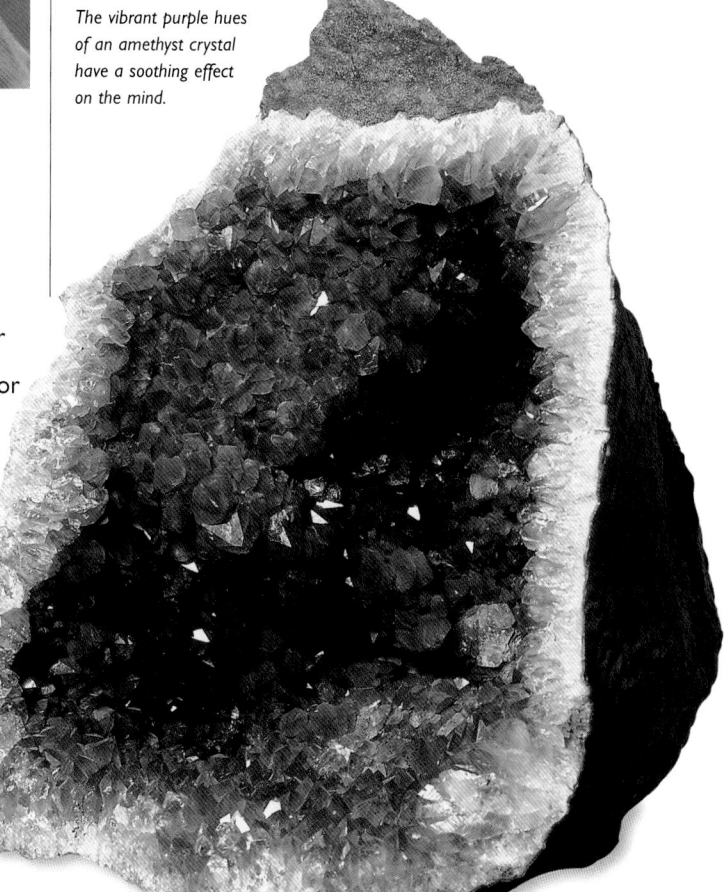

Mother Earth: Planet of Rebirth

Our story starts with the creation of the Earth – with the origin of minerals in the very structure of the planet on which we live. Minerals are natural, inorganic chemical substances. Approximately 2500 different types exist.

The mineral kingdom provides the chemical building blocks for everything on the Earth: rocks, plants, animals – and humans. About 90 per cent of each of us is made of water, and the rest is minerals!

The Earth is Always Moving

The Earth originally formed out of clouds of gas and the dust of other stars. Heavy elements like nickel and iron sank to form the hot core, which is still molten, made of liquid

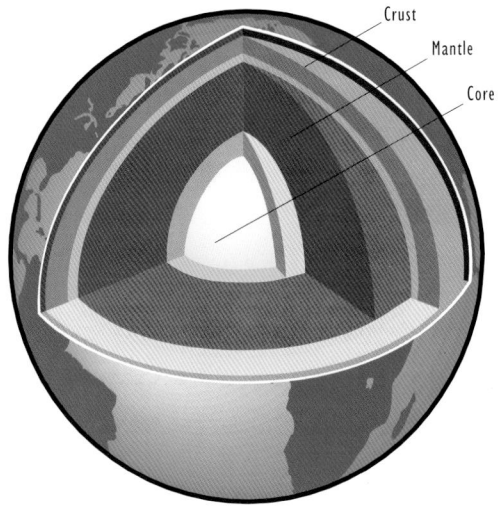

The Earth is made up of different layers. These are liquid at the core and solid on the surface.

Crust

Mantle

Core

minerals that are slowly pushed up to the surface. Lighter minerals such as silicon and oxygen, the ingredients of quartz, form part of a thicker, sometimes semi-molten layer called the mantle. Finally, the very lightest minerals float up to the surface of the Earth. This part, which is where we live and walk, is called the crust. Earthquake zones or volcanic areas like

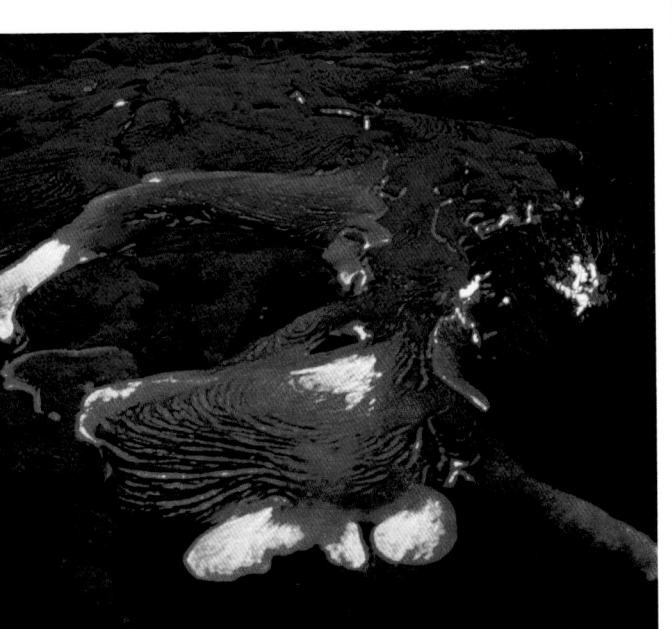

Flowing red-hot lava spills onto the Earth's surface after a volcanic eruption.

The Three Main Types of Rocks

Igneous: these layers originally formed as a mass of molten rock (called magma) deep inside the Earth's core. They rise to cover the crust through cracks or volcanic eruptions. Combined with water in the upper layers just below the surface, magma may form quartz crystals in large gaps called veins. Depending on the other minerals present, gems like emeralds or aquamarine may form.

Metamorphic: these are rock layers that have been changed after their original formation, usually by increases in pressure, heat, water vapour or chemical reactions. For example, layers of clay and sand sinking into the crust under pressure can form the mineral compound corundum, otherwise known as sapphire or ruby.

Sedimentary: these are layers of soft rock on the surface, formed by the actions of wind and water on surface minerals. The most common is limestone.

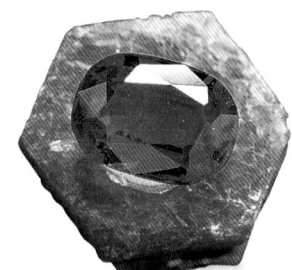

Rubies are one of the most precious gems that can be found in the world.

Mount Etna in Sicily show how thin the crust actually is. As heat from the Earth's core pushes minerals upwards, cooler rocks sink, melt at the core and are pushed up to the surface again. The Earth is constantly shifting and recycling minerals.

The Earth's Floating Crust

The Earth's crust literally floats on the mantle. It is made up of different sections or 'plates'; wherever these collide with each other, the pressure folds rocks into mountains or bursts open volcanoes. Deep in the oceans, cracks in the crust allow new mineral masses to grow, pushing continents sideways. This movement happens because of the cycles of rising heated minerals and sinking cooler layers. New sources of precious stones and gems continue to be found because the Earth's surface is never static, and the location of stones and gems is always changing. Even though this process takes millions of years, new mineral layers are continually being formed within the Earth's structure.

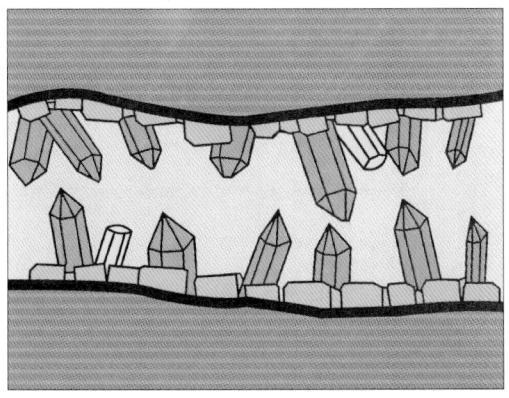

Crystals form in pockets or areas of space between rock layers. Mining techniques have developed to harvest these treasures.

The Making of Crystals

The many compounds of minerals that are found in the Earth's crust have been classified into different groups. Here are some of the most significant categories, which include many of the stones that you are likely to encounter.

Crystal Shapes and Inclusions

A crystal is a chemical compound that has changed naturally from a liquid to a solid with a regular geometric form and smooth sides. Crystals follow geometrical principles as their molecules arrange themselves. Quartz crystals divide and subdivide themselves along a hexagonal axis, meaning they typically have six sides called 'faces'. The points are called 'terminations' and crystals with points at both ends are 'double terminated'. It is also possible for twin crystals to form like mirror images of each other. Some crystals contain specks that look like flaws, but which are simply air bubbles or specks of other minerals; these are called 'inclusions'. Rutilated quartz contains many hairlike strands of rutile, a mineral sometimes called 'Venus' hair'.

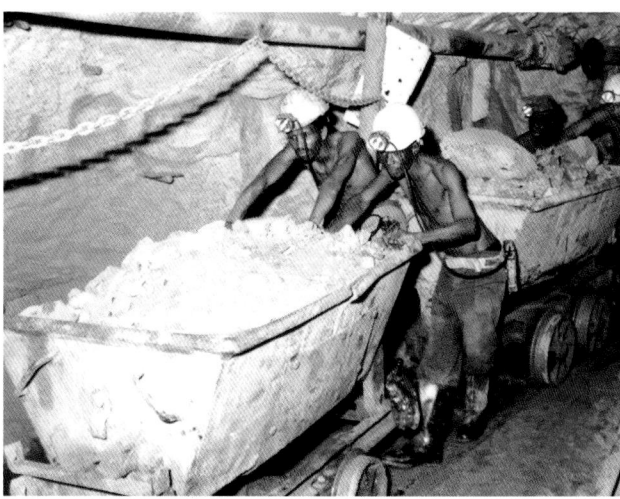

Crystals are mined from deep inside the Earth's crust. This is not a modern phenomenon – mining has been carried out for centuries.

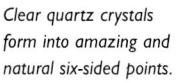

Clear quartz crystals form into amazing and natural six-sided points.

Crystal Extraction Methods

In ancient times, our ancestors gathered crystals from the surface of the Earth quite spontaneously, and even today mineral enthusiasts still do this. Mining for metals and crystals has been happening since the Stone Age, with very well established workings in the Middle East during Roman times. Modern industrial mining for many kinds of precious stones takes place extensively in countries such as Sri Lanka, Brazil and South Africa. When you buy a crystal it is worth remembering it has come via the miner, the wholesaler, the retailer and others before reaching you. This is why cleansing the crystals you buy is so important (see pages 146–147).

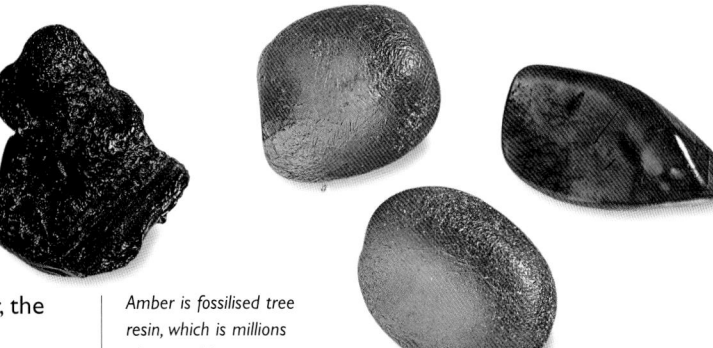

Amber is fossilised tree resin, which is millions of years old.

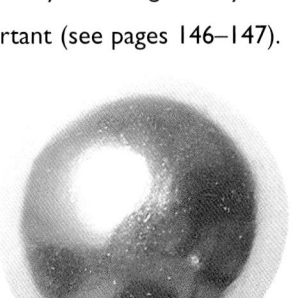

Pearls are another example of an organic material. In this case, the origin is animal.

Organic Minerals

'Organic' in this context means something with plant or animal origins. A few such minerals exist. Amber, for example, is the fossilised resin of an ancient pine tree. Pearls form when a grain of sand irritates the inner lining of the pearl oyster.

Main Groups of Metals and Crystals

Native elements *(uncombined with other elements)* gold, silver, platinum, copper, carbon (as diamond).

Sulphides *(metal plus sulphur)* iron plus sulphur makes pyrite (fool's gold).

Oxides *(main group is silicon dioxide, making quartz)* clear quartz, amethyst, rose quartz, smoky quartz; also microcrystalline forms called chalcedony, the name given to crystals such as carnelian and tiger's eye because of their waxy or translucent appearance. Opals are similar to quartz but are made of silicon dioxide and water. Aluminium oxide forms the compound corundum, whose red and blue forms are rubies and sapphires respectively.

Silicates within this group are feldspars comprising a huge number of crystals, very common in the Earth's crust. Moonstone and labradorite are varieties of feldspar made up of sodium and calcium. Another large silicate group are garnets, which may be rich in aluminium, iron or chromium depending on their location. Other silicate minerals are tourmaline and the beryls, including aquamarine and emerald.

Royal Crystals

Crystals and precious stones have long been valued as hunting tools, carvings, jewellery or icons. They were used as badges of royalty and power, symbolising the unique status of kings and queens. They are so precious that wars have been fought over them.

The Ancient Egyptians were mining emeralds, peridot, lapis lazuli and other precious stones over 3000 years ago. They were highly skilled in polishing and setting in gold and their work can still be admired in their relics, especially the treasures of the Pharaohs. For thousands of years, diamonds and other gems have been mined in India, Sri Lanka and Burma (now called Myanmar), as well as countries in South America and Africa. The ancient Mayan and Chinese civilisations produced exquisite carvings of jade and emerald.

Queen Elizabeth II wearing the Imperial State Crown, one of the most important items of regalia in the Crown Jewels.

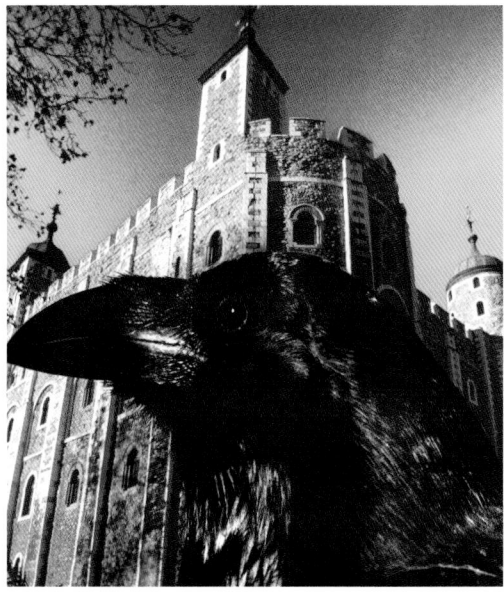

The Tower of London, surrounded by the famous ravens, is where the British Crown Jewels can be seen.

The British Royal Family's Crown Jewels

The Jewel House in the Tower of London contains all of the British Royal Family's regalia. The most famous element of this collection is St Edward's Crown, which is worn by the reigning monarch. The first Crown Jewels were assembled by King Edward the Confessor in the eleventh century. In

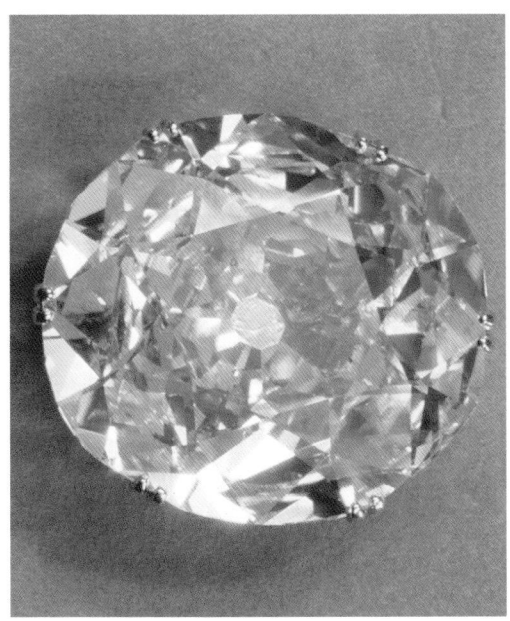

The Koh-i-noor, one of the largest diamonds in the world, is set in the crown of Queen Elizabeth the Queen Mother.

1216, King John Plantagenet subsequently lost them in quicksand in East Anglia. The next collection also had a rather chequered history. During the Civil War in 1649, Oliver Cromwell ordered them to be broken up; however, remnants were saved and later incorporated into the new regalia fashioned for King Charles II when he ascended the throne in 1661. Today, the collection is priceless. In the early twentieth century, the largest diamond ever found, the Cullinan, was cut into four segments. One segment, known as the 'Star of Africa' is carried in the Sovereign's Sceptre. It weighs more than 530 carats and has 74 facets, making it the world's largest cut diamond.

The History of the Koh-i-noor

The Koh-i-noor is one of the largest single diamonds in the world and was first owned by the Rajah of Malwa in India in 1304. It has a weight of 186 carats. To put this weight into perspective, most modern diamond engagement rings weigh approximately 0.25 to 1 carat. For several hundred years, the jewel belonged to various Indian emperors. In 1739, the Shah of Persia invaded Delhi and pillaged the city to find the legendary diamond. He was told that the defeated emperor had the jewel hidden in his turban. He invited his captive to exchange turbans. Unrolling the cloth the Shah found the jewel. He cried out 'Koh-i-noor', or 'Mountain of light!' – which remained its name.

When Lahore, the capital of Punjab, was annexed to British India in 1849, the stone passed to the East India Company, who presented it to Queen Victoria in 1850. It was displayed at the Crystal Palace exhibition, disappointing viewers because it did not appear to sparkle enough. Queen Victoria therefore had the diamond re-cut, reducing it from 186 carats to 108.93.

In 1911 the stone was set in the crown of Queen Mary. In 1937 the diamond was reset, this time in the crown of Queen Elizabeth the Queen Mother.

Crystals Today

In the early twentieth century, fabulous jewels began to adorn famous Hollywood movie stars and be seen regularly on the screen and in magazines. It is not surprising that these legendary bejewelled icons have become as admired as royalty.

Famous Women and their Gems

The screen goddess Marlene Dietrich loved emeralds, especially those carved into smooth-domed cabochons. She once lost a 37-carat emerald ring in a cake mixture and found it again in a piece of the cake! Elizabeth Taylor has been one of Hollywood's greatest stars, with an amazing jewellery collection. The Taylor–Burton diamond given to her by Richard Burton weighs almost 70 carats. She also has a collection of dazzling emerald jewellery that once belonged to a Russian Grand Duchess. Jacqueline Kennedy Onassis also collected dazzling pieces, especially from her second husband Aristotle Onassis. His engagement ring to her was auctioned at Sotheby's for $2.6 million in 1996. When Princess Diana's fine sparkling sapphire and diamond engagement ring was originally shown to the world's press, it sparked a fashion for copies of the design.

Marlene Dietrich, the legendary screen icon, adored emeralds, especially when they were cut into smooth, rounded cabochons.

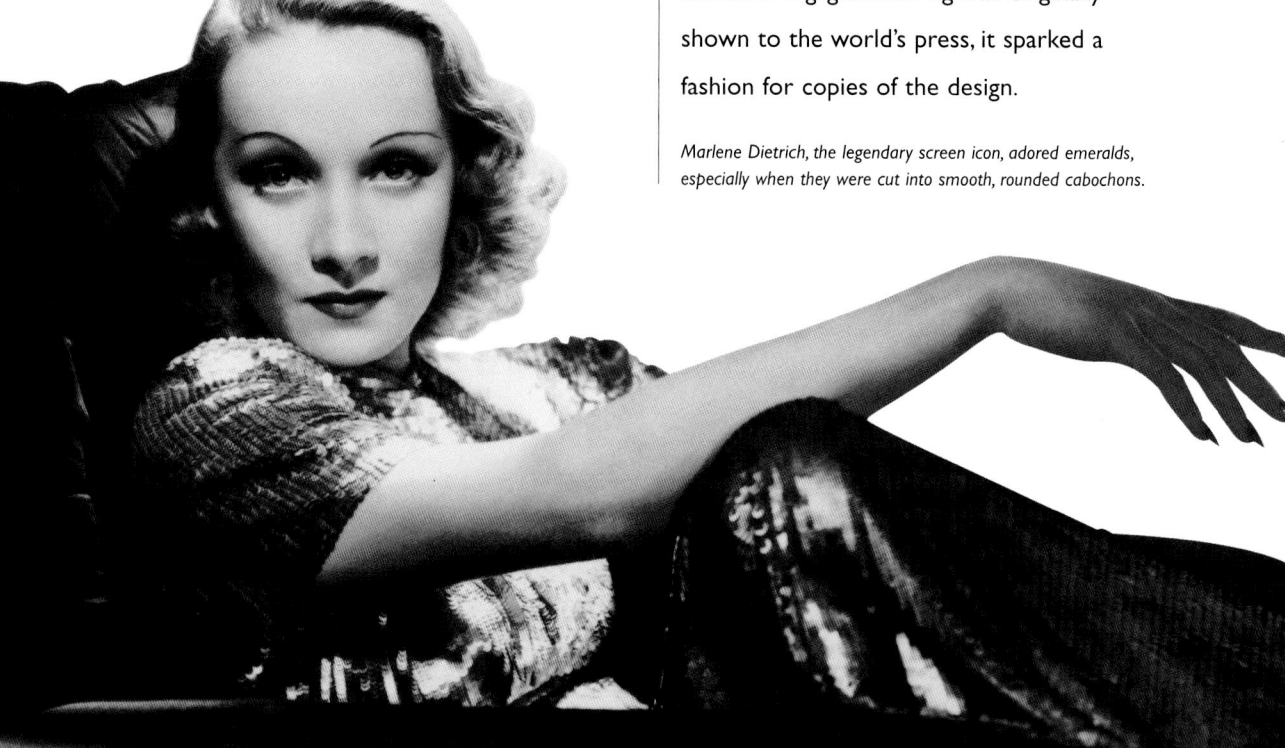

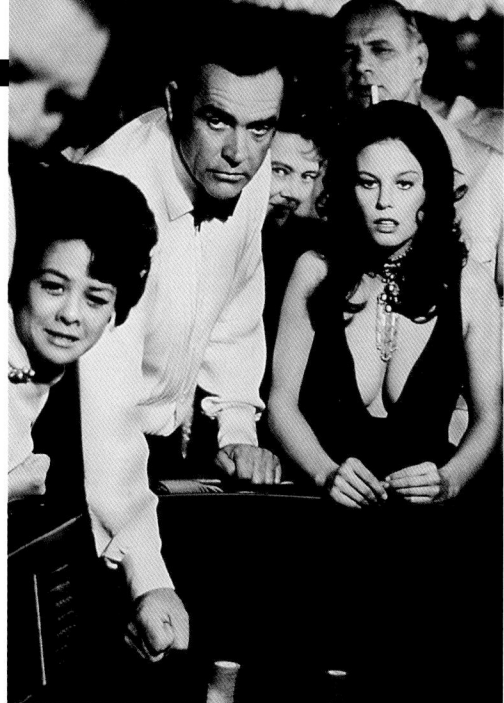

In the film Diamonds are Forever, *James Bond discovers the power of diamonds and what others will do to get them.*

Crystal Movies

Even in our sophisticated age, nothing beats a good adventure story, as film-makers know very well. The idea of a dangerous hunt for a huge, priceless emerald inspired the film *Romancing the Stone*, and the James Bond epic *Diamonds are Forever*, as well known for the song as for the story, deals with diamonds as a source of staggering wealth and power. In the 1970s and early 1980s, the 'Superman' movies introduced new ideas: namely that crystals could hold energy and even power spacecraft! It also explored the idea that diamonds could hold information – a idea realised in the development of the silicon chip. This interesting shift in presentation coincided with a general interest in crystals for healing.

The New Age – Expanding Crystal Awareness

Since the 1960s, crystals have been used increasingly as healing tools. Many writers have linked this awareness to the New Age, a rise in spiritual consciousness, particularly towards the dawn of the New Millennium. In fact, crystals have been used for healing since before Egyptian times. However, with advances in geology and quantum physics, the structure and energy of crystals is beginning to be understood in different terms. People are made up of the same elements as crystals. We are made of the same minerals that are recycled by the Earth in spite of the fact that we are organic beings, and minerals are inorganic. Perhaps one way of explaining the response to crystal energies is to say we subtly recognise elements that are in us all.

A rose quartz crystal placed on the body can enhance relaxation and feelings of well-being and happiness.

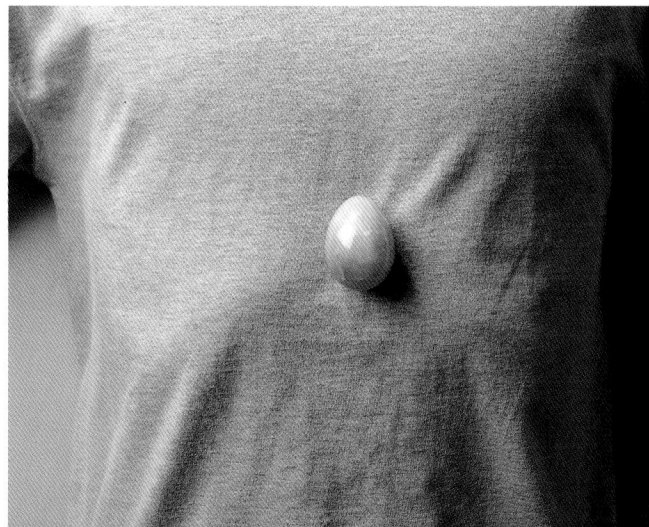

Crystals, Colours and Chakras

One of the most striking things about crystals is their colour. This is often what first attracts us, such as when our eye is drawn to the vivid green of emeralds or the deep purple of amethysts. Different colours can affect us physically and emotionally – for example, the blue-green colour of the sea is calming to the eyes and the spirit.

The colour spectrum can be used as a model for understanding the different energies at work in our bodies.

Colour Healing

If you take a cut-glass pendulum and hang it in a sunny window, your walls will be covered in many dancing rainbows showing the seven pure colour shades of the spectrum – red, orange, yellow, green, blue, indigo and violet. The white light that splits into all these colours is the only part of the spectrum we can see, although insects and some animals can see infrared and ultraviolet waves too.

In ancient Egyptian times, healers chose ingredients for their patients on the basis of the colour of the problem. For example, red was for blood, purple for bruising, yellow for jaundice. The wearing of

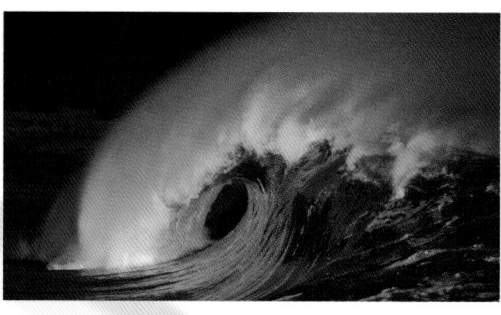

When we see blue or green shades, in nature or elsewhere, these act as a relaxant and have a calming effect on us.

clothes or jewellery of that colour came to be associated with the prevention of the condition; if you had poor circulation you were advised to wear red. (This was because cold feet could became warmer more quickly in red socks than in any other colour.)

By the twentieth century, scientists were beginning to experiment with light waves, noting that the properties of the red and orange rays were 'warmer', and the blue and purple rays 'cooler', with the colour green in the middle as a balance. These days, light frequencies directed through lasers are being used in surgery and for healing wounded tissue.

The rainbow colours to be found in crystals show all the colours of the spectrum. Specific colours are used in different healing methods.

The Chakra System

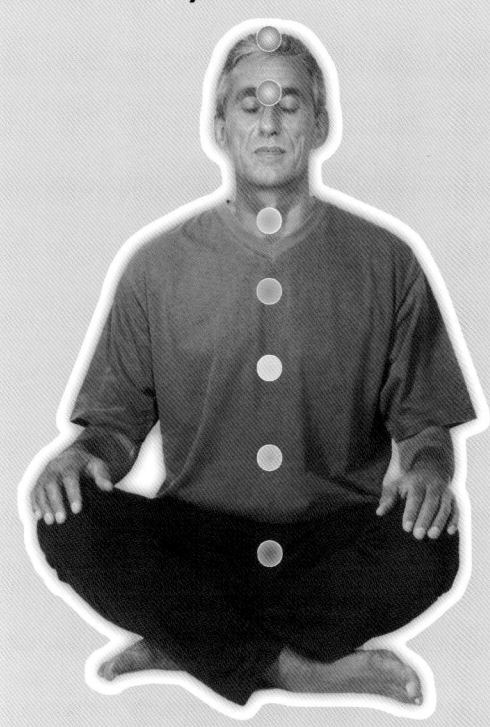

Several thousand years ago, in India, the energy frequencies of the body were perceived as being on seven different levels, each corresponding to an area in the body, centred in a 'chakra' or 'wheel'. The white light of universal energy was considered to enter through the crown of the head and then modulated in frequency through each of the colour levels from violet at the crown to red at the base of the spine. This ancient model is widely used in healing work and yoga practice today.

Meditating on the colours of the rainbow can bring strong feelings of relaxation and calm.

Chakra	Colour	Gland	Body Area
crown	violet	pineal	top of head
third eye	indigo	pituitary	mid-forehead
throat	blue	thyroid	throat
heart	green	thymus	centre of chest
solar plexus	yellow	spleen	under diaphragm
sacrum	orange	ovaries/testes	lower abdomen
root	red	adrenals	base of spine

Within each colour, shades are possible. Green can vary from yellow-green to emerald to dark green, but all shades relate to the heart chakra.

Small crystals can easily be placed on your body and around your living and working environment.

The way universal energy passes into the body is through the breath. As you breathe in – not just air but life force – the energy levels are maintained at appropriate levels. However, if there is disharmony, then other help may be needed. Colours and crystals can be used to rebalance diminished chakra energies.

Colour Healing Chart

This colour healing chart is designed to suggest links between colours, body energies, colour effects, chakra centres and crystals. The original seven colours of the spectrum have been expanded to include shades, as well as rays like silver. This chart corresponds exactly with the Crystal Index (pages 147–179), where individual stones are discussed in detail. Guided by the way you feel, you will be able to choose the appropriate colours to help you, as well as select useful crystals. You will find some simple crystal healing methods described on pages 180–181.

Some of these correspondences may be surprising. Black, for example, often has an undeserved negative association, but it can

have quite a different meaning. In many healing traditions such among the Native Americans, for example, black is simply seen as the complement to white. Observing the night sky, the darkness creates the shadow that allows the light of the stars to appear like diamonds on black velvet. Native American teachings revere the darkness as the source of mystery, the place from which all new things are born. Every creation myth on Earth relates the origin of the planet to a time of dark formlessness, out of which came light.

Here are some examples showing how you can use the chart. If you feel cold and lacking in energy, you will see that red is a warming colour and garnets are suggested. You can either find some red in your wardrobe, or try wearing the crystal or meditating on it (see pages 184–185). If you are afraid of change, try wearing or meditating with labradorite. If you want to expand a relationship, wear amber colours or the stone. You will discover your own favourite colours and stones very quickly. If you find yourself using a lot of one particular stone or colour, then that chakra clearly needs energising.

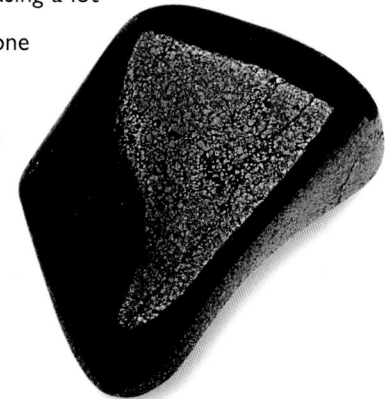

Tumblestones are examples of small polished crystals that are very easy to carry around with you.

The Colour Healing Chart

Colour	Energy	Effect	Chakra	Stone	
Red	action	warming	root	garnet	
Orange	relationship	expanding	sacrum	amber	
Yellow	mental alertness	clearing	solar plexus	topaz	
Light Green	spontaneity	refreshing	heart	peridot	
Rich Green	love	harmonising	heart	emerald	
Turquoise*	protection	strengthening	heart/thymus	turquoise	
Pale Blue	communication	soothing	throat	celestite	
Dark Blue	intuition	connecting	third eye	lapis lazuli	
Violet	insight	inspiring	crown	amethyst	
Pink	unconditional love	releasing	heart	rose quartz	
White	universal energy	healing	all chakras	clear quartz	
Black	universal mystery	visioning	root	obsidian	
Brown	rootedness	grounding	root	smoky quartz	
Iridescent	change	flowing	third eye	labradorite	
Gold	self-worth	revitalising	crown	gold	
Silver	inner knowledge	calming	third eye	silver	

* Turquoise (blue-green) is often seen as corresponding to a minor chakra point, at the thymus gland in the upper chest, which supports the immune system.

Choosing and Caring for Crystals

Selecting the crystals you want and taking care of them is an important part of building a collection. This can become a very rewarding pastime as well as having interesting subtle effects on you and your living space.

Choosing Crystals

You will be attracted to stones because of their colour, their shape or size, or even for more subtle reasons. Remember, we have discussed that you and crystals share mineral elements in common. Crystals have their own 'frequency' thanks to the arrangement of their

To clean crystals and get rid of any negative energy that might be lingering, hold them under clear running water.

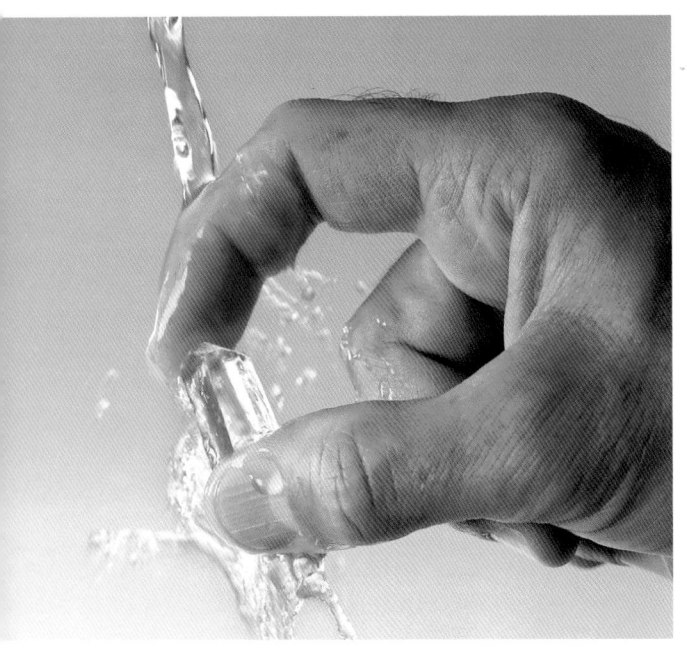

molecules – and so do you. This means that if a crystal jumps out at you or you feel sensations of tingling when you pick up a particular stone, then this is the one for you. It has been demonstrated with willing subjects that human electromagnetic energies change when crystals are brought near the body; you are simply reacting to the stone. You should trust that feeling and go with it (and just hope you are not drawn to the most expensive ones!). Remember there is a difference between a naturally terminated crystal point such as quartz and a stone that has been polished, cut or shaped. One is in a natural state and the other has been worked by human hands. They are equally beautiful, but they have different energies.

Cleansing Crystals

Having purchased your crystals, it makes sense to clean them. They have been mined, extracted, possibly tumbled or cut, sold to a wholesaler, transported, brought to sale and

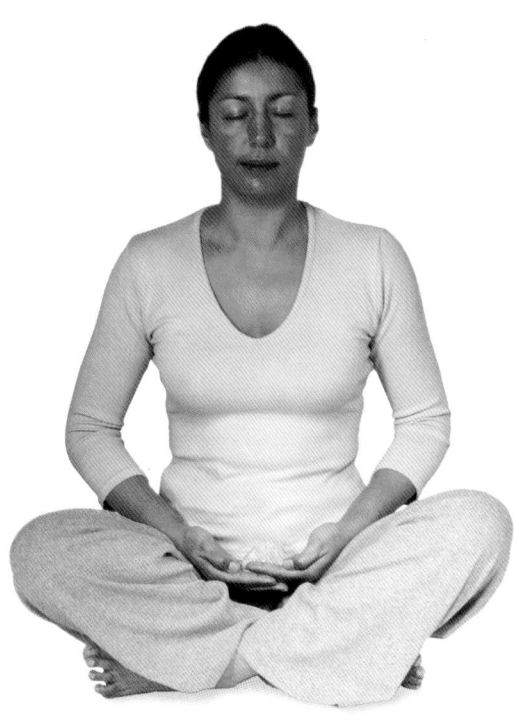

If you sit quietly and hold your crystal in your hands, you can 'programme' it with positive energy.

'Programming' Crystals

Programming a crystal means allowing new energy to flow into the crystal from you, making it uniquely yours. You could choose to charge it with the pink ray of unconditional love or visualise pure white universal light flowing down your arms, into your hands and filling the crystal. You can then ask the stone to continue to reflect that love in your personal space, and place it carefully wherever you think it needs to sit.

The Crystal Index

handled by many people before you. Cleansing is not just about removing dirt, grease and dust, it also clears previous energies from the stone. Simply hold your crystal under flowing cold water for several minutes and visualise all other energy traces being dissolved. If you are not sure if the crystal is fully clear, ask in your mind and intuit the response, and repeat until you feel the stone is clear. Crystals should be cleaned regularly, especially if they are used for healing.

The Crystal Index covers the next 32 pages. You will find the stones arranged by colour, corresponding to the chart on page 145. The colour ray is further explained, and then each stone is given a profile showing geological, geographical, historical and healing information. As well as reading them all, try flipping the pages and stopping at a colour that attracts you on a particular day. You may need that energy!

Amethyst reflects the colour violet and brings inspiration into our hearts and minds. It is a very popular crystal for healing work.

Red

Red is the bright stimulating colour of action. Wearing red is very energising, and red gemstones help you feel dynamic and confident.

Ruby

Geology: Ruby is a variety of corundum, the second hardest known mineral, coloured red by the element chromium. The most precious rubies can be rarer and more valuable than diamonds. Fine rubies glow like red-hot coals. Pinkish or darker red examples also occur. Some very rare stones show a six-pointed star effect in bright light due to bands of rutile in their structure. These are called star rubies.

Sources: In Myanmar, some ruby mines date from the Stone and Bronze Ages. Today this country is still the most famous source of rubies. Thailand produces rubies of a darker colour and is the most important ruby trading centre in the world.

History: 'Ruby' comes from the Latin word *ruber* meaning red. Similar words are found in Persian and Sanskrit for both the stone and the colour red. Rubies have been venerated for thousands of years. In the Old Testament,

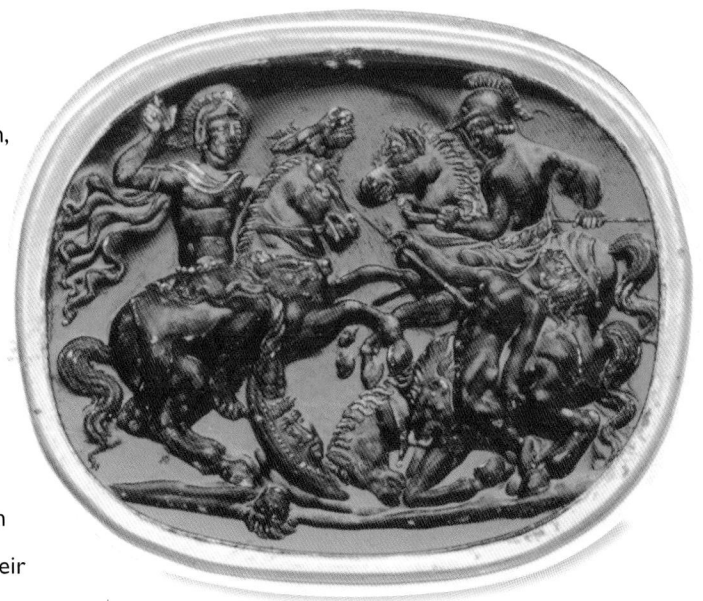

Exquisitely carved rubies have been used as personal signet rings to seal documents for centuries.

God places this 'lord of gems' on Aaron's neck. The Bible also states that wisdom is 'more precious than rubies'.

Healing uses: Ruby lights a fire of courage within you, encouraging you to step beyond yourself to new possibilities. It increases your physical vitality and your physical energy, boosting your circulation and bringing strength to you. It is a stone that symbolises power, leadership and integrity.

Garnet

Geology: Garnets form in igneous and metamorphic rocks under high pressure, and occur in very precise symmetrical crystals with twelve diamond-shaped facets. They are mostly known for their deep red colour, but can be found in pink, orange and even green shades. Pyrope garnets have a dark ruby-red colour, and rhodolite garnets are also popular, with a pinkish to purplish red sheen.

The rich red hues of garnets mean that the stones make very attractive jewellery.

Sources: Pyrope garnets are mined in South Africa and also the USA, specifically in Utah and Arizona, where the common name for them is 'anthill garnets'. This is because tiny examples are excavated by ants when building their nests. The rhodolite variety are obtained from Africa, India and Sri Lanka.

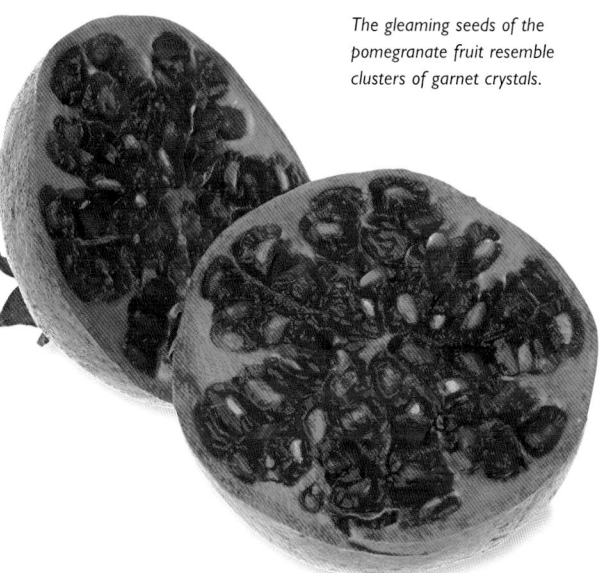

The gleaming seeds of the pomegranate fruit resemble clusters of garnet crystals.

History: The name 'garnet' derives from the pomegranate, a fruit with dark seeds in bright red flesh resembling garnet clusters! Legend has it that Noah's Ark was lit up at night by a garnet lantern, and garnets have traditionally been used as a protective talisman when travelling.

Healing uses: Garnet provides a calm, grounding strength to the physical body. It helps you feel centred with a reservoir of inner strength and confidence. It is used to strengthen and regenerate the physical body, boost the circulation and the reproductive energies.

Garnets can be quite large stones and look particularly beautiful when they are set in simple silver or gold.

Warning

Wearing red stones is not recommended for people with high blood pressure or heart problems.

Orange

Warm sunny shades of orange are very positive colours. Orange removes fear and replaces it with optimism, improving your relationships with others.

Amber

Geology: Amber is fossilised resin or tree sap from the ancient pine tree *Pinus succinifera* and has taken approximately 25–50 million years to harden. Amber is also called succinite. Thousands of samples have been found containing whole insects, pollen grains and ancient plants. Amber is organic because of its plant origin. It is usually found in yellow, gold or orange shades, but red, brown and green varieties also exist.

Amber has been worn as an ornament for thousands of years.

Sources: Fine amber is mainly found in the Baltic states and the Dominican Republic.

History: Archaeological finds reveal that humankind has used and revered amber since the Stone Age. In ancient Greece, amber was considered to be the juice or essence of the setting sun. In the epic poem the *Odyssey*, Homer mentions amber being given as a princely gift. In Roman times, amber artefacts were regarded as being more valuable than slaves.

Healing uses: Amber helps lift your spirits. It builds your physical vitality and positively charges your energy levels. It shields you from negativity from other people or from your environment. It is used to clear and rebalance the heart, the abdomen and lower back areas.

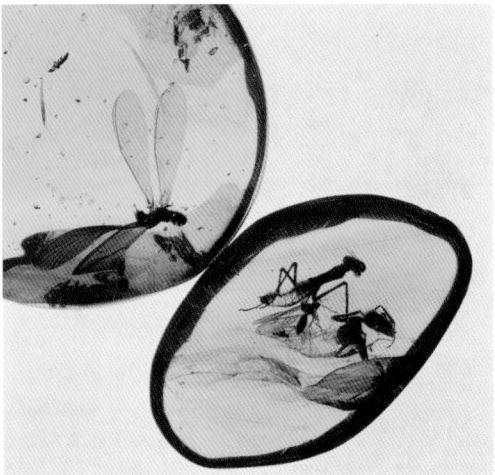

Some examples of amber contain whole insects preserved within them. These make interesting pieces of jewellery.

Carnelian

Geology: Carnelian is a variety of chalcedony, a kind of quartz made up of tiny finely grained microcrystals. It is found in shades of apricot, deep orange and even red-brown, and good quality stones have a translucent sheen. It is easily carved and has often been used for seals or signet rings.

Sources: Carnelian comes from Brazil, Uruguay and also from India. Indian carnelian grows redder on exposure to the sun. It is readily available in the form of small polished tumblestones.

History: As far back as 3000 BCE, carnelian and other gemstones were used in Mesopotamia and Egypt as amulets for protection. Carnelian was also reputed to be used as one of the twelve sacred stones set in the breastplate of Aaron. In the Middle Ages, powdered carnelian mixed with water was taken as a remedy against the plague. In medieval times, gemstones were often identified with different emotional states, and carnelian was seen as a healer of anger.

Carnelian stones have a deep warm colour. They also have an attractive mellow sheen.

Healing uses: Carnelian helps to ease depression and gives you a sense of inner stability. It can also help to balance the mind when you are trying to tackle difficult mental tasks. Carnelian warms and stimulates the appetite and balances the female reproductive system, easing menstrual pain. It promotes a sense of attunement with oneself. Its energy is warm, joyful and opening, particularly when it is placed on the lower abdominal area.

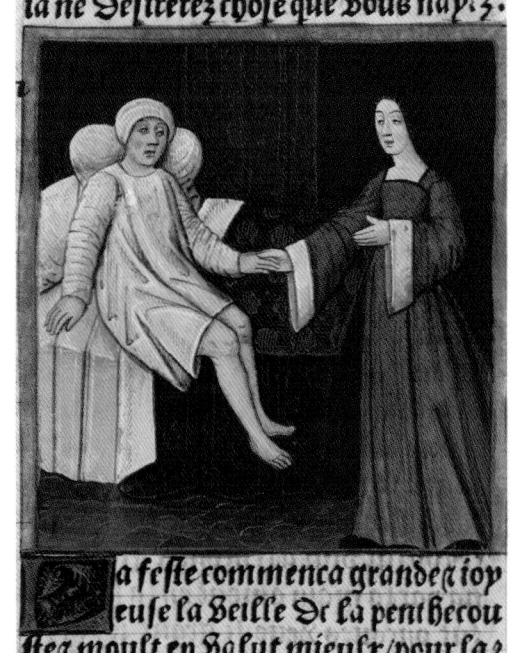

Carnelian was a popular healing gem in medieval times. It was used as a remedy against the plague.

Yellow

Yellow is a bright colour that is stimulating to the mind; a positive radiance full of energy and zest. Yellow gemstones sparkle against the skin like sunlight.

Citrine

Geology: Natural citrine is a pale yellow quartz with a gentle sparkle and sheen. True citrine tends to be light in colour. Darker yellow or orange examples are very likely to be artificially heat-treated amethyst or smoky quartz. Such stones can often be detected by their reddish sheen. It is possible to obtain very large pieces of citrine as well as delicate crystal clusters and the six-sided terminations that are typical of quartz crystals in general.

Golden yellow citrine is a beautiful stone to place in your environment.

Healing uses: Citrine clears your mind of conflicting thoughts and provides space to think. It is used to detoxify the body and has a beneficial effect on the kidneys, liver and gall bladder. It tones the digestion and the circulation. It attracts abundance into your life, whether in the form of money or relationships. Try placing it beside your bed to help you sleep.

Sources: Today most citrine is mined in Brazil in the state of Rio Grande do Sul. Some deposits also exist in Madagascar.

History: The name citrine derives from the French word *citron* (lemon), alluding to the pale yellow colour. In the past, the stone was thought to protect against the venom of poisonous snakes.

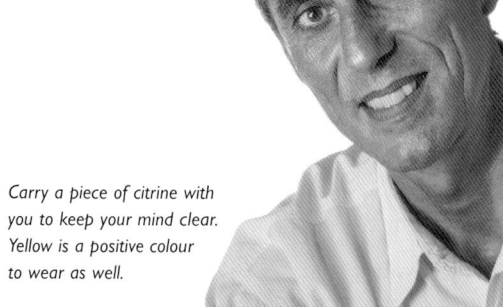

Carry a piece of citrine with you to keep your mind clear. Yellow is a positive colour to wear as well.

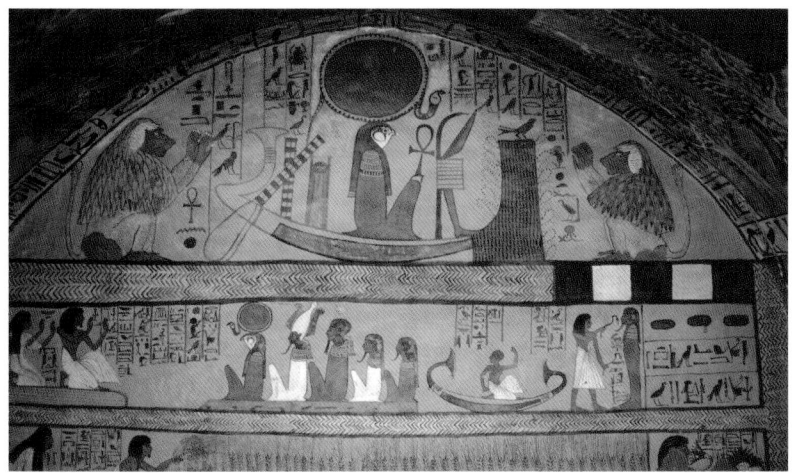

The ancient Egyptians associated yellow topaz with Ra, the sun god. In this wall painting, Ra is the figure sitting in the boat flanked by two baboons.

Topaz has a very effective cleansing effect on the body when it is used in healing.

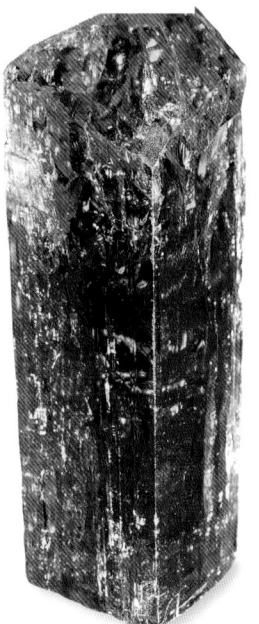

Topaz

Geology: Topaz is a yellow gemstone that has been used for jewellery for centuries. It is mostly yellow in colour, but it can also be found in orange, red, blue and even green shades. It can form massive clusters of up to a hundred kilograms in weight and is one of the hardest minerals in nature. Its colour has often caused it to be confused with the less valuable citrine, yet it has a beautiful transparent lustre all of its own.

Sources: Brazil is known for high-quality yellow topaz, with other deposits occurring in Sri Lanka, Myanmar and the USA. Russian topaz is pale blue in colour.

History: Ancient Egyptians associated the yellow gemstone with Ra, the sun god, and the Romans with Jupiter, the king of the gods. It was used in protective amulets. A gem thought to have many mystical properties, topaz was said to change colour in the presence of poisons in food or drink – it was even used to detect these. A stunning giant topaz is set in the Portuguese royal crown.

Healing uses: Yellow topaz is useful for focusing your mind on complex problems and generating fresh new ideas. Topaz is valued in healing as a detoxifying stone. It has particularly beneficial effects on the liver, gall bladder and the whole body in general. Topaz also has a toning effect on the nervous system. It helps to enhance overall energy levels and brings inspiration and creativity.

Light Green

Light green is a gentle shade like new golden-green leaves in springtime. It is a youthful energy, fresh and subtle.

Peridot

Geology: Peridot is a variety of olivine, with a lovely pale-green colour provided by iron, nickel and chromium. It is a volcanic gem. In Hawaii on the island of Oahu, you can find volcanic olivine grains on the beaches. Peridot has also been found in meteorite deposits.

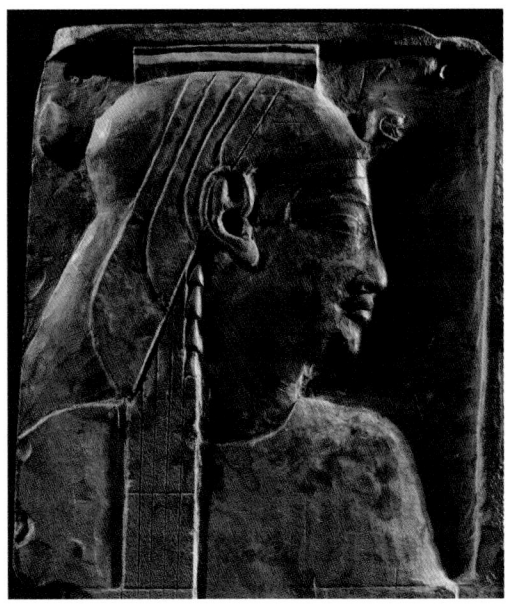

Peridot is said to have been a favourite stone of Queen Cleopatra, who must have appreciated its pale green colour.

Sources: More than 3500 years ago, the Egyptians used a peridot from a mine on an island called Zeberget in the Red Sea. This continued to yield gems until after the First World War. Today, most peridot is mined in Arizona, with specimens also found in Myanmar, Brazil and Hawaii. In the 1990s a new deposit was discovered in the Pakistan-owned region of Kashmir.

Peridot stones have a gentle fresh green colour, which is very lightening to the mind and spirit. It is used in healing to reduce stress and tension.

History: Legend has it that peridot was a favourite gemstone of Queen Cleopatra. Peridot is found decorating many medieval churches, including the Shrine of the Three Kings in Cologne Cathedral in Germany. Set in gold, the stone was traditionally credited with the power to drive away evil spirits. Some stones were large enough to be carved into drinking goblets.

Healing uses: Peridot has a light, revitalising effect on your mind and reawakens your appreciation of beauty. It is used in healing to revitalise the heart, spleen and adrenal glands, toning the body and mind, reducing stress and tension. It activates a sense of joy within you.

Jade

Geology: Jade is the name applied to two ornamental stones from China and Central America, nephrite and jadeite. These are very similar in structure and used in similar ways. Jade is a beautiful stone mostly found in various shades of pale to vivid green. Jade is usually cut into smooth dome shapes called cabochons, as well as carved into bangles, beads and statues. Dealers have to gamble when buying jade. They purchase a boulder with only a tiny opening visible from the outside. On splitting, the interior may be found to reveal fine stone or be worthless.

Sources: Top quality jade (jadeite) now comes mostly from Myanmar and Guatemala. The main deposits of nephrite are found in Canada, Australia, the USA and Taiwan.

History: Jade has been the royal gemstone of China for more than 4000 years. Priceless jade artefacts were placed in the tombs of emperors as a symbol of their power and wealth. In Central America, jade was sacred to the Olmec, Mayan and Toltec peoples, who carved it into masks and sacred relics. Jade

Jade occurs in soft and beautiful shades of green. It looks particularly lovely when carved into statues.

became popular in Europe in the sixteenth century when beautiful artefacts began to be brought over from Central America.

Healing uses: Jade helps to balance emotional states, particularly in highly sensitive individuals. It can calm the heart and soothe away anxiety. Jade is often used in healing to bring the energy of unconditional love and peace into the heart, as well as nurturing and caring for the spirit.

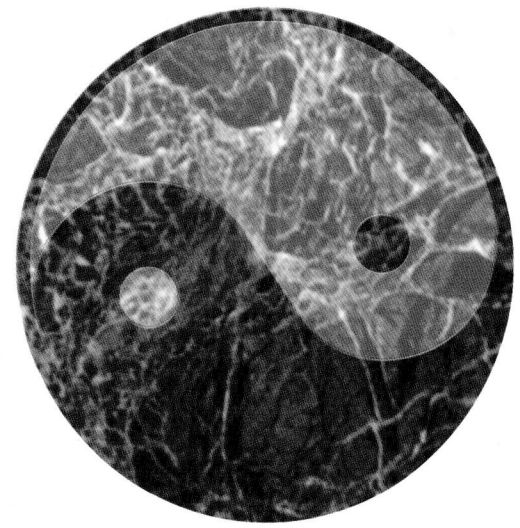

The energy of jade is balancing and harmonising, as suggested by this yin and yang symbol.

Rich Green

Vivid shades of green are soothing to the eye, restful and calming. Green blends yellow and blue, balancing warm and cool energies. Green stones are very beneficial to the heart chakra.

Emerald

Geology: Emerald is the green variety of beryl. Its colour is caused by chromium and iron. True emeralds contain tiny inclusions and other flaws. Because emeralds grow in metamorphic layers of rock under pressure, the size of the gems is usually small, with larger examples being very rare.

Darker green shades are very calming — they are particularly useful when working with the heart chakra.

Sources: Colombia, the producer of the astonishing emeralds associated with the Aztec empire, is still the main producer of fine stones today. Zambia and Brazil also produce top-quality emeralds, as do Zimbabwe, Pakistan and Madagascar.

History: The Aztecs yielded up treasure to the conqueror Hernán Cortes, notably emeralds carved into fish and flowers, with some examples the size of a fist. The colour of the stone made it particularly sacred to the ancient peoples of South America. Emeralds were also found in ancient Egypt — Cleopatra had her own mines near the Red Sea.

Healing uses: The energy of emerald can help to connect you with your creative source. The green colour links you to Nature. In healing, emerald is used to balance the heart and open it up to divine love.

True emeralds have a dramatic effect when set in jewellery. Here they are partnered with gold in a pair of stunning earrings.

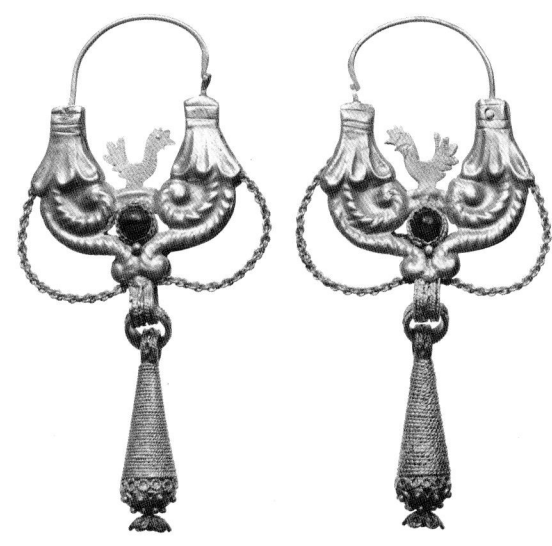

Moldavite

Geology: Moldavite is a dark-green form of tektite, which is a kind of fused glass formed when meteor showers hit the Earth millions of years ago. Moldavite is not crystalline in structure; it has swirls, bobbles and craters and forms unusual shapes due to its molten origin. Black and brown tektites exist, but rare dark-green moldavite is the most collectable.

Sources: Moldavia in Eastern Europe is considered to be the best source of green tektite. Fine examples are also found in Moldau in former Czechoslovakia, Thailand and South East Asia, Australia and the USA.

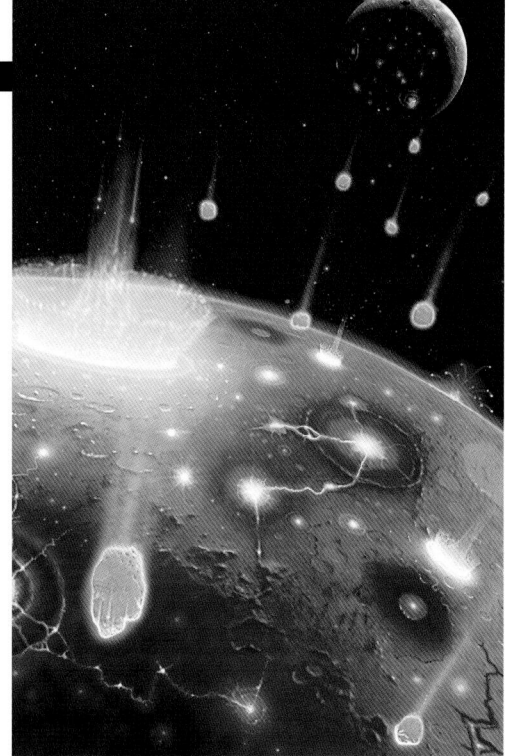

Moldavite falls to Earth from space in meteor showers. Meteorites containing moldavite fuse with geological deposits on the Earth.

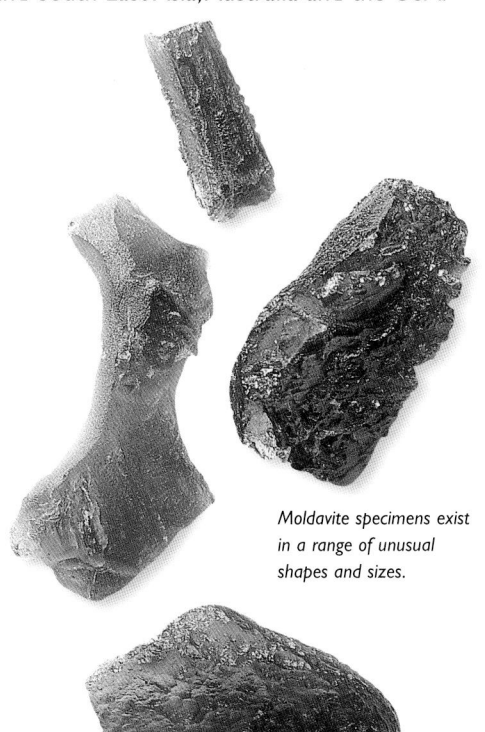

Moldavite specimens exist in a range of unusual shapes and sizes.

History: Moldavite is fascinating because of its extraterrestrial origin. It is a fusion of elements from space with geological deposits on the surface of the Earth. It has sometimes been used for making jewellery.

Healing uses: Moldavite can be used to help connect you to deeper levels of spiritual awareness, from the earthly to other dimensions and realms of being. The stone reminds us that we are all travellers through space – even as we go about our daily lives. Our planet is sailing on a continual journey. In healing, the stone can be placed on the forehead to enhance spiritual awareness of our place in the cosmos.

Turquoise

This shade is a fusion of green and blue, a cool and soothing balm to the heart and the emotions. Turquoise stones show up particularly well against darker skins.

Turquoise

Geology: Turquoise is a valuable mineral known scientifically as hydrated copper aluminium phosphate. Its colour ranges from sky blue to various shades of blue-green; the more iron is present, the greener the shade. True specimens contain tiny crystalline deposits that can be seen only with a microscope. There are many fake turquoises on the market that have been stained or dyed. True turquoise is very porous and should not be cleaned with chemicals, just warm soapy water.

Sources: Iran produces very pale sky-blue turquoise with no green tinges and veins; Arizona and New Mexico also yield fine examples. Afghanistan and the Middle East are other sources of the mineral.

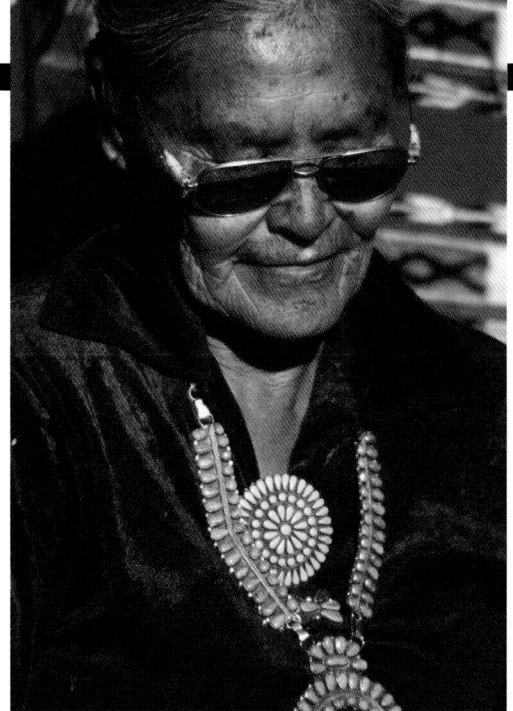

Fine turquoise jewellery is still made by talented Navajo craftspeople. The stone looks stunning when set in silver.

History: For thousands of years, Persia was the main source of turquoise. At Sinai in Egypt turquoise was being mined over 5000 years ago. In Mexico, turquoise was revered as a stone fit only for the gods. In the south-west USA, the Native American Navajo continue to make fine turquoise jewellery set in silver.

Healing uses: Turquoise ignites courage in your heart and strengthens your awareness of all life forms. It is used in healing to tone the whole body, as well as easing the lungs, chest and throat areas and boosting the immune system.

Turquoise is a protective stone that benefits and tones the whole of the immune system.

Aquamarine

Geology: Aquamarine is another variety of beryl, with a pale blue-green colour like sea water – the meaning of its name. The purer the blue shade, the more expensive the stone.

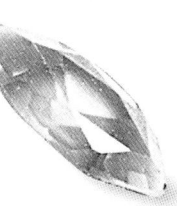
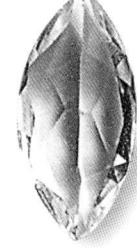

Aquamarine forms hexagonal crystals and is found in coarse granite rocks. Some aquamarines are heat-treated to increase the blue colour. The rough stones have a similar appearance to tourmaline.

Sources: Brazil is the leading producer of aquamarine, with the USA, Zambia, Mozambique and Pakistan also yielding wonderful specimens.

History: Perhaps not surprisingly, there is a great deal of sea folklore and legends associated with aquamarine. It was said to be treasured by mermaids, and was carried by sailors to ensure their safety while at sea. The stone was also seen as a traditional guardian of marriage and it remains an appropriate token to give as an anniversary gift.

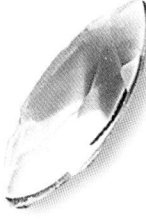
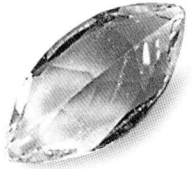
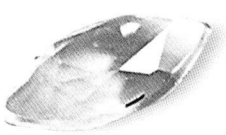

Aquamarine is a popular stone and is most commonly set in silver. This shows off its delicate colour to perfection.

Healing uses: Aquamarine expands and uplifts your spirits and helps you think clearly. It is seen as enhancing self-expression and self-worth, particularly in the sphere of your chosen line of work. It has a gently purifying effect on the mind and body, particularly helping the energies of the thyroid, spleen, liver and kidneys. In healing, aquamarine can be placed on the throat to balance the emotions and aid their clear verbal expression. Meditation with aquamarine can help to instil peace and calm in you.

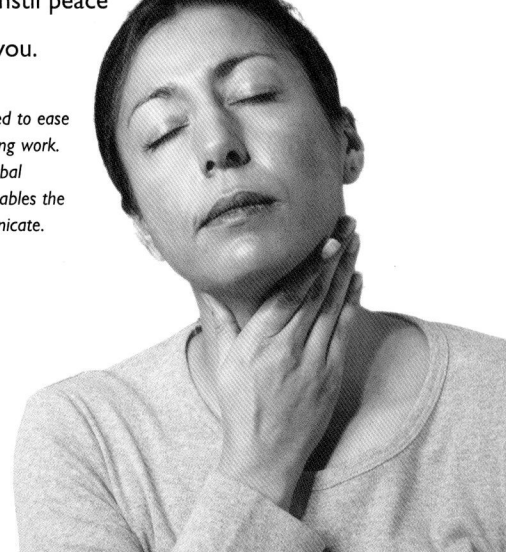

Aquamarine is used to ease the throat in healing work. This aids clear verbal expression and enables the patient to communicate.

Pale Blue

Pale blue is very gentle and soothing to the nerves, the sight and the emotions. Pale-blue stones emit a soft healing energy, which is very much needed in our mad, overexcited world.

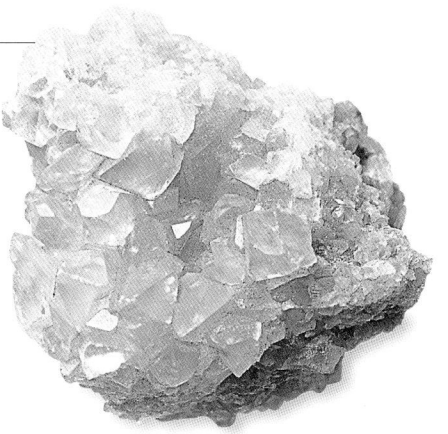

Celestite

Geology: Celestite is a form of strontium sulphate. It is a clear transparent mineral with a very pale blue colour deepening to blue-grey, a shade that is unique in the mineral kingdom. It forms larger clusters with pronounced bladed crystals, as well as smaller nodules with tiny inward-growing crystals.

Sources: The most abundant sources of celestite tend to be found in sedimentary rocks in the USA, particularly in New York, Michigan and Ohio. Specimens also occur in Germany, Madagascar and Sicily.

Celestite is also known as the stone of heaven, symbolising the sacred energy of angels and celestial beings.

The soft grey-blue of celestite can be used in your environment to soothe and calm the emotions.

History: Celestite is highly valued among mineral collectors, and over the past few years has become more prominent in New Age shops because of its healing uses.

Healing uses: Celestite is the blue of a summer sky. It brings about expansion, open-heartedness and room to breathe. Placed in a room, celestite calms the energy and is a wonderful focus for meditation. Some healers see it as a stone that symbolises sacred personal space. In healing, it is used to enhance thyroid balance and reduce stress. If placed on the throat, it aids self-expression. It is also useful for healers to use on themselves to replenish their energies.

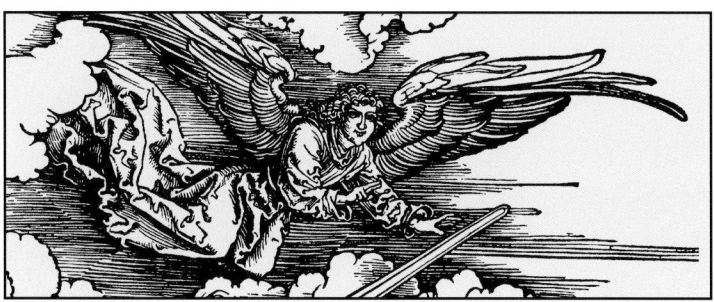

Blue Moonstone

Geology: Moonstone is a member of the feldspar family of minerals. It is a colourless or pale milky stone and when turned in the light, it shows a shimmering translucent blue sheen. This can be a silvery milky white in some specimens, but the blue stones are seen as more valuable. The stone contains layers that reflect light back at each other, creating the shimmering coloured effect. The most effective way of enhancing this property is to cut and polish the stones into cabochons, so they are smooth, rounded domes.

Sources: Some of the best examples of moonstone are to be found in Madagascar, Sri Lanka, Australia, Brazil and the USA.

The changing light of the moon is reflected in the soft lustre of moonstone.

Blue moonstone has a special gentle sheen. No wonder it is considered a sacred stone!

History: In India, moonstone is considered sacred and is dedicated to the goddess in her lunar forms.

Healing uses: Moonstone is associated with feminine energy and the cyclical nature of feminine rhythms. It brings balance and harmony to your emotions. It is a wonderful stone to mark changing feminine cycles though girlhood to puberty, motherhood and wise-womanhood. It is seen as hormone-balancing and brings equilibrium to the senses. Worn as jewellery set in silver, it is one of the most attractive of the semi-precious stones.

Dark Blue

Rich dark-blue shades are cool and contemplative, bringing a meditative state of calm to the spirit. Deep-blue stones are often associated with loyalty and high ideals.

Sapphire

Geology: Sapphire is a variety of corundum, which is the second-hardest known mineral, in the same family as ruby. Mostly known as a source of rich blue stones, sapphire can also be found in other shades like pink, gold, white or even black. Star sapphires contain needles of rutile that reflect a six-pointed star in bright light. Most sapphires have been heat-treated to deepen the colour. Generally sapphires are cut in oval or rounded rectangular forms to display their blue hues.

Sources: Historically, Myanmar and Kashmir are the most famous sapphire producers. However, Sri Lanka produces most of the stones found today, ranging from pale sky-blue to rich, deep shades.

Sapphires have been cut and set in fine jewellery for hundreds of years. Here, diamonds set off an amazing large stone.

Deep blue sapphire is a very 'royal' shade of blue. It is a favourite stone for engagement rings.

History: Traditionally, sapphire was seen as a symbol of fidelity, making it a favourite for engagement rings. It also has an extensive history as a jewel of royalty and high priesthood. The British Crown Jewels contain very large sapphires of 'royal' blue.

Healing uses: Blue sapphire connects you to your highest ideals and spiritual essence. It enables you to communicate your own inner truth. Allow the colour to guide you to your own path of awareness. In healing, sapphire may be applied to the forehead to bring emotional balance and guide your thoughts to the present moment. Sapphire is also said to strengthen the kidneys and the heart.

Lapis Lazuli

Geology: Lapis lazuli is made up of the blue mineral lazurite with golden strands or microcrystals of pyrite and white calcite. The colour of lapis lazuli is always deep blue, and the pyrite crystals help to distinguish it from its cousin sodalite, which is also blue but lacks the pyrite. Lapis tends to be opaque in character. It is porous and should be cleaned only with warm soapy water. It is also fairly brittle and needs careful storage.

Lapis lazuli is a deep blue stone with gold and white strands running through it.

Sources: Lapis lazuli has been mined for over 6000 years. Afghanistan is an ancient source still used today. Lapis is also mined in Chile, the USA, Siberia and Myanmar.

History: The tomb of Tutankhamun yielded up many astonishing treasures, most notably the famous mask of the young king fashioned in gold and lapis lazuli. The Pharaohs were adorned with the stone in life and death. In medieval and Renaissance paintings, enamelling and stained glass, particularly rich shades of blue were obtained by using lapis lazuli ground to a powder.

Healing uses: Lapis lazuli assists with spiritual purification, turning the mind away from earthly concerns. It links you to your higher guidance and opens your inner awareness. With its golden pyrite inclusions, it activates the fire of spiritual illumination, especially if placed on the forehead over the third eye. It is said to bring strength and vitality to the whole body.

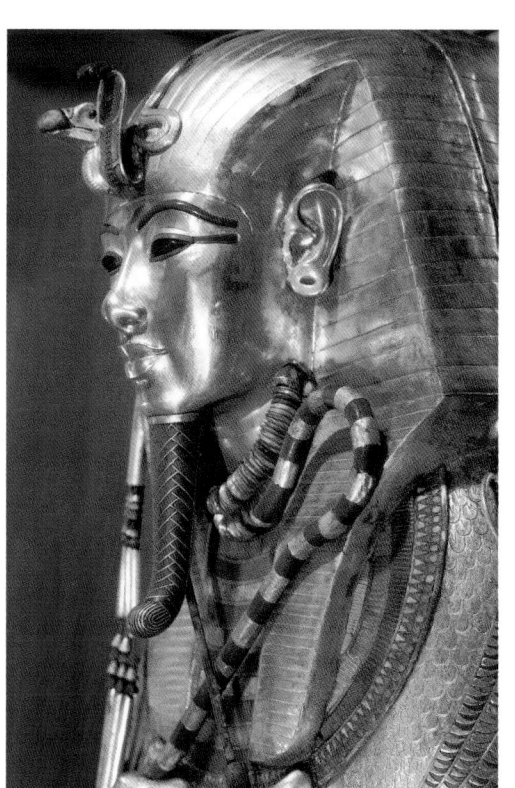

Superb jewellery and gold funeral masks inlaid with lapis adorned the body of the young boy king Tutankhamun.

Violet

Purple and violet shades are beneficially stimulating to the brain – as a mixture of energising red and cooling blue, they bring wisdom into action.

Amethyst

Geology: Amethyst is purple quartz that can occur in many forms, ranging from tiny crystals to points, clusters and geodes, which are rocks with inner cavities of varying sizes where the crystals grow inwards. Large geodes are sometimes displayed cut open to show the amethyst formations. Amethyst varies in colour from dark purple to paler lavender shades.

Sources: Amethyst is found in Brazil, Uruguay, Bolivia and Argentina, Namibia, Zambia and other African countries. The Ural Mountains in Russia produce very fine amethysts cut for jewellery.

History: The Russian monarch Catherine the Great was passionate about amethysts, and there are also many examples found in the British Crown Jewels. Bishops

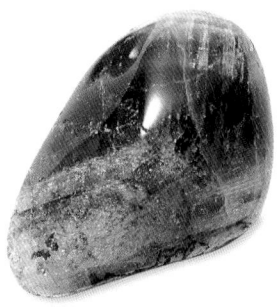
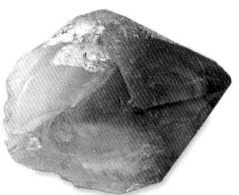

Small amethyst tumblestones are easy to carry with you when you need them.

traditionally wear amethyst rings. The stone has long had a religious connection and it is found decorating many churches and cathedrals.

Healing uses: Amethyst is one of the most popular stones for healing. It will help you to feel spiritually open and aware, purifying and cleansing your energies on physical, mental, emotional and spiritual levels. Placed either on the forehead or above the crown of the head, amethyst energy feels like a shower of cool gentle rain through the whole body. Amethyst can also be used to shield you from negativity.

If you meditate with amethyst, the energy of the stone can clear the whole body.

Iolite

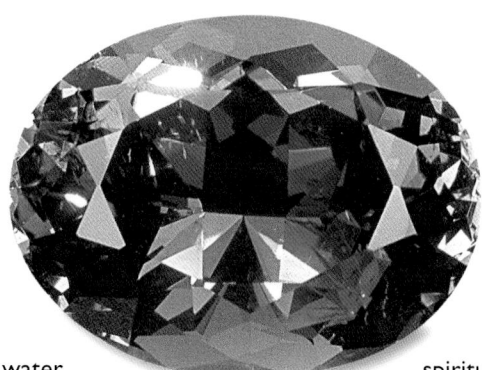

Iolite shimmers with its own special reflections. It makes really stunning jewellery.

Geology: Iolite is a violet variety of the mineral cordierite, which can also be found in brown or black shades. In the past, iolite was sometimes known as water sapphire because of its beautiful violet-blue hues. It makes very attractive jewellery. Its structure creates a display called pleochroism, where reflections of violet, clear and golden lights appear from different angles within the same stone, making a shimmering effect.

Sources: Iolite deposits are found in many parts of the world, including Sri Lanka, India, Mozambique, Madagascar, Brazil and Myanmar.

History: The Vikings obtained iolite from sources in Norway and Greenland and used thin pieces of the stone as lenses to look up at the sun so they could navigate successfully. The name iolite comes from *ios*, the Greek word for violet.

The Vikings used iolite that was found in Norway and Greenland.

Healing uses: Iolite can be used to focus your meditation on higher dimensions of spirituality. As human beings, we have the capacity to connect with much wider energies than we are aware of in our everyday life. Awareness of our true spiritual home can help us to behave more responsibly and caringly in the physical world. Iolite can be placed above the crown of the head when lying down to meditate or to receive healing. Iolite is also used when trying to balance the energies of the physical body.

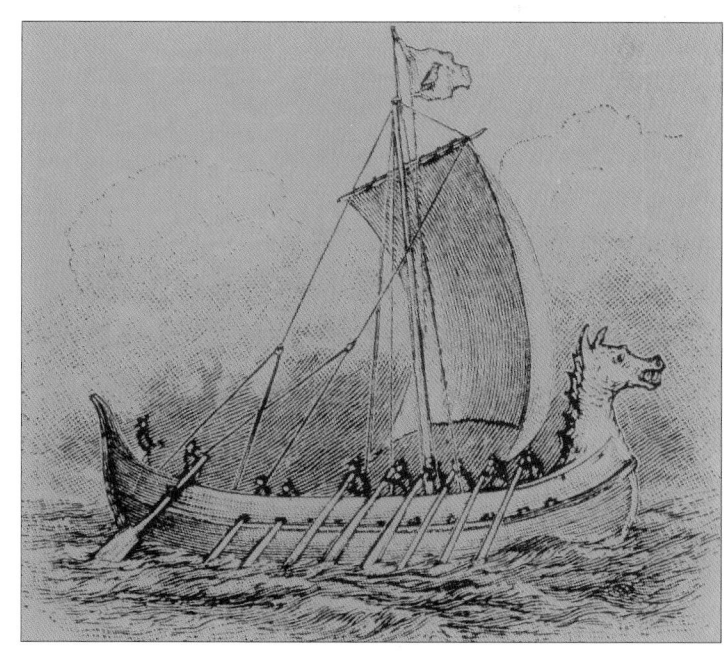

Pink

Shades of pink are linked to delicate gentle feelings of unconditional love, soothing to the eye and nurturing to the spirit. Pink stones are attractive against all skin types.

Rose Quartz

Geology: Titanium and iron traces give rose quartz its pink colour. It occurs in massive pieces and rarely in well-formed crystals. Brazilian rose quartz is used for carving figurines, spheres and obelisks. In jewellery, the preferred way of presenting rose quartz is as cabochons, smooth rounded stones polished to show the fine pink shade. A rare variety contains golden threads of rutile, giving a sparkling pink appearance.

Soft rose quartz has a gentle effect on the body and mind.

Sources: Brazil is a main producer of massive rose quartz slabs, as well as flat-faced crystals. India, Madagascar and the USA are other notable sources.

History: Rose quartz is very popular with mineral collectors and is also one of the favourite stones of New Age healers.

Healing uses: Rose quartz brings you a gentle sense of warmth and wellbeing in the heart. It is a good stone to have beside your bed if you have difficulty sleeping or if you feel anxious. It soothes physical, emotional and environmental stress. It helps balance the emotional and sexual energies, clearing anger, jealousy or misunderstanding. Meditation with rose quartz brings emotional clarity and peace and the return of a childlike trust. Rose quartz is often placed over the centre of the chest in healing sessions to balance the energies of the heart.

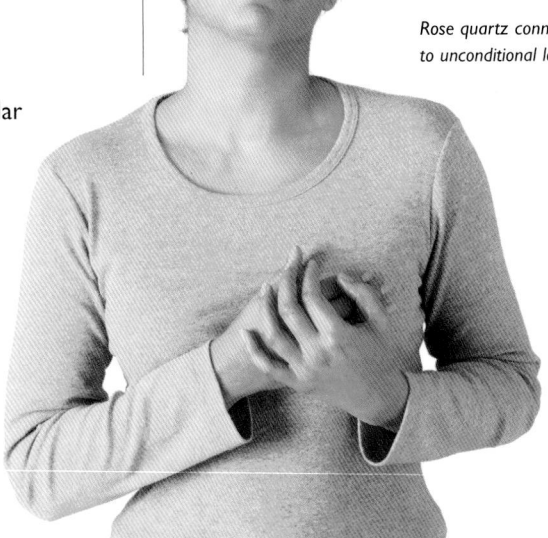

Rose quartz connects you to unconditional love.

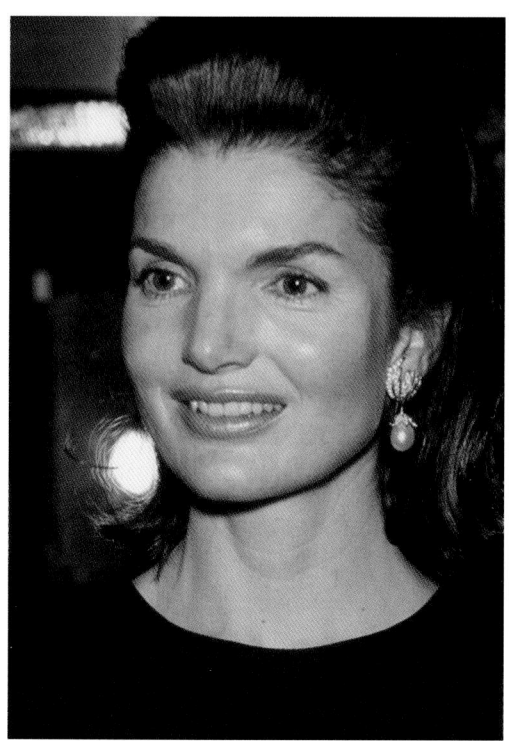

Jackie Kennedy had an outstanding jewellery collection and wore many accessories, including a fabulous kunzite ring.

Kunzite

Geology: Kunzite is a very attractive lavender-pink stone, formed from lithium aluminium silicate, a pink variety of spodumene. Like iolite, kunzite is pleochroic, meaning that it will show different shades of pink and violet when turned in the light. Although it is as hard as quartz, it is a challenge for gem cutters to bring out all the pink delicacy of this stone, as it can break easily if struck in the wrong direction. It is often found with beryl and tourmaline.

Sources: Kunzite was first discovered in Connecticut, USA, then commercially extracted in California. Today Brazil, Madagascar and Afghanistan produce most of the gems on the market.

History: Kunzite was named after a famous gemologist and scholar called George Kunz, who was a gem buyer for Tiffany & Co. in the early twentieth century. Kunz was a collector not just of stones but also of legends about gems and jewels.

Healing uses: The combination of violet, a deeply spiritual hue, and pink, relating to the heart, make kunzite a useful stone for helping you connect to the wider perspective of love as the creative energy behind all things. It can be placed on the chest area in tandem with a rose quartz crystal to support and expand the energy of the heart.

Kunzite has a gentle lavender-pink colour, which is very soothing to the eye. It is used to open the heart and its energy.

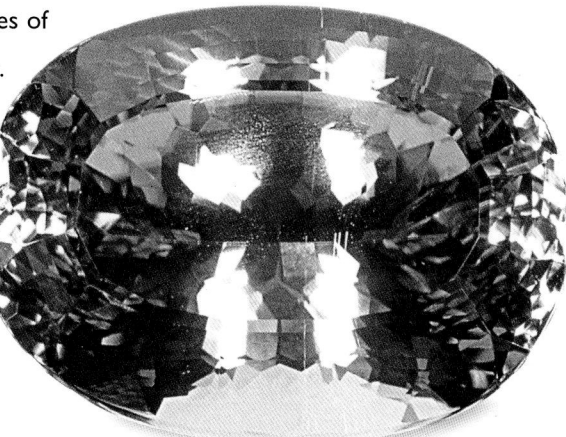

White

White is a combination of all the colours in the spectrum. Rays of sunlight passing though cut diamonds cause a brilliant rainbow effect. Colourless gems represent unity and perfection.

Diamond

Geology: Diamonds are forever – made of pure carbon, they are the hardest known substance on the Earth, have the highest melting point and atoms packed more densely than any other mineral. Though they are well known as jewellery, diamonds are also used in industry as excellent electrical insulators. Despite their hardness, they have to be handled very skilfully by jewellers because they will split if they are wrongly struck. They occur in clear, pink, pale yellow, blue, green, reddish and even black specimens. Diamonds form in pipelike gaps in a host rock called kimberlite.

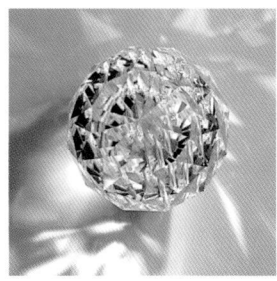

Exquisitely cut diamonds reflect all the colours of the spectrum.

Sources: Diamonds are found in South Africa, India, Brazil, Russia, Australia and the USA.

History: There are many famous diamond stories. When the world's largest diamond, the 3106-carat Cullinan was discovered in 1905, workers were seen to play with it like a lump of glass at the edge of a mine shaft in South Africa. The Cullinan was presented to King Edward VII on his sixty-sixth birthday and was cut up into four diamonds that now form part of the British Crown Jewels.

Healing uses: Diamond brings out your unique qualities. This aspect is at the root of its use in rings to mark engagements and long marriages. It is a master healer, activating the purest energy all around and within.

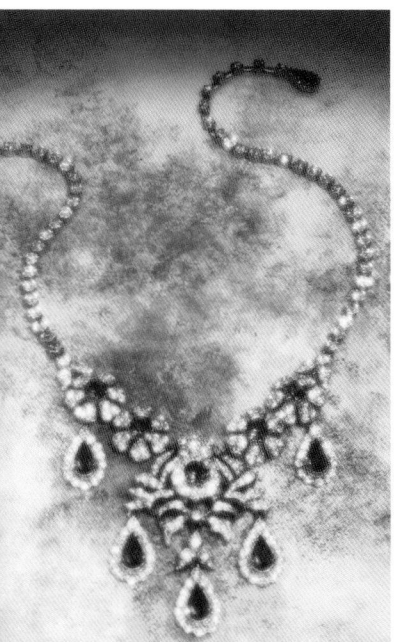

The energy of diamonds is said to bring out your own unique personality.

Clear Quartz

Fine quartz clusters form in a huge variety of shapes and sizes.

Geology: Quartz is one of the most common minerals found in the Earth's crust. It is found in countless varieties of clusters, points, masses, colours and forms. Clear quartz is also known as rock crystal. Though the stone may be cloudy white, the best quality points are completely clear with an icelike appearance. These stones are well defined, and may be single- or double- terminated. Clear quartz with tiny golden needles of rutile is also called rutilated quartz.

Sources: Brazil, the USA and Africa are among the main sources of the better quality clear quartz.

History: The original meaning of the word 'crystal', usually applied to quartz, is from the Greek word for frozen. Clear quartz is the original crystal ball, with its patterns and milky inclusions providing inspiration for seers. In South America and other locations around the world, large lumps of clear quartz have been found carved into the shape of crystal skulls by ancient peoples.

Healing uses: Clear quartz is one of the most commonly used stones in healing. It help to focus and amplify physical, mental and emotional energy. Quartz points can be placed on any areas of the body that need energising. Quartz can also be used protectively in challenging environments. Rutilated quartz eases depression and clears negativity.

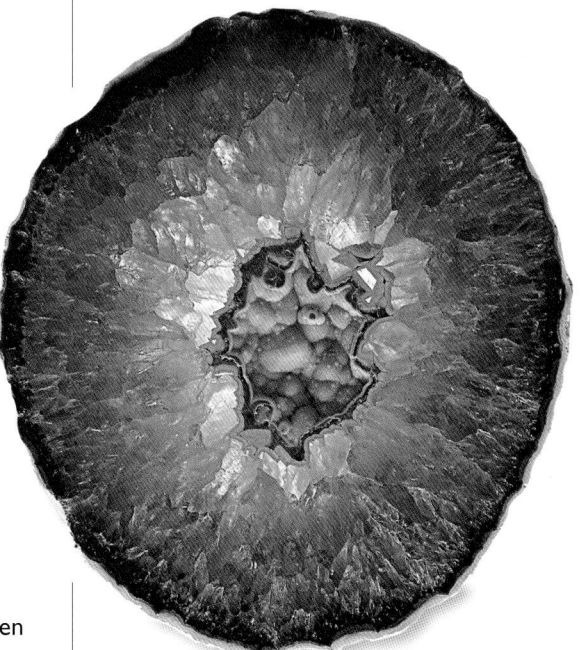

Quartz crystals are shown here growing into the available space. Stones like these are often cut in half and polished.

Black

Black absorbs all colours within it, like the rainbow sheen of a starling's wing feathers. Black simply holds all the colours of the spectrum in density. Rather than being negative, black stones have mystery in their depths.

Obsidian

Geology: Obsidian is a glassy-textured silicon dioxide, formed from rapidly cooled volcanic lava. Iron and magnesium give the stone its black or very dark green colour. Bubbles of long-trapped air may create rainbow or golden reflections. A particularly attractive form of the stone is snowflake obsidian, which contains white speckled inclusions of cristobalite.

Sources: Obsidian is found in many states of the USA, such as Arizona, Colorado and Texas, as well as in Mexico, Italy and Scotland.

Snowflake obsidian is a particularly attractive version of the usual black obsidian.

History: Another name for obsidian is 'Apache tear', showing its links to the Native American tribes of the south-western USA. There have been notable archaeological finds of ancient arrow heads chipped from obsidian, indicating its use in hunting and the tooling of leather for at least 10,000 years.

Healing uses: Obsidian has a strong masculine affinity. It affects the energies of the lower abdomen and the root chakra. Meditating with obsidian activates warrior energy when you face uncertainty. It is a very grounding stone, helping to prepare for action, and is said to disperse fear.

This stone turtle, with the white speckled inclusions of cristobalite, is an example of snowflake obsidian.

Native Americans have been hunting with obsidian-tipped arrows for thousands of years.

Black Tourmaline

Geology: The long rectangular shapes of tourmaline and its varied colours make it one of the most popular stones to collect. It occurs in a range of colours, including black, pink, green and blue, as well as forms with more than one colour, such as 'watermelon' with pink inside and green outside. Black tourmaline is called schorl and is the most common opaque form of the stone, very rich in iron. An unusual property of tourmaline is that it can be electrically charged by heating, so one end is positive and the other negative, giving it a kind of magnetic pull. The stone is cut and set in jewellery, carved into figurines and sometimes mounted in uncut form.

Black tourmaline forms into regular shapes and is very popular to collect.

Sources: Kenya, Madagascar and other African countries produce the stone, as well as Brazil, Sri Lanka, Pakistan and the USA.

History: The many colours of tourmaline have made it a favourite with jewel collectors for centuries – the name comes from an old Sinhalese word *turmali*, which means 'mixed'.

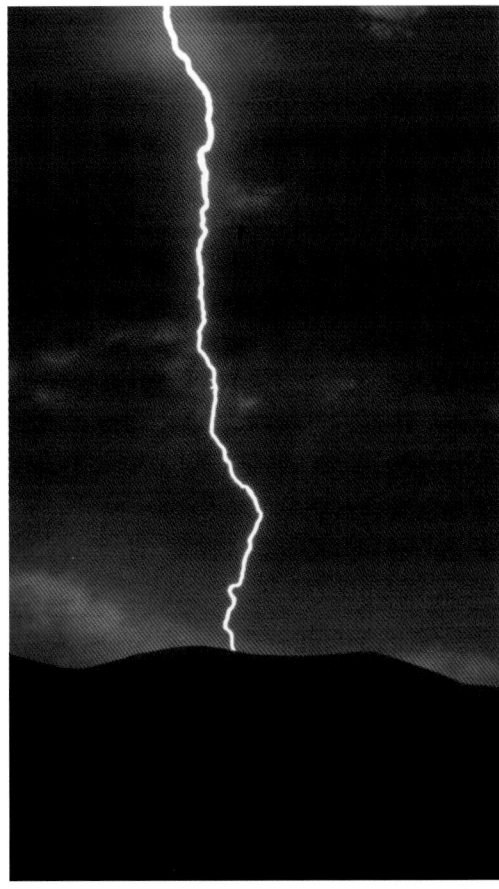

The power of a lightning charge crackles through the air. Tourmaline can be electrically charged by heating.

Healing uses: Black tourmaline has a powerful, dense energy that helps to anchor you if you feel unfocused or pulled in different directions. It has a strong protective influence, which can help you when you are emotionally or physically vulnerable. It strengthens and vitalises you and makes you aware of the electromagnetic energies of the Earth. It can be placed on the base of the spine to help stabilise and 'root' your energies.

Brown

Brown is the colour associated with earth, the soil, the dense matter from which all growing things take root; it has a comforting and centring energy. Brown stones are regarded as 'earthing' in healing work.

Smoky Quartz

Smoky quartz occurs in tawny shades of soft brown. It is a very hard mineral.

Geology: Smoky quartz is the brown or black variety of quartz, which is thought to have undergone exposure to radiation during its formation. Smoky quartz is often found in granite rocks that still show a tiny amount of natural radioactivity. Most smoky quartz has been heat-treated to deepen the colour even further. It is often carved into spheres, pyramids, eggs and figurines. Smoky quartz forms well-defined six-sided points and is a mineral as hard as clear quartz. Some specimens also contain golden needles of rutile.

All brown crystals remind us that we come from the Earth, and have a positive grounding effect on the body.

Sources: The world's largest supplier of smoky quartz is Brazil, with the Cairngorm Mountains in Scotland, Colorado in the USA and the Swiss Alps also producing fine specimens.

History: Brown stones like smoky quartz were popular in jewellery in the 1920s and 1930s, particularly in brooches and pendants of neo-Celtic designs.

Healing uses: Smoky quartz helps to strengthen and ground your energies and clear away negativity. Meditation with the stone helps to transform turbulent emotions. It can help to build sexual vitality when used on the lower abdomen and the base of the spine. If you work on a computer, smoky quartz protects against electromagnetic radiation – place a piece on top of your monitor.

Tiger's Eye

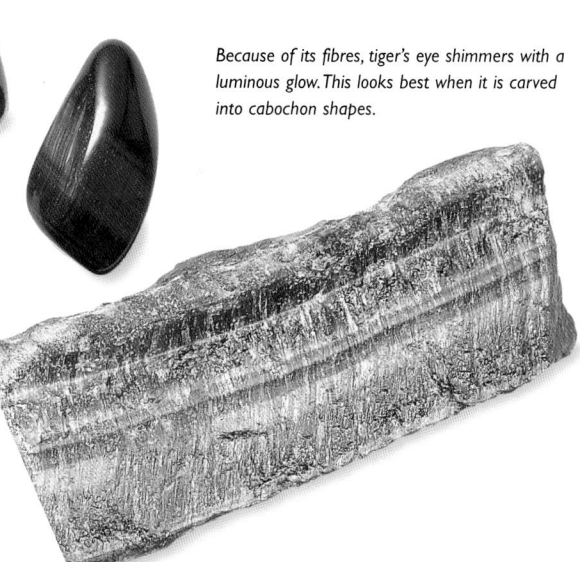

Geology: Tiger's eye is a variety of chalcedony, which is quartz containing tiny microcrystals. It is made up of lustrous brown and yellow fibres in layers that reflect the light in an unusual way, causing a phenomenon called 'chatoyancy' (like a cat's eye) when the stone is moved from side to side. It is normally found in shades of brown and gold. However, blue varieties also exist and some heat-treated specimens may have a reddish tinge. Tiger's eye is very attractive when cut and polished in cabochons, smooth rounded shapes that demonstrate the chatoyancy more clearly.

Because of its fibres, tiger's eye shimmers with a luminous glow. This looks best when it is carved into cabochon shapes.

Sources: Large deposits are found in Myanmar, India, Australia and South Africa.

History: In medieval times, tiger's eye was often used as a protection against the evil eye.

Healing uses: With a combination of earthy brown and radiant gold shades, tiger's eye is useful to help spirit into matter, bringing ideas into reality. When you embark on a new path of expansion, it stabilises you and makes sure you that have your feet on the ground. It is thought to be a relaxing and calming stone, which can be helpful for inducing sleep. Used over the solar plexus or the abdomen, it helps to balance and harmonise both physical and emotional energies.

Use tiger's eye to relax and calm your mind. It is a stone with very calming energies.

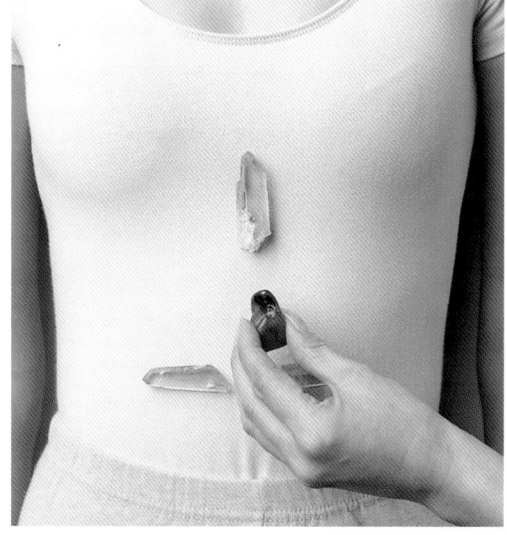

Iridescent

Iridescence is not so much a colour as a quality, a sudden appearance of shimmering colours as light moves over a surface. Iridescent stones have long been regarded as having magical properties.

Labradorite

Geology: The beautiful mineral labradorite may show iridescent flashes in a whole variety of shades across its surface – deep blue, violet, green, gold and orange. It is quite dull in appearance until light plays upon it in the right direction. The effect is caused by different intergrowing layers in its structure, which reflect light waves back against each other, creating the play of colours. Labradorite with many thin layers will show the best effects. As a mineral, it is a variety of feldspar, and forms in chunks embedded in host rocks.

Sources: It is mostly found in Labrador, Canada – from where it gets its name – and also in Scandinavia, where it is sold under the name 'spectrolite'. Some deposits occur in the USA and Russia.

History: The beautiful variety of colours and changing appearance of labradorite have caused it to be used as a magical talisman since ancient times.

Healing uses: Labradorite reminds you of the changing nature of life moment by moment. Flashes of deep blue within the stone help you to recall that spirit is behind and within all matter. Labradorite expands the third eye and the crown, opening you up to deeper perceptions of reality, and encouraging you to see with new eyes. Its gently shimmering colours may also help to bring you interesting dreams.

Shimmering labradorite displays many hues. It can bring you vivid dreams and enable you to see beyond reality.

Opal

Geology: Opals are not true crystals. Classed as mineraloids, they have a unique structure. They formed millions of years ago as a solution that settled in the cracks and layers of sedimentary rocks, and opals still contain between 6 and 10 per cent water. Packed with miniscule spheres of silicon and oxygen molecules, opals flash with many tiny shimmering rainbows as light bounces in these microscopic spaces – the effect is known as 'opalescence'. The stone's background may be clear, milky white, pale yellow, black or even the orange-red that is found in fire opals. Black opals contain the brightest colours and are also the most expensive.

Sources: Ancient opal came from mines in Eastern Europe, but for the past one hundred years the main producer has been Australia. Fire opals are found in Mexico and in the state of Oregon in the USA.

History: Few stones have had such a varied and fascinating history as opals. There have been many archaeological finds of opal artefacts that are thousands of years old. Opals were adored by the ancient Romans; used as an eye tonic in the Middle Ages;

Opals look very good in simple jewellery settings and look particularly attractive when they are set in rings.

celebrated by Shakespeare; and were a favourite gemstone of Queen Victoria.

Healing uses: Opal is alive with gentle shimmers of iridescent colour. The most common background is a milky white. This makes the stone very much in tune with the third eye and the crown chakras. The stone can be used to enhance psychic awareness as well as energising all levels and areas of the body, because of the rainbow of colours that are contained within it.

Opals shimmer with their own beautiful rainbow colours. They can be used to energise the whole of the body.

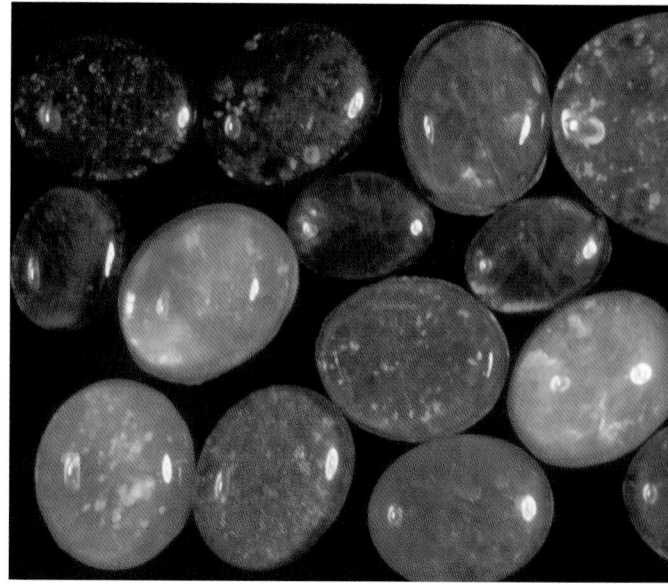

Gold

Gold as a colour ray is radiant, and as warm and bright as the sun itself. The precious metal has been treasured as a setting for gemstones and jewels since the beginning of humankind, and gold minerals are strongly attractive.

The Metal Gold

The hues of the metal gold have mesmerised humankind for thousands of years.

Geology: Gold is a rare and noble metal. Its chemical symbol is Au, which comes from *aurum*, the Latin word for gold. Gold is soft enough to be beaten into fine leaves, and 28 grammes can make a gold wire 80 kilometres in length. Its purity is measured in carats, a word derived from Italian, Greek and Arabic words for carob seeds, which were used to balance the scales in ancient trading practices. Pure gold is 24 carat. A combination of yellow gold with copper is often known as red gold, and with platinum, white gold.

Sources: Today, gold is extensively mined in California, Mexico, Colorado and Canada.

History: Examples of gold jewellery date back thousand of years. The art of smelting and working gold produced amazing Egyptian, Sumerian and South American artefacts. It has traditionally been a symbol of nobility and royalty. The would-be conquerors of the New World sought El Dorado, the fabled city made entirely of gold.

Healing uses: Gold is seen as cleansing to the whole body, but particularly to the brain and the nervous system. Wearing gold helps to attract positive energy and abundance. In medicine, gold is used to treat rheumatoid arthritis, ulcers, certain types of cancer and to repair damaged tissues in surgery.

Pure gold in bars is one of the most valuable commodities to be found. It is immediately associated with wealth and power.

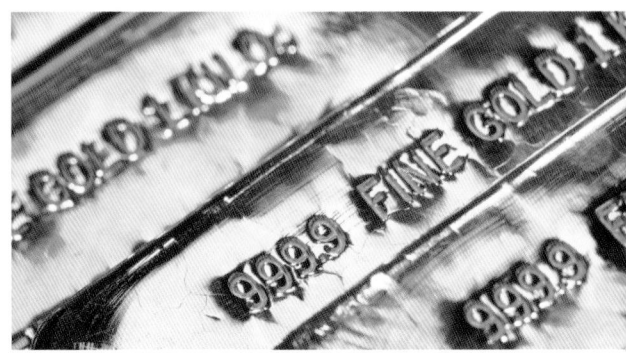

Pyrite is twice as hard as gold and cannot be worked in the same way, although the variety from Italy can be faceted for jewellery.

Sources: Significant quantities of pyrite have been found in the states of Missouri and Illinois, USA. Other sources have also been discovered in South Africa, Peru, Germany, Russia, Italy and Spain.

History: Although the mineral has a high iron content, pyrite has never been used as a source of iron. However, during the Second World War, pyrite was mined as a source of sulphur for industrial purposes. Any jewellery that is labelled as marcasite is in fact more likely to be pyrite, because marcasite slowly deteriorates over time.

Healing uses: Pyrite is seen as an overall cleanser of the body, and if brought into your environment it helps to dispel negativity and clear your electromagnetic field. Place it on your desk when working to improve your energy levels. In healing, pyrite can be placed at the base of the spine or on the lower abdomen to boost your energy.

Pyrite has a different sheen to gold – it is paler and looks more like brass.

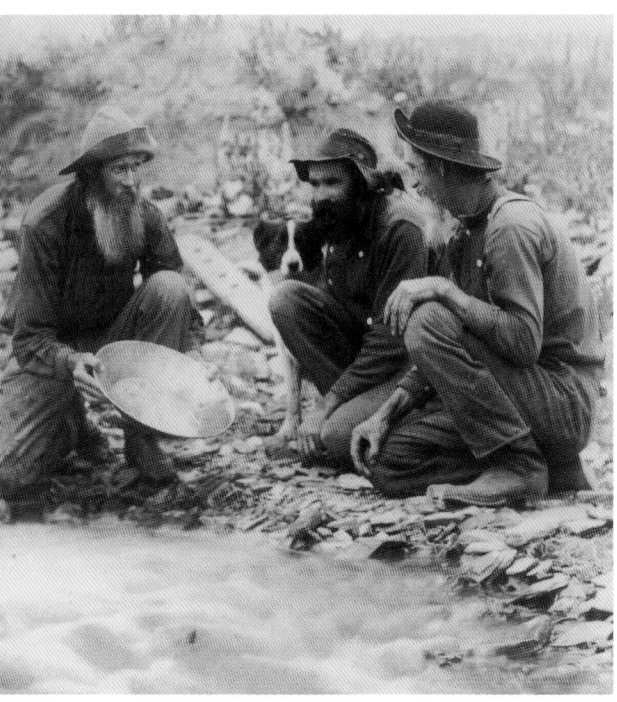

Early gold panners often mistook pyrite for gold. Although it looks very similar, pyrite has to be worked in a different way.

Pyrite

Geology: Pyrite is a beautiful mineral with a yellow sheen like brass. It is also known as 'fool's gold' because it has often been mistaken for the real thing. It is very common and forms opaque crystals with precise, geometric, often cuboid formations. It has a high percentage of iron and sulphur in its composition. Pyrite has the same chemistry as marcasite, and the two are difficult to distinguish from each other.

Silver

The changing energy of the silver ray is like the moon shining on water, delicate and pure, with a fluidity that is cooling and soothing to the senses. Silver as a metal and silver-grey stones have a subtle sheen against the skin.

The Metal Silver

Geology: Silver is a metal with the symbol Ag for *argentum*, the Latin word for silver. It can occur alone in nature and is also often found with gold, copper or mercury deposits. It is extremely soft, like gold, and is the most electrically and thermally conductive metal, making it very useful in the photographic, watch-making and computer industries. It can be drawn without breaking into fine wire the thickness of human hair. Fine silver is 999 parts per thousand pure; most jewellery is set in sterling silver, which is 925 parts silver with 75 parts copper.

The soft silver glow of moonlight encases the Earth in a silver radiance. Silver connects you to this moon energy.

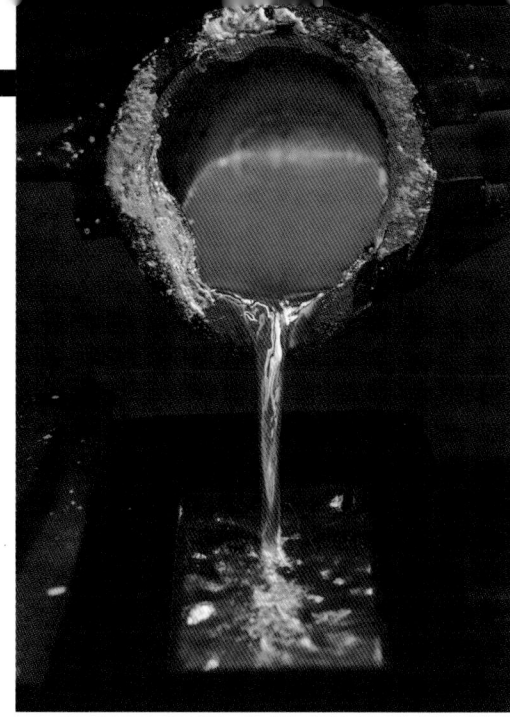

Red-hot silver ore pours into a waiting mould. Like gold, silver is extremely soft and can be worked very easily.

Sources: Silver is widely distributed all over the globe. The most notable deposits today are situated in Mexico, Canada and in Arizona in the USA.

History: Many examples of stunning silver jewellery and artefacts can be found in ancient Celtic, Roman and Indian civilisations. Silver has often been associated with the moon because of its silvery shimmer.

Healing uses: The energy of silver is cool, as opposed to the bright radiance of gold. Silver is subtle, seen as linked to the unconscious, bringing intuitive impulses. Silver connects you with your dream-self, the part of you that is mysterious and knowing.

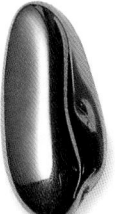

Haematite has an attractive matt sheen to it. It is used to warm and strengthen blood circulation and increase physical energy.

Haematite

Geology: Haematite is iron oxide, a mineral that is a source of opaque, silver-grey crystals. The host rock and its dust are blood-red in colour, providing a natural source of red pigment. Haematite may form crystals in a number of shapes and masses – rounded kidney-shaped stones as well as bladed crystals can be found.

Sources: Notable specimens can be found in the Lake District in Northern England, Mexico, Brazil, Australia and Canada.

History: In ancient times, the red rocks of haematite were said to be formed from the blood of warriors who died in battle. The word 'haematite' comes from the Greek root *haem*, which refers to the blood. Traditionally it was held by women in childbirth. For centuries and even until recently, finely ground particles of red haematite dust were used in make-up formulations as blusher!

Healing uses: Haematite is a grounding and strengthening stone, which helps to centre you very much in the body, particularly when your energies are overstretched. It has a calming and soothing effect on the nerves. It can be worn to strengthen courage and energy when facing difficult challenges. Haematite also counteracts negative energy in your environment, for example, when placed near a computer. In healing, it is considered to balance blood circulation.

Haematite powder is blood red and is therefore used in healing work to treat blood disorders and the circulatory system.

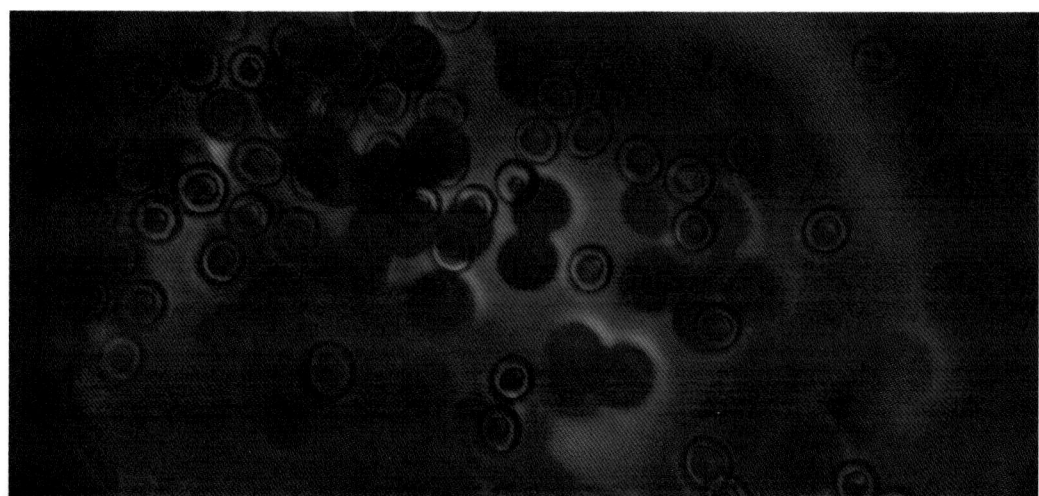

Simple Crystal Healing Methods

Working with crystal energies involves fine-tuning your intuition and sensitivity to your environment. You can use the chart on page 145, or choose a crystal from the Crystal Index because of its colours or associations. Alternatively, you can simply work with a stone because you feel that it is the right one for you.

What is Healing?

The word 'healing' is derived from an old Germanic root *hael*, which can mean 'complete', 'whole' or even 'holy'. It is a process by which the body, mind and spirit are gently balanced to bring a sense of wholeness, oneness with all life. Anyone can benefit from healing, provided they

Crystals can be hung on a chain so that you can use them as pendulums for dowsing work.

Gently laying a crystal over your heart area can soothe any troubled emotions.

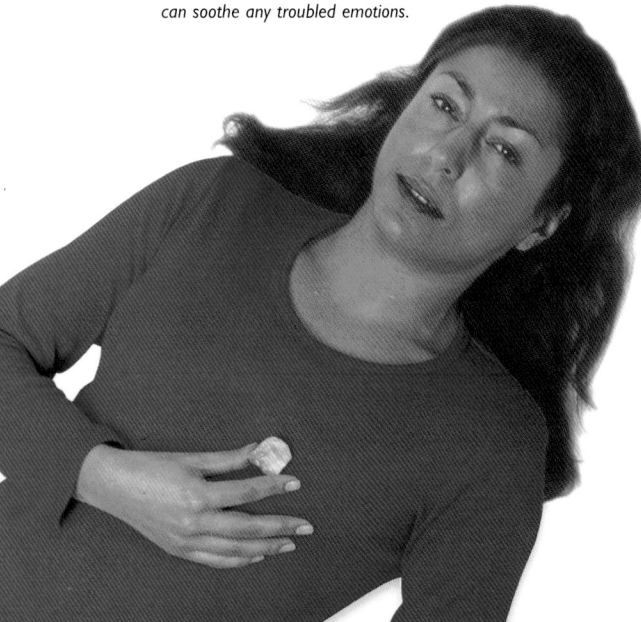

are open to receiving it. If you have complex physical problems or deep emotional issues, you are advised to seek the help of a suitably qualified practitioner. For general balancing and opening your own awareness, you can benefit from working on yourself. After any exercises it is useful to make notes or drawings you can come back to at a later date – healing is an ever-unfolding process.

Using a Pendulum

A pendulum can be made of a balanced quartz or cut-glass point suspended on a chain or a string. Dowsing, as this is called, is an ancient art. If you hold the pendulum still and say your real name, it should respond by turning clockwise. If you say a false name, it should swing from side to side or anti-clockwise. With practice, you will get used to how your pendulum shows 'yes' and 'no'. You can then sit and touch each chakra area from base to crown with one hand, asking if that level needs energy, and watching the pendulum swing in response. You can also simply hold the pendulum over a stone and ask if it is the right one to use at this time.

Working with a Single Crystal

Prepare your space: clear away everyday clutter, light a candle and perhaps some incense. Select a suitable stone for yourself – by intuition, dowsing or by consulting the chart or Crystal Index – and sit quietly holding it in your hands. Breathe deeply and relax. Take your awareness into your body and note any tensions. Using your breath, simply dissolve them like clouds in a blue sky. Then take your awareness to your stone – to its colour, shape and feeling in your hands. Relax and see what impressions or feelings come to you for a few minutes. To come out of the process, take a few deep breaths and gently stretch your arms and hands.

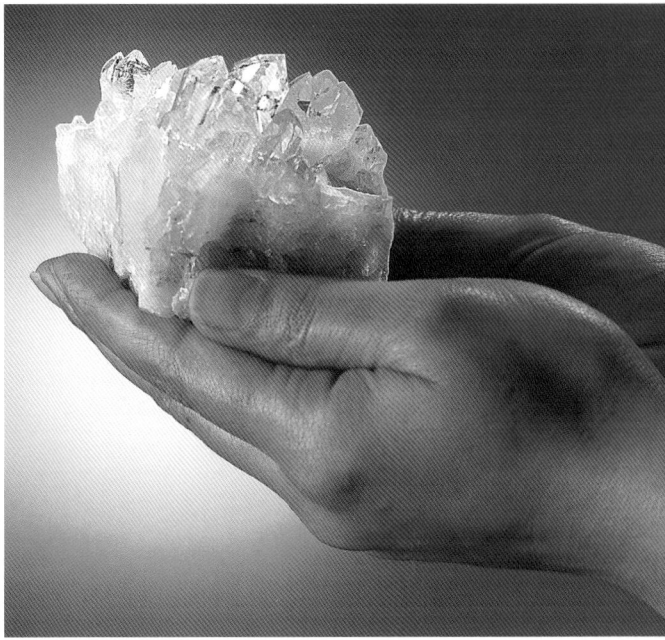

Holding a crystal in your hands can help to fine-tune your intuition. What exactly are you expecting from this mineral?

Using Crystals on the Body

Lie down comfortably on a mat on the floor. Place a piece of rose quartz over your heart and then relax, slowly breathing away any tension in your body. Silently and gently focus your intention on opening and expanding the energies in your heart chakra. Breathe into the heart area and visualise the rose quartz crystal shining the light of unconditional love into your whole being. Now visualise that rosy ray expanding beyond you to include all life forms. To end the exercise, take a few slow, deep breaths and then flex your fingers and toes before slowly getting up.

Living With Crystals

Crystals can play a vital part in making your environment beautiful wherever you are. You may choose them for their beauty, or for a particular function that is relevant to you or your living space. Here are some ideas for placing and using crystals in your space.

Bedroom

It is worth saying here that too many crystals in the bedroom may not be such a good idea: you mostly want to relax and sleep in there, so too many amplified energies may not help! Having said that, stones like tiger's eye, amethyst and rose quartz are said to be gentle and restful to have around you, perhaps at your bedside. If you want to enhance the energy for love-making, don't forget Cleopatra's favourite green stones like peridot or the expansive warm energy of amber. In a child's bedroom, a gentle blue stone like celestite brings a sense of peace and calm.

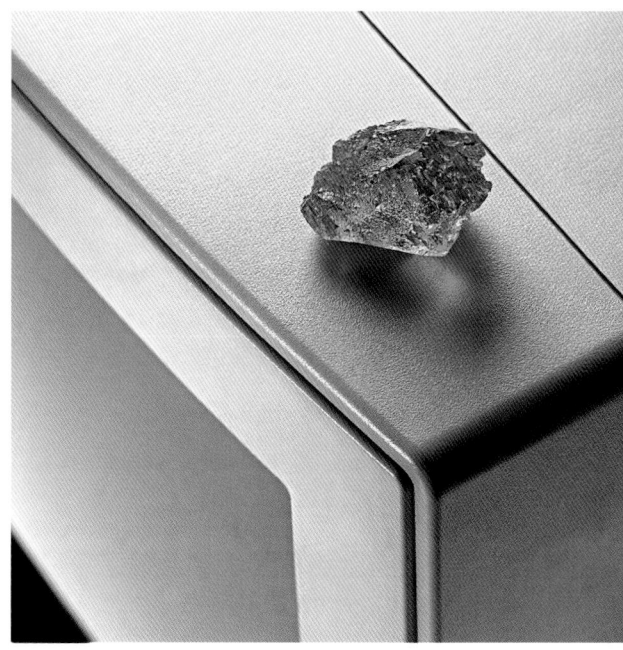

Try placing a crystal on your computer monitor to balance your environment and disperse negative energies.

Study or Office

Here electromagnetic radiation from computers is the main issue. Stones like smoky quartz or amethyst can be used to help maintain a balanced environment. Try placing a stone on top of your monitor. If you are to have a meeting you feel may be challenging, you can place a large piece of rose quartz in the middle of the table to calm the energies. If you need inspiration, a beautiful clear quartz cluster is a wonderful,

Focusing on your chosen crystals can help clear away negativity and generate new ideas. Remember that stones constantly used for this need regular cleansing.

complex, light-filled shape to concentrate on, clearing your mind for new ideas. Stones that sit constantly in an electronic environment will need regular cleansing.

Bathroom

It can be very restful to put little smooth polished crystals in the bath with you. Water is a great conductor, so the bath will be gently energised by them – and so will you. Rose quartz, carnelian, citrine, amethyst or tiger's eye are fun to try. Place the crystals in the bath, run the water, and add three to four drops of an essential oil like lavender or frankincense, light a candle on the window sill and lie back for a lovely mystical soak.

Crystals really come into their own when they are placed in water. Try bathing with crystals in the bath for a really restful soak.

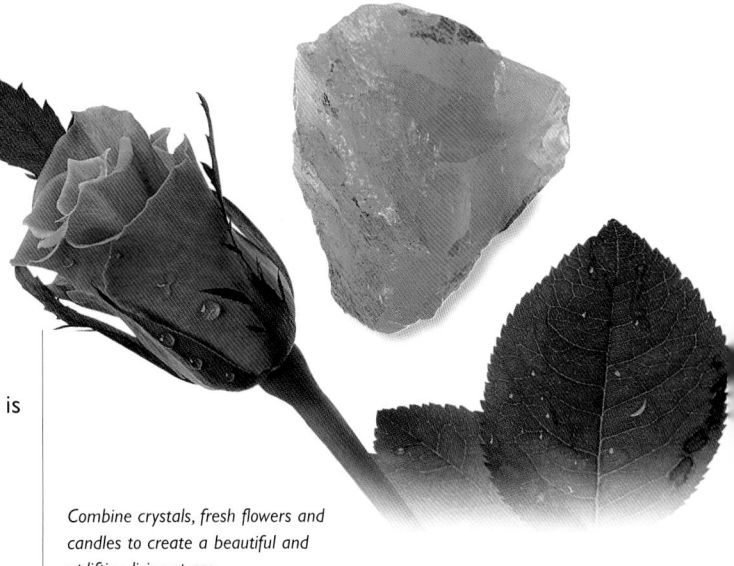

Combine crystals, fresh flowers and candles to create a beautiful and uplifting living space.

Living Room

Here you may wish to create a special space for your crystals. A good idea is to set aside a particular table covered with a silk cloth, with a beautiful candle in a holder, a vase for fresh flowers, and an incense holder, as well as your stones. In India, and other countries, many houses have their own small shrines, which are tended daily. A beautiful arrangement of crystals, candles and fresh flowers is an attractive focal point and helps to provide a wonderful energy in your living room. Even the intrusive presence of a television set can be enhanced by an amethyst cluster placed on it, which helps balance electromagnetic rays as well.

Meditating with Crystals

Meditation is a way of accessing a state of deep stillness, which is health-giving in this fast-moving modern age. In a meditative state, you experience deep peace and relaxation. This allows your body to restore itself on a cellular level, and your mind and spirit to be regenerated.

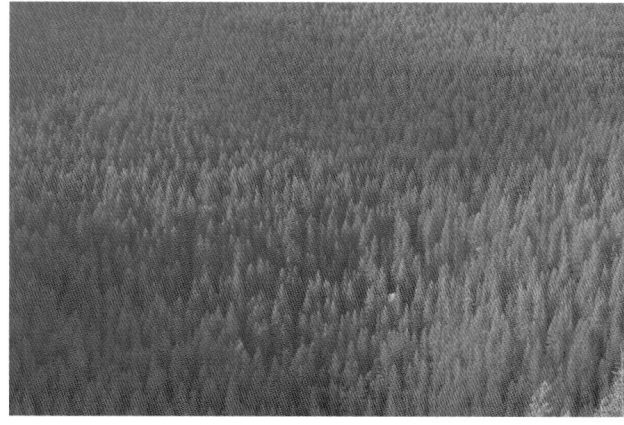

Meditation aims to create in your mind the stillness and peace that is found in nature. It can be very energising.

Making Time and Creating Space

Meditation is not 'doing nothing', it is allowing yourself time to just 'be', releasing yourself from daily demands for a short and beneficial time. Try to arrange a regular fifteen-minute slot each day for yourself and see how it works for you.

Crystals as a Focus

For meditation, crystals can be contemplated as a fixed object, held in the hands, or placed on the body. To develop the earlier exercises, you can add in visualisation, allowing the power of your creative imagination and intuition to respond to the crystal. After these exercises, try writing notes or drawing your experiences and keep them as a reference.

Clear Quartz Exercise: Inner Cleansing

Using a clear quartz cluster or point, sit holding the crystal in your hands. Breathe deeply and release all tension from your body for a few moments. Now imagine a fountain of white light that begins just above the crown of your head and enters

Sit and relax and allow your creative imagination to run free. If you also hold your crystal you can allow your imagination to work on that too.

Use a crystal that feels right to you at the time. You will know instinctively which one is right for you.

your skull, flowing down your face, neck, back, shoulders, arms, hands and into your crystal. As the energy builds in the crystal, allow it to flow on down your abdomen, hips, legs and into the Earth. Thank the Earth for her gifts. Imagine yourself to be a conduit between Earth and Heaven. To end the exercise, breathe deeply and flex your feet and hands.

your head, up the tree, and out into the universe. Relax and feel yourself to be a part of all Nature. Breathe deeply and stretch your arms to come out of the exercise – and thank the tree for allowing you to do this.

You can work with any stones that seem appropriate to you – with time, you will develop your own favourites. Try to be aware and thankful at all times for the gifts of the mineral kingdom and the Earth.

All stones, minerals and precious gems come from the Earth. Try to remember this at all times.

Amber Exercise: Connecting to the Plant Kingdom

Amber is an organic gemstone made up of fossilised tree resin, often containing tiny pollen grains or other ancient life forms. For this exercise, take a piece of amber with you on a walk. If possible, find a tall pine tree, or if none is nearby, let your intuition guide you to a tree. Stand with your back to the trunk and hold the amber in your hands. Breathe deeply and feel the upright strength of the tree. Imagine you are drawing warm earth energy up though your feet, your legs, hips, abdomen and into the amber in your hands. Allow the energy to continue flowing up through your back, heart, shoulders and up out of

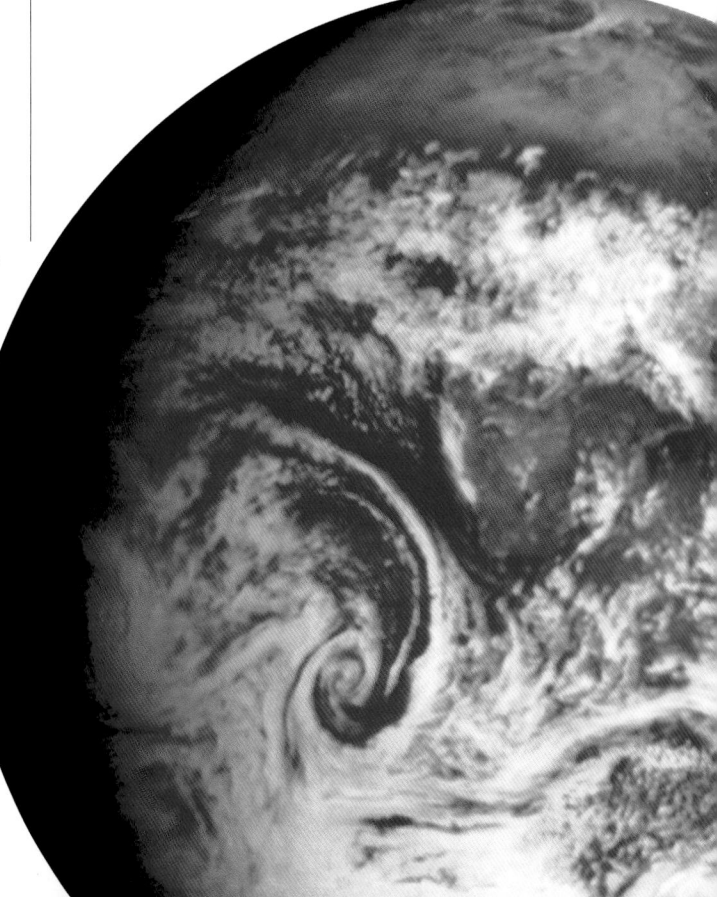

Buying Crystals

Obtaining crystals for your collection can be a lot of fun; however, a little preparation is a good idea. Use these guidelines to help you make informed and appropriate choices so you are happy with your purchases and feel they are right for you.

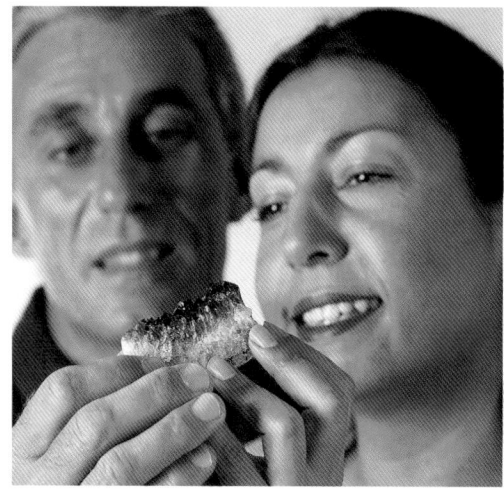

Buy your crystals from a supplier who will give you helpful advice and important information.

Today crystals are widely available from a variety of sources. You can buy inexpensive stones that are both aesthetically appealing and are useful for healing purposes.

Finding a Supplier

When you are buying crystals, it really helps to do your research. Your local telephone directory may contain listings of crystal shops and outlets. If you know a crystal healing practitioner, ask them where they source their stones – perhaps they will sell to you. The main thing is, visit as many of these people and places as you can. Feel the atmosphere: are the stones housed and displayed with care? If you ask questions (as you should), are you given helpful answers and advice? Many stones on the market are heat-treated, dyed or grown artificially in a laboratory. Ask the supplier where their stones come from. If they are unwilling to discuss it, think twice about buying. Many fairs and trade shows supply crystals, and the same guidelines apply here. Get to know your retailer and trust your intuition. There are mail order crystal companies, but the disadvantage is that you do not see or handle the stones before you buy. Your personal experience of the stones is important, particularly if you want them for healing work.

Try out crystals in the shop and feel which ones are right for you. This is a vital part of buying your stones.

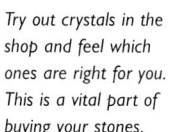

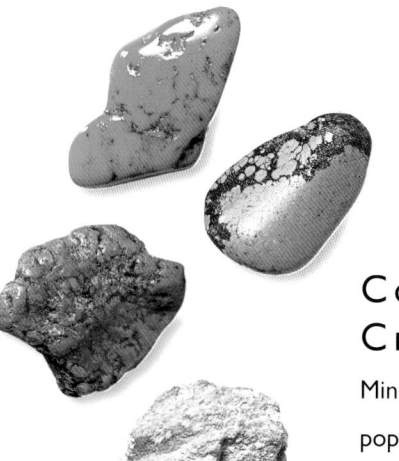

Natural minerals can be collected from beaches or other locations. Be sure that you have permission to do this.

Collecting Crystals

Mineral collecting is a popular hobby. Even collecting stones from the beach or rivers is a fun pastime. Your local museum may know of a geological group who go out collecting, and it is a wonderful experience to see rocks in veins in a natural setting. If you live in a granite area, for example, it will be possible to find stones with small quartz crystals embedded in them. It is best to join a group so that you do not get into trouble for trespassing or for doing any environmental damage.

Buying for Other People

Some crystal healing books suggest you should choose your own stones rather than choose them for other people – again, because of the personal interaction between the holder and the stone. To choose for someone, you really need to ask your intuition, visualise the person and ask if the stone is right for them.

The beauty and variety of crystals means that you will always find something to suit your purpose and your price range.

Birthstone List

This may also help when choosing crystals for other people. Birthstone lists became very popular in the eighteenth and nineteenth centuries and do vary, but here is a general selection.

January	garnet	
February	amethyst	
March	aquamarine	
April	diamond	
May	tourmaline	
June	moonstone	
July	carnelian	
August	peridot	
September	lapis lazuli	
October	opal	
November	topaz	
December	turquoise	

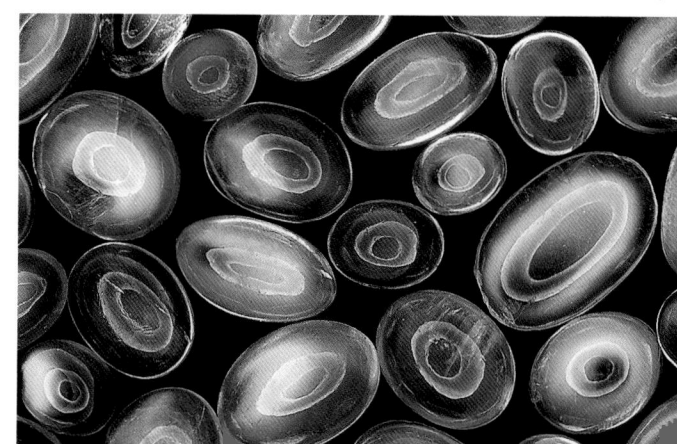

Glossary

Here is a list of terms that occur in the text with explanations.

Cabochon

a gem cut and polished into a smooth, domed shape.

Chakra

an energy centre in the body.

Chatoyancy

a shimmering light-effect like a cat's eye, e.g. in tiger's eye.

Cleansing

the practice of cleaning crystals physically and energetically.

Conductor

an agent that allows the free flow of heat or electricity.

Crystal

a mineral with a precise geometrically arranged structure.

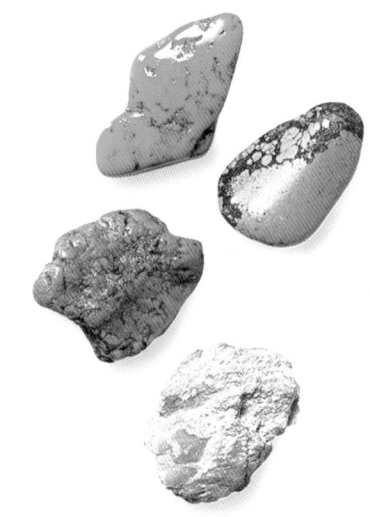

Element

one of the basic building blocks of matter, e.g. carbon or hydrogen.

Face

one of the sides of a crystal.

Geode

a hollow lump of rock with crystals growing inward.

Geology

the science of the history and development of the Earth and its minerals.

Inclusion

specks, bubbles or other minerals showing up in crystals.

Inorganic

a substance of inert origin like a mineral.

Iridescence

a shimmering multicoloured play of light.

Magma

molten rock at the Earth's core.

Mineral

a natural inorganic chemical compound.

Molten

melted or in liquid form, e.g. volcanic lava.

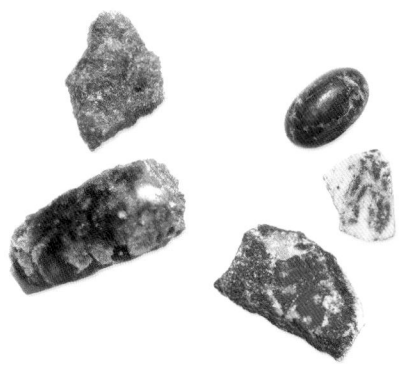

Nodule

a small lump of rock.

Opalescence

a milky, soft, luminous sheen, as in opals.

Organic

a substance with a plant or animal origin.

Programming

conscious intent directed into a crystal for healing purposes.

Rutile

strands of golden mineral appearing in clear quartz and other stones.

Setting

the art of placing gemstones in precious metal.

Termination

the pointed end of a crystal.

Tumblestones

small, smooth, crystal pebbles rounded off in a machine.

Useful Addresses and Websites

United Kingdom

The International Association of Crystal Healing Therapists (IACHT)

PO Box 344, Manchester, M60 2EZ, UK

www.iacht.co.uk

Publishes a list of accredited therapists in the UK and details of training in crystal healing.

The European College of Vibrational Medicine

Unity, Hall Green, Rectory Road, Gissing, Diss, Norfolk, IP22 5UX, UK

Tel: +44 (0) 1379 677869

www.raven.org.uk

An online distance learning college with courses on crystal healing.

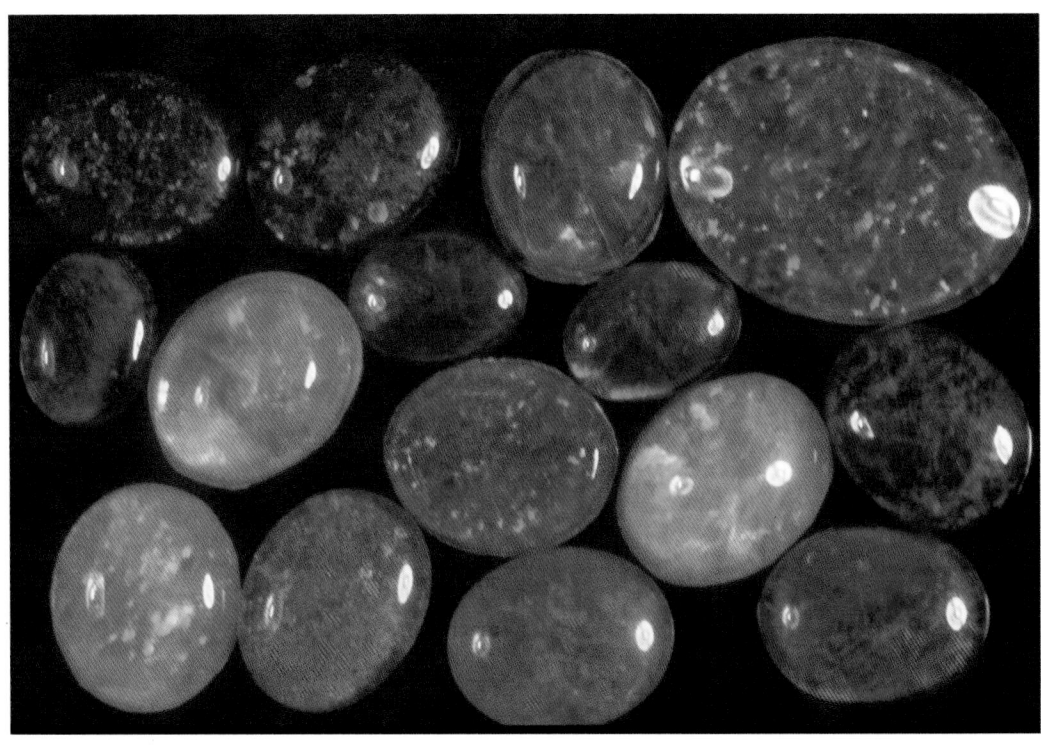

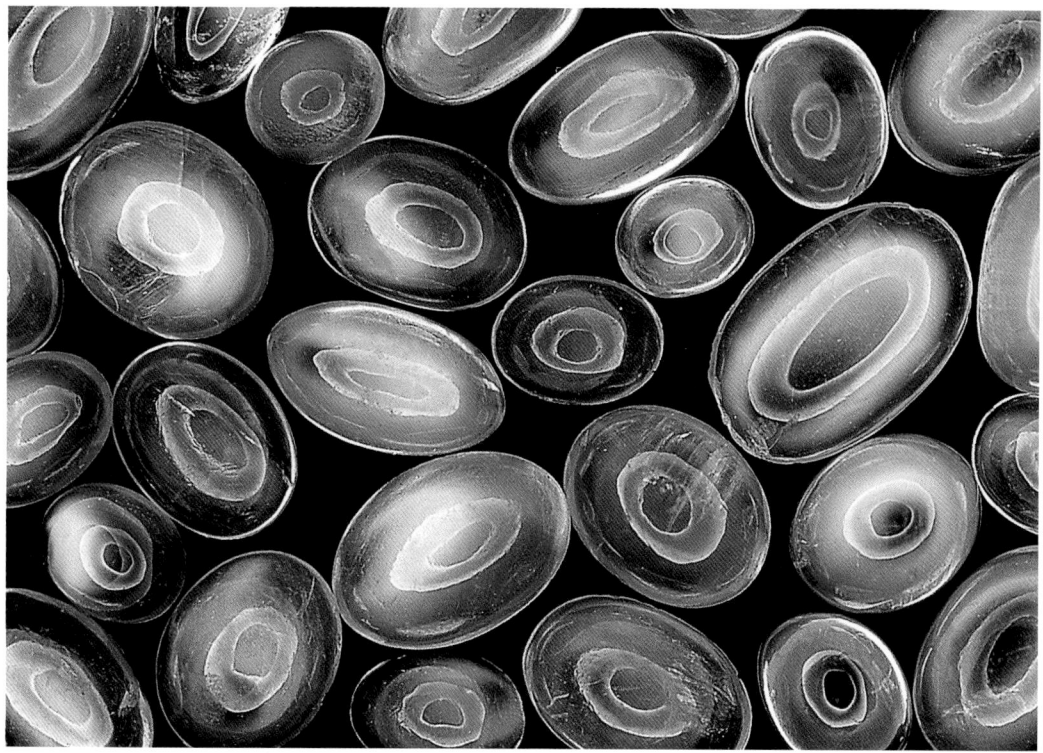

USA

The Crystalis Institute

440 Bayley Hazen Road, Walden,

Vermont, USA

www.crystalisinstitute.com

Set up by Naisha Ahsian in the USA and offers

courses in crystal healing.

Association of Melody Crystal Healing

www.taomchi.com

Information on crystology, crystal healing,

courses and instructors.

The Internet is full of amazing and informative

websites on crystals. Here are a few:

International Colored Gemstone Association

www.gemstone.org

Geological information

www.mineralgalleries.com

www.nationalgeographic.com (good for superb

photographic material)

www.nhm.ac.uk (The Natural History

Museum, London, UK)

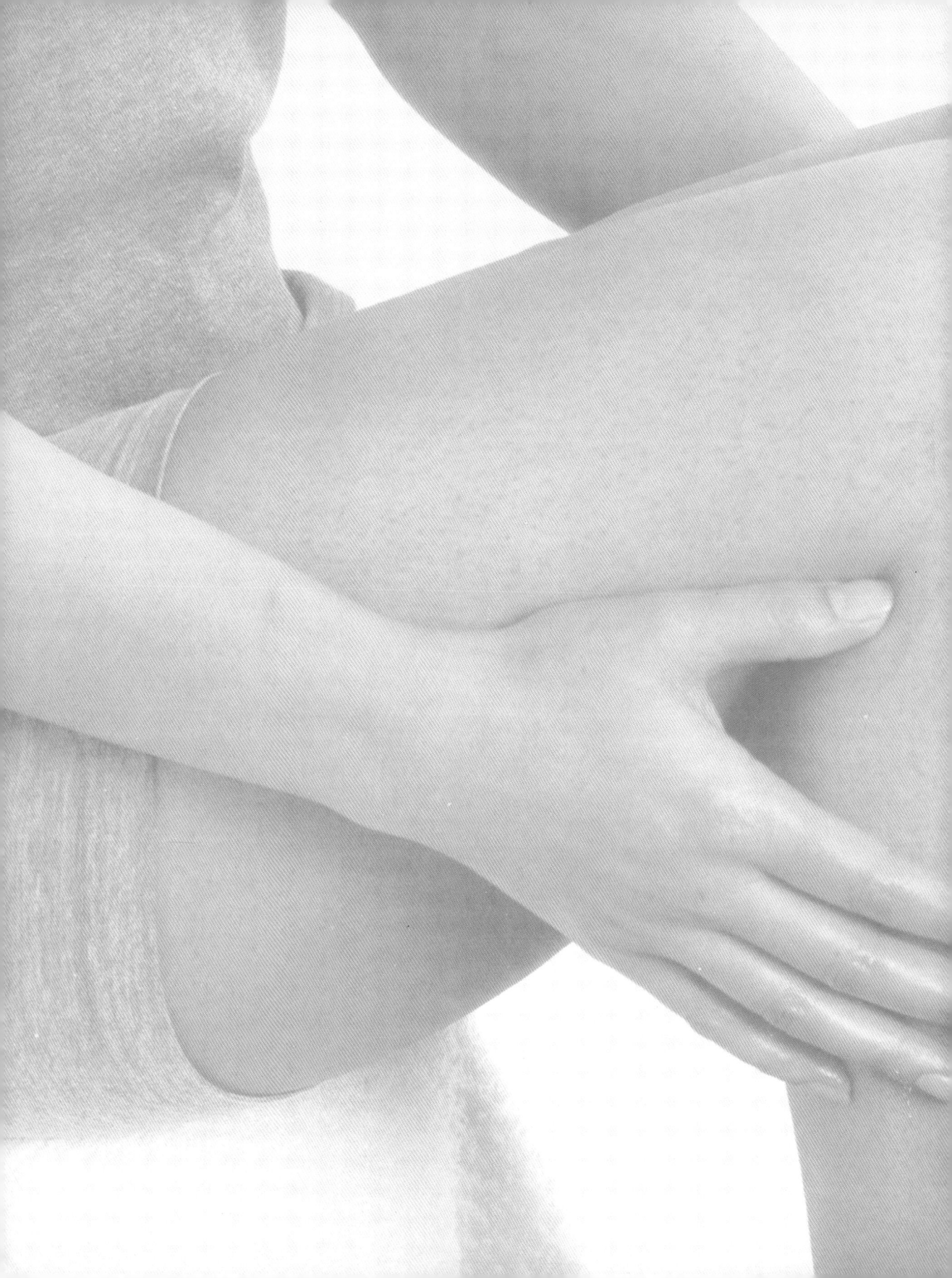

home remedies

Introduction

In the old days, when you had a sore throat your first reaction was probably not to call out the doctor but to head for the kitchen cabinet. There you would find the honey jar, spoon a liberal portion into some boiling water, add the juice and rind of two or three lemons and sip the warming concoction slowly. Honey and lemon is one of the best known and best loved home remedies and is still used today as a basis for many of the most famous over-the-counter medicines and throat sweets.

A cupful of honey, lemon and hot water will help to ease the symptoms of a cold such as sore throat.

Nowadays, however, new technology and increasingly sophisticated medical advances have all but banished the old-fashioned home remedy to the archives of history. Most are dismissed as 'old wives' tales' and yet many of these ancient remedies have been the subject of rigorous clinical trials. The humble garlic, for example, has probably been the subject of more scientific studies than any

other herb. We now know it is excellent for thinning blood, lowering cholesterol levels and even curing the common cold. It is marketed as the new cure-all for myriad complaints.

Modern drugs can be life savers but they often have too many side effects to warrant their use for every little sniffle or tummy upset. Home and herbal remedies tend to heal without suppressing symptoms, and used in the correct dosage are perfectly safe and have no side effects. Herbs are easy to find and can be used in cooking or in salads. Some, which you can grow in your garden, can be ground up and used as inhalants or to perfume a bath. Others – which are more likely to be in your

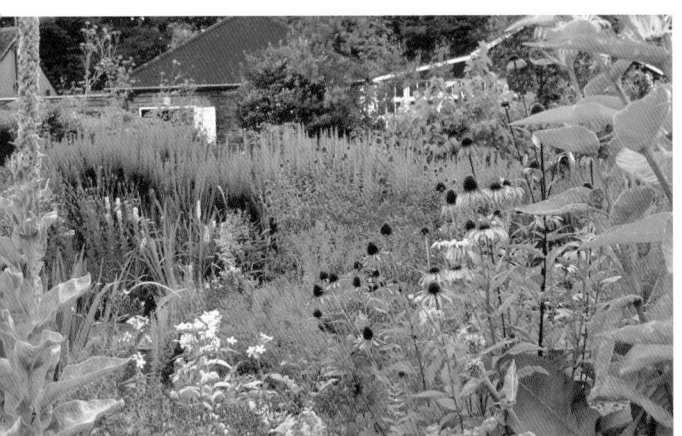

The modern herb garden can provide many home remedy possibilities. Herbs can be added to food or used as a treatment.

kitchen cupboard – can be added to cooking or made up into poultices and muscle rubs.

As the methods of testing the compounds contained in many natural remedies become more sophisticated, many cynics are beginning to sit up and take notice. And as more and more of our so-called 'wonderdrugs' prove only to suppress symptoms rather than get to the root cause, it is little wonder that more and more people are now looking for a healthier option for everyday complaints. The beauty of home remedies is that they are accessible and easy to prepare. Many of the remedies contained in this section have been passed down through the generations by word of mouth – others have surpassed all expectations in clinical trials. Some you will remember from the old nursery rhymes. Remember when Jack fell down and broke his crown and Jill fixed it with vinegar and brown paper? It may have sounded a strange remedy for a bad head, but in fact this used to be a remedy for headaches and migraine!

Garlic has been the subject of many scientific studies.

How to Make Home Remedies

Compress

A compress is simply a piece of cloth soaked in a bowl of hot or cold herbal extract. It eases the strain of painful joints and muscles and can help to soothe skin rashes. Almost any herbs can be applied as a compress if you need to treat a problem locally. All you need to do is soak a piece of muslin or lint in the herbal infusion of your choice and apply it to the affected area, renewing it as and when necessary.

Steam Inhalation

For steam inhalations, which are best for stressed or inflamed lungs, make up an infusion of the herb you want to use (essential oils can also be used) and add it to a basinful of hot water. Drape a towel around your head and the basin so that you keep the steam in, and inhale slowly and deeply for a few minutes.

Tincture

To make a tincture, put 500g (1lb 2oz) of fresh herbs or 200g (7oz) of dried herbs in a jar and add 500ml (18fl oz) of vodka (it acts as a preservative). Add 200ml (7fl oz) of water, seal the jar and store in a cool place for 2–3 weeks, checking and shaking it occasionally. Strain the liquid through a muslin bag into a jug and then into sterilised bottles.

Infusion

To make an infusion to drink hot or cold, warm a teapot and add about 25g (1oz) of dried herbs or 50g (1¾oz) of fresh herbs. Pour 500ml (18fl oz) of hot water on the herbs. Cover the pot until the herbs have infused (about 10 minutes). Strain the infusion through a plastic tea strainer. Add a little honey or unrefined sugar. Drink a cupful. You can keep the remainder in a jug and store in the fridge for up to 48 hours to be taken as necessary.

History of Home Remedies

Home remedies have been around for thousands of years. Even these days about 30 per cent of prescription drugs are still synthesised from plants. In fact, the word 'drug' comes from an old Dutch word, *drogge*, which means 'to dry' – which is how many plant medications were prepared.

Honey is one of the oldest remedies known to man – in the days of the ancient Egyptians it was used as a remedy for high blood pressure. Honey contains a huge range of vitamins, enzymes, proteins and amino acids; it can actually be classified as a complete food. Honey not only lowers blood pressure but is also a key factor in transmitting nerve impulses.

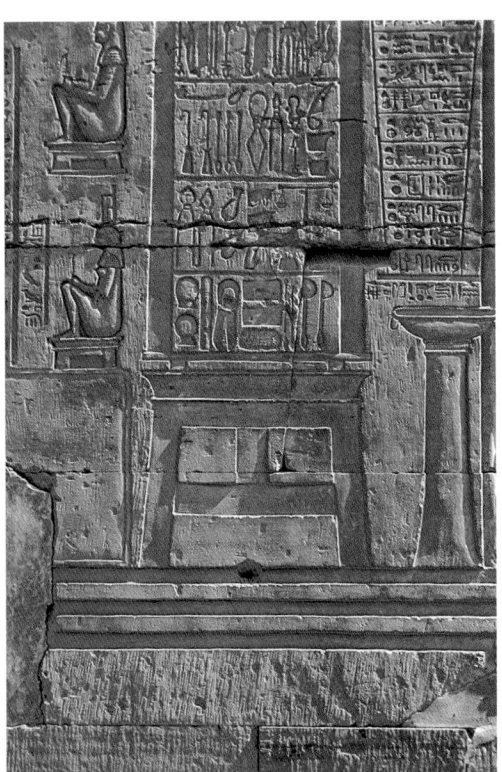

Vinegar is another ancient remedy which has stood the test of time. Cider vinegar was used for treating ailments long before the expression 'an apple a day keeps the doctor away' came about. Apples contain pectin – a soluble fibre – as well as all sorts of vitamins and minerals. Cider vinegar is rich in potassium, which promotes cell growth, and for many years vinegar was believed to be the 'fountain of youth'. It can help high blood pressure and is excellent for curing cramp. Vinegar was also used by the ancient Assyrians to cure earache, and during the American Revolutionary and Civil Wars it was used as both an antiseptic and disinfectant.

The Chinese were big on home remedies and were one of the first civilisations to recognise ginger for its therapeutic properties. It was and still is used to combat nausea, boost the immune system and reduce inflammation.

The ancient Egyptians used honey for high blood pressure centuries before the full range of its benefits had been scientifically analysed. It contains a raft of vitamins and may be classified as a complete food. No wonder it is so useful in the battle against colds.

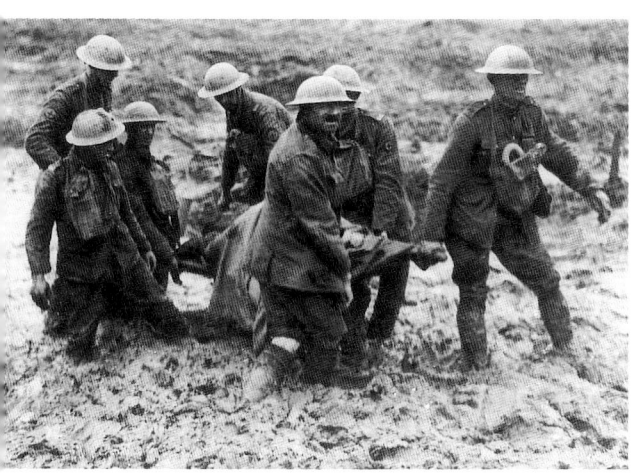

Some of the best home remedies were discovered on the battlefield. Garlic was used to dress wounds in the First World War.

For more than 2000 years celery was another remedy used by Oriental healers to treat high blood pressure. Recent research has shown that celery does contain compounds that reduce high blood pressure by relaxing the smooth muscle lining the blood vessels.

Some of the best home remedies were discovered on the battlefield. During the First World War, for example, garlic was pounded in water and applied to wounds on a bed of moss as an accepted field dressing, while during the eighteenth century sailors used to thrust a piece of shag tobacco into a wound to staunch the bleeding!

So you can see that home remedies are an excellent form of first-line treatment. And although this book is not in any way intended to replace the advice of your GP, by being more aware of the benefits of home remedies

Vinegar has many uses as a natural home remedy. It is rich in potassium and can help with cramp and high blood pressure.

you can begin to understand how to heal yourself.

Naturally, if symptoms persist, or you are in any doubt whatsoever about a health problem, you should always consult a professional. But before you pick up the telephone, you should use this section as a reference point for everything from smelly feet to the common cold. You will be surprised at what may be lurking in your kitchen cabinet that might just do the trick!

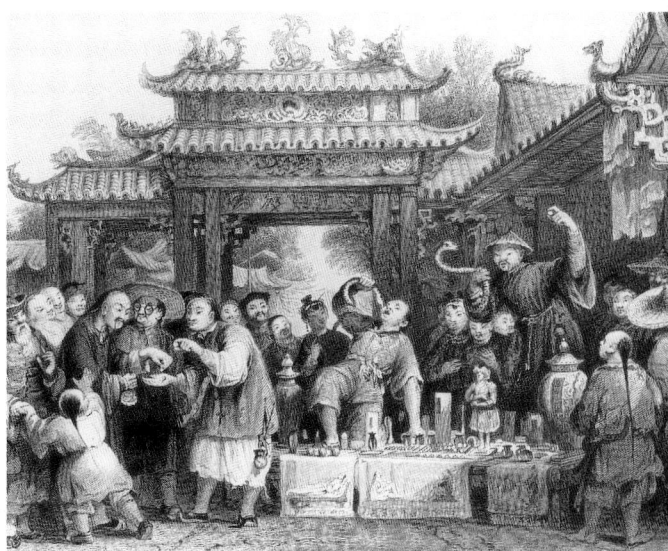

China has a long history of natural home remedy use, including ginger to combat nausea and celery to reduce high blood pressure.

Burns, Scalds and Sunburn

Although second- and third-degree burns require hospital treatment, mild first-degree burns are often superficial and can be treated at home. Any burn needs cooling down, so run tepid water directly onto the wound for at least five minutes to reduce the heat and give pain relief. For a chemical burn it is vital to keep flushing the skin with cold running water until well after the pain has subsided. Clean the burn of any grit or dirt very carefully, avoiding breaking the skin or blistered areas.

Olive oil can bring effective relief to a painful scald.

Remedies for Burns

Plain yogurt applied to a burn will keep it cool, or you can make up a soothing poultice from honey and yogurt. Adding crushed elderberries to the poultice will make it more effective or mash the leaves of the elder with a little butter and use it as a mild cream for the affected area.

Cucumber mashed to a pulp and mixed with glycerine makes a particularly wonderful moisturising balm.

Cool the whole area with a cider vinegar splash and make sure the person who has been burned has plenty of fluids.

Try making a tea using lemon balm, which will both calm the patient and provide further pain relief.

Flush the skin with cold running water for a while after a chemical burn – even after the pain has subsided.

Remedies for Scalds

Olive oil can bring immediate relief to a painful scald and will improve the chances of healing without blisters or scars. If you have any lavender or peppermint essential oils to hand, add these to the olive oil to help ease the stinging sensation around the wound.

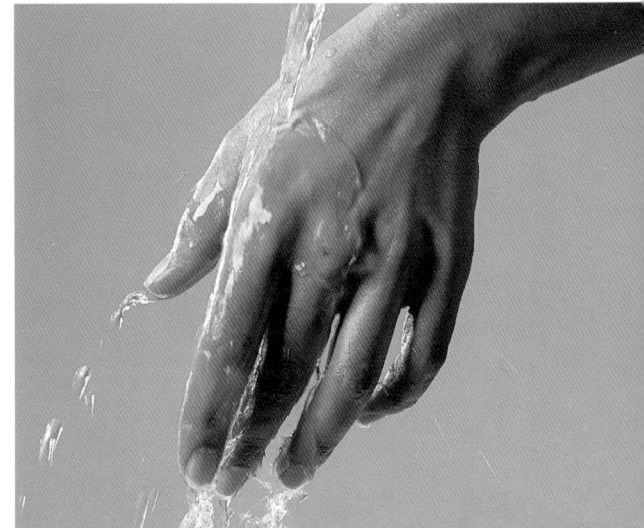

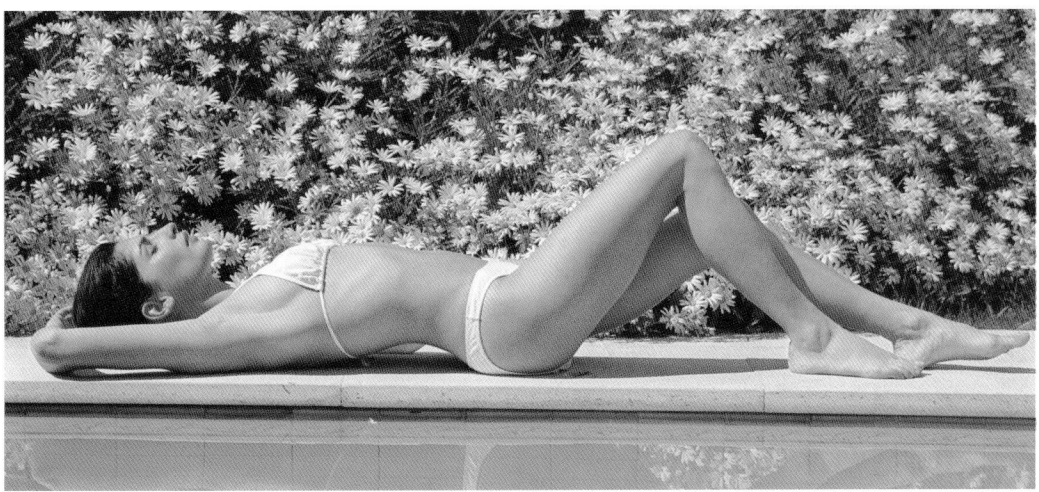

When sunburn spoils a holiday, natural home remedies made from lemon, cold tea and bicarbonate of soda can come to the rescue.

Remedies for Sunburn

For instant relief from sunburn, dab on a little lemon juice or soak a flannel in cold tea and place it over the affected area. For the kind of all-over sunburn that keeps you awake at night, try adding two tablespoons of bicarbonate of soda to a cool bath and immerse your whole body in the water. You can also mash the pulp of a ripe avocado and smooth over the sunburnt area for a soothing effect.

Bathe your face in buttermilk or grate up some potatoes and apply to the sunburned area. The starch will cool and soothe the burn. Use cold peppermint tea as a mild wash to ease the stinging. Or you can try dissolving Epsom salts or baking soda in cold water and draping a cloth soaked in the solution over the affected area.

Milk of magnesia has been successfully used to treat sunburn, and mud or clay can ease the stinging pain.

Remedy for Chapped Skin

Fill a muslin bag full of oats, then tie it up at the top and drop it in a cool bath, or soak it in warm water, squeeze it out and rub it over the chapped area during the day to ease the pain.

A muslin bag filled with oats and soaked in a cool bath can be rubbed over areas of chapped skin to help relieve the pain.

FIRST AID
Bites and Stings

There is nothing more painful and irritating than being stung by an angry wasp or bitten alive by mosquitoes. It is vital that you have identified what has bitten you before using a home remedy, and if you are travelling abroad and are stung by an unknown flying creature it is always safest to seek medical advice. However, for the everyday type of insect bite or sting, ice cold water or witch hazel are good first-line remedies.

Remedies for Bee Stings

Remove bee stings with tweezers (grasp the sting below the poison sac). Apply a paste of bicarbonate of soda and cold water. A mixture of parsley juice and honey will also help to ease the irritation – crush the parsley leaves and stems to release the juice.

A cold wet tea bag makes a great poultice for bites and stings. Tea contains tannic acid, which helps to reduce swelling.

It helps to identify what you have been bitten by before using a home remedy.

Remedies for Wasp Stings

Cider vinegar or lemon will help to stop the irritation and itching. In the rare event of swallowing a wasp, drink a glass of cold water mixed with a teaspoon of salt. If you have been stung in the mouth, suck on ice cubes until the pain subsides. Mix cider vinegar with baking soda to make a poultice and apply directly to a bite. A cold, wet teabag makes a great poultice – the tannic acid helps to reduce swelling. A paste of ground cloves and cold water can also help.

Remedies for Mosquito Bites

Rub neat garlic directly onto mosquito bites to prevent infection – and mosquitoes loathe the smell of garlic, so eat the rest of the clove raw! Honey and baking soda mixed together

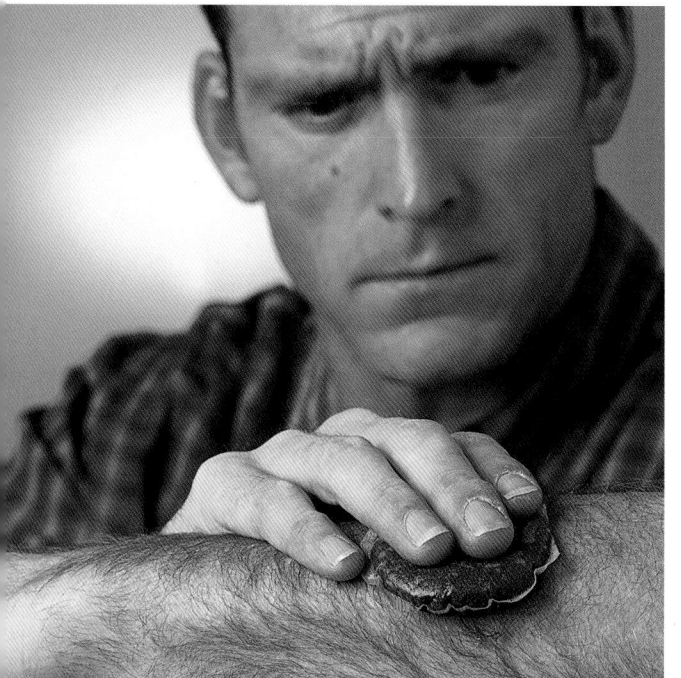

The pain of a jellyfish sting can be reduced by pouring seawater over the affected area for at least ten minutes.

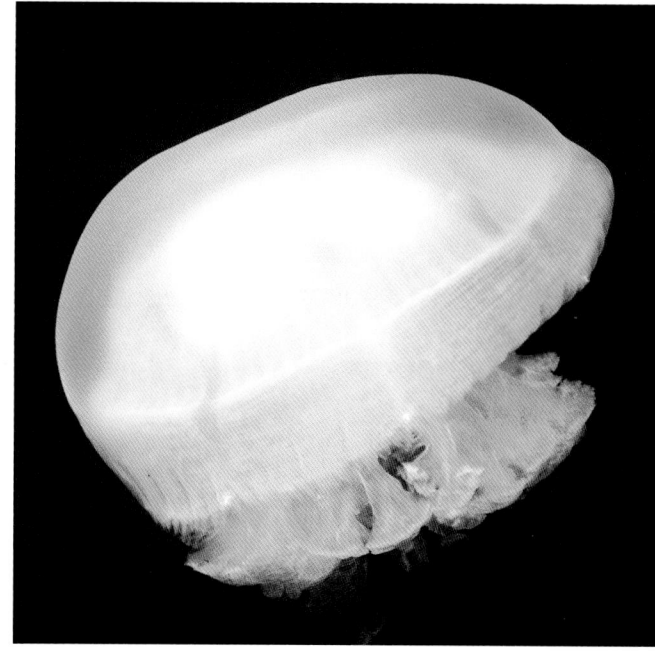

can help the itchiness around the bite, or rub the rind of a lemon neat onto the site of the bite. Sprinkle dried lavender along your window sill to stop further attacks – the smell of lavender also instantly repels mosquitoes!

To make another mosquito repellent, tie together some dried lavender, peppermint and catnip and secure it with a piece of thin wire. Light the bundle and keep it in a jar nearby. The smoke will mask your own smell and literally put the bugs off the scent!

If you are covered in bites, you need to break down the toxins which have been released into your body. Try drinking herb teas made from dandelion root, red clover or burdock.

Make a tincture of horseradish using half a cup of grated horseradish root and 600ml (1 pint) of rubbing alcohol. Steep the root in the alcohol for 2–3 days. Shake the mixture up twice every day. Strain off the grated root and bottle the liquid. You can use the tincture for most bites and stings, minor skin wounds and any superficial infections.

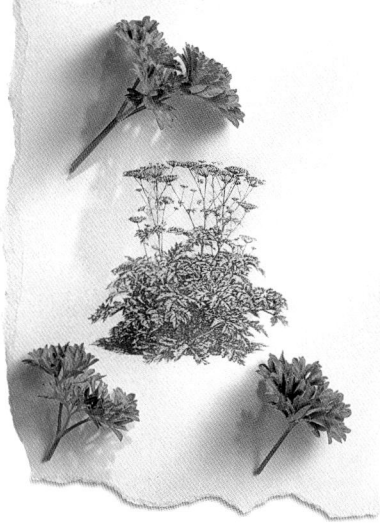

Parsley juice combined with honey can help to ease the irritation caused by bee stings.

Remedies for Stinging Nettle Stings

Apply the juice from the stems of the nettles. Dock leaves, which often grow nearby, can also be wrapped around the affected area to ease the pain.

Remedies for Jellyfish Stings

Pour seawater over the affected area for ten minutes. The water releases the remaining toxins. Cold cider vinegar, ice, alcohol or diluted ammonia applied to the sting are all effective.

FIRST AID
Cuts and Grazes

Cuts and grazes have a habit of looking far worse than they really are, but once minor injuries are cleaned up there are several remedies which can be used to help. If a cut is bleeding profusely, elevate the injured part and press a clean cloth directly onto the wound. The most important thing with any cut or graze is to get the affected area as clean as possible before applying any covering.

Remedies for Cuts and Grazes

Wash cuts and grazes with diluted witch hazel to prevent infection. You can also use Friar's balsam or a few drops of calendula in warm water. If none of this is to hand, warm, soapy water with a few drops of lemon juice or a teaspoon of salt added will do the trick. If you are really out in the sticks, then plain spittle can be a great healer.

Parsley juice or thick cream can be placed directly onto a wound and covered with a gauze dressing.

Washing cuts and grazes with witch hazel can help to prevent infection.

Crush up some parsley leaves and apply the juice directly onto a cut or graze.

Change it every two hours to make sure the wound is cleansed efficiently. Try washing the wound with the water from boiled parsnips and apply the warm pulp as a poultice.

Garlic acts as a marvellous natural antiseptic, so make up a mixture of crushed garlic and honey for a healing poultice and apply it directly to cuts and grazes. Use honey neat and cover with a bandage to prevent air or moisture penetrating the wound.

For a gravel graze, apply bread mixed with egg yolk and warm milk directly to the graze in order to gently draw out any small pieces of grit. Mash up raw avocado and cover with sterile gauze to prevent infection and promote healing.

Honey is particularly effective at drawing out the tiny pieces of gravel that tend to be found in children's cuts and grazes. Lemon is one of nature's most powerful astringents, so use it raw on cuts and grazes to stop bleeding. It will sting like mad but it really does the trick.

Drinking a cup of peppermint tea will immediately help to clot blood. It is particularly useful for nosebleeds.

Garlic wine made from chopped garlic steeped in white wine for several hours will cleanse and prevent infections in wounds and cuts.

In order to protect the area after cleaning, you should apply a paste of garlic and honey and cover with some fine gauze.

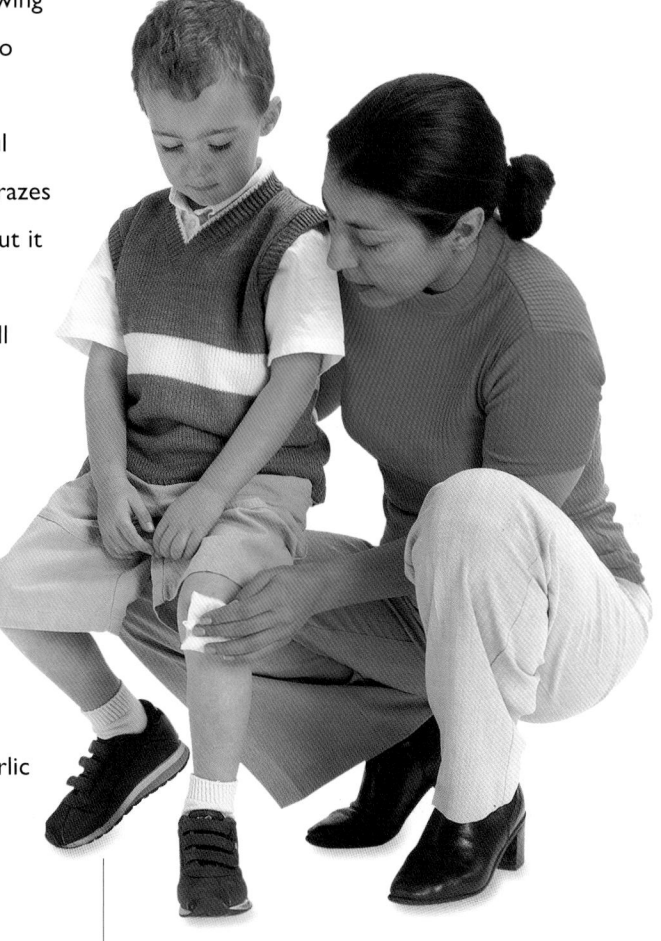

Apply a poultice of bread mixed with egg yolk and warm milk directly to a gravel graze to draw out any small pieces of grit.

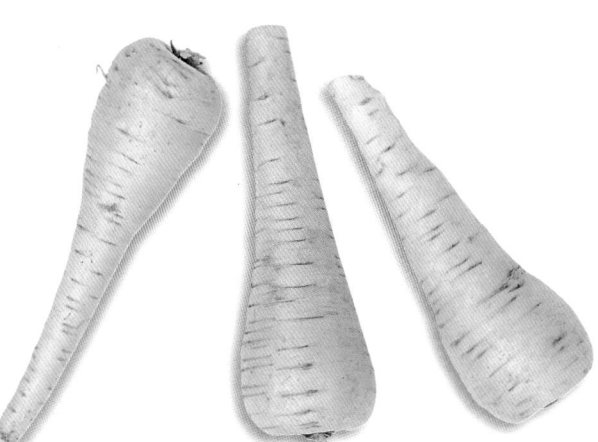

You can wash a wound with the water from boiled parsnips and apply the warm pulp as a poultice.

Washing Wounds

Use the following for washing wounds:

- Witch hazel (diluted)
- Friar's balsam (diluted)
- Calendula (diluted)
- Water with salt or drops of lemon juice
- Water in which parsnips have been boiled

Bruises, Sprains and Shock

Old wives used to recommend cold steak be placed directly onto a bruise. Nowadays, ice-cold water is the best cure, or a gentler method is to swab the bruise with a warm compress and massage it gently to stimulate the circulation. Injuries that cause bruises or sprains may lead to shock and even fainting, and caution is needed in these cases.

Remedies for Bruises and Sprains

If you have no ice, try a packet of frozen vegetables. Soak a sprained hand or foot in a bowl of warm water into which you have grated an onion and a potato.

Massaging a bruise or sprain with onion will bring pain relief to the affected area.

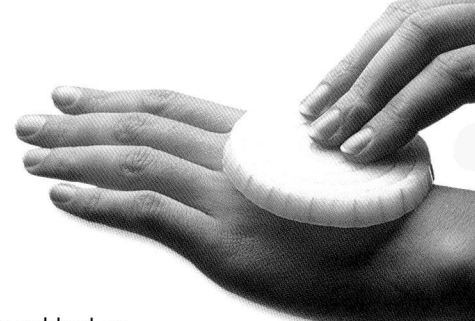

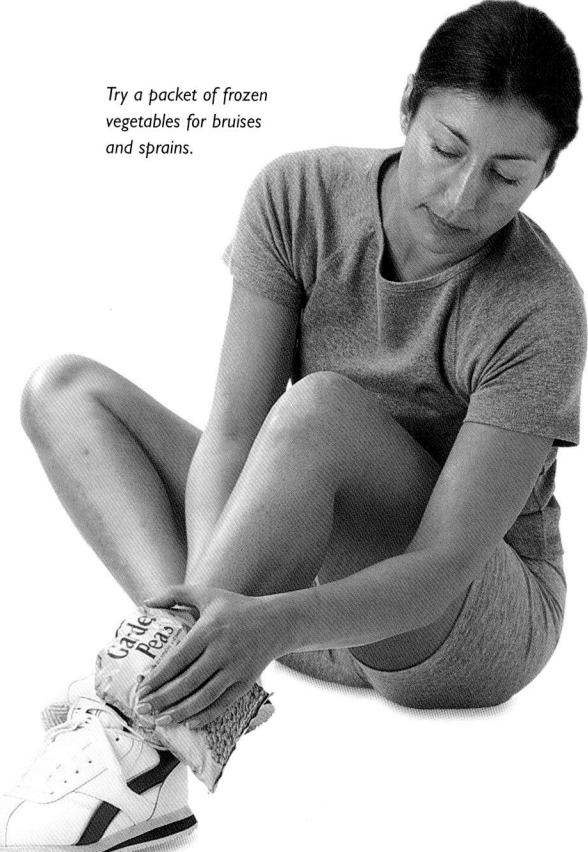

Try a packet of frozen vegetables for bruises and sprains.

Half an onion rubbed on the affected area will quickly soothe it. Black eyes can be miraculously cured with a cold comfrey teabag placed directly over the offending area. Witch hazel will also help to soothe swellings and also to reduce inflammation and bleeding.

Apply hot or cold compresses of vinegar, particularly the type that is made from astringent fruits such as blackberry, raspberry and rose, because they will help to reduce swelling and inflammation.

An old cook's remedy is parsley butter or oats mixed to a paste with boiling water and applied on a cloth to the affected area.

Remedies for Shock

Hot, sweet tea was always thought to be a restorative remedy for shock, and in fact honey added to any hot drink is a great healer. Basil and sage tea sweetened with honey is a great cure for someone who has experienced a mild shock.

Chamomile tea is also useful in this situation because it acts as a gentle sedative and therefore eases tension.

Orange blossom in hot water is believed to relieve anxiety. Not only can it be given to a patient as a kind of infusion, orange blossom water has a further point in its favour; a flannel can be steeped in the liquid to cool a patient down. Its soothing and refreshing properties will help to restore calm.

Cinnamon and honey dissolved in boiling water will help to pep someone up after they have fainted.

Remedies for Fainting

A hot tea made from peppermint, sage, lemon balm or rosemary will quickly revive someone coming round after fainting. Cinnamon and honey dissolved in boiling water is also good for this. Angelica was believed by ancient wise women to be the elixir of life and can be an excellent tonic.

Caution

- If you receive a blow to the head it may cause concussion, and you should always be seen by a doctor.

- Any injury that causes bruising or a sprain may also cause shock and fainting.

- There is a big difference between clinical shock, which can kill, and the sort of mild shock people suffer when they receive bad news or minor injuries. Again, it is best to seek medical advice.

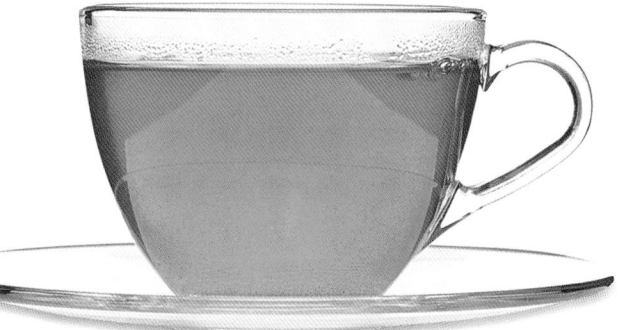

Chamomile tea and basil and sage tea are very effective means of restoring calm and will help in the management of shock.

Colds, Flu and Coughs

Plenty of garlic or the herb echinacea will help boost the immune system and stop colds and flu from getting a hold. If you should be unlucky, however, at the first sign of a cold and fever make up a mustard footbath by adding one teaspoon of dried mustard to a bowl of very hot water. Mustard has a warming effect and inhaling an infusion will clear phlegm and draw infection and congestion away from the chest.

Remedies for Colds and Flu

Lemon and honey are traditional remedies for colds and flu – lemon because of its high vitamin C content and because it improves the body's ability to expel toxins, and honey because it can help to soothe a sore throat. You could make up a hot drink with the juice of two to four lemons and stir in a dessertspoon of honey for a comforting home remedy.

Add fresh ginger or peppermint, or their essential oils, to a hot bath or footbath. They both help you to perspire, which gets rid of toxins from the body. A ginger footbath also draws away blood from the head to the feet and in this way can reduce the heat congestion you so often feel in the rest of the body when you are suffering from a cold or flu.

Echinacea, available in tablet form, helps to boost the immune system and keep colds and flu at bay.

Garlic is a natural antibiotic and is good for all bronchial problems and lung complaints. If you eat garlic neat, try eating a sprig of parsley or dandelion leaf afterwards to freshen your breath.

Onions are excellent for colds. Put a thick slice of onion into boiling water and add half a teaspoon of cayenne pepper. Strain and drink the liquid hot at bedtime.

Pour 600ml (1 pint) of hot water over a handful of fresh pine needles, put a towel over your head and inhale the vapours deeply to counteract congestion.

You can even add a little lemon and

Garlic can act as a natural antibiotic and is good for all bronchial problems.

Pine needles can provide relief from chestiness. Pour hot water over some pine needles in a bowl, place a towel over your head and the bowl and inhale the vapours.

honey to the remaining water and drink it so that you increase your levels of vitamins C and A, which will help to speed up your recovery from illness.

Eat plenty of yogurt, which can kill bacteria on its own. It will also help your body to produce more antibodies that will kill any invading organisms.

Remedies for Coughs

If you have a persistent cough, try a poultice of roasted onion applied to the chest every two hours. Onions can also be drunk as a warm broth to cleanse the airways and to reduce congestion.

Try an infusion of grated fresh ginger root with spices such as cloves and cinnamon to help ease a chesty cough.

In Romany medicine, nettles are believed to rid the lungs and stomach of excess phlegm. For asthma and bronchitis, add a handful of young nettles to 300ml (½ pint) of boiling water. Strain and drink the juice.

A cabbage leaf poultice works well when the chest is tight from coughing. Cabbage has an extraordinary ability to draw out toxins.

Crush the leaves with a rolling pin until the juice starts to appear. Place three or four leaves over the chest area and cover with gauze. Then place a warm blanket over to keep in place. You can also drink the juice of the cabbage sweetened with a teaspoon of honey.

If you have a cold, you could try a bedtime drink of onion and cayenne pepper in hot water to soothe the symptoms.

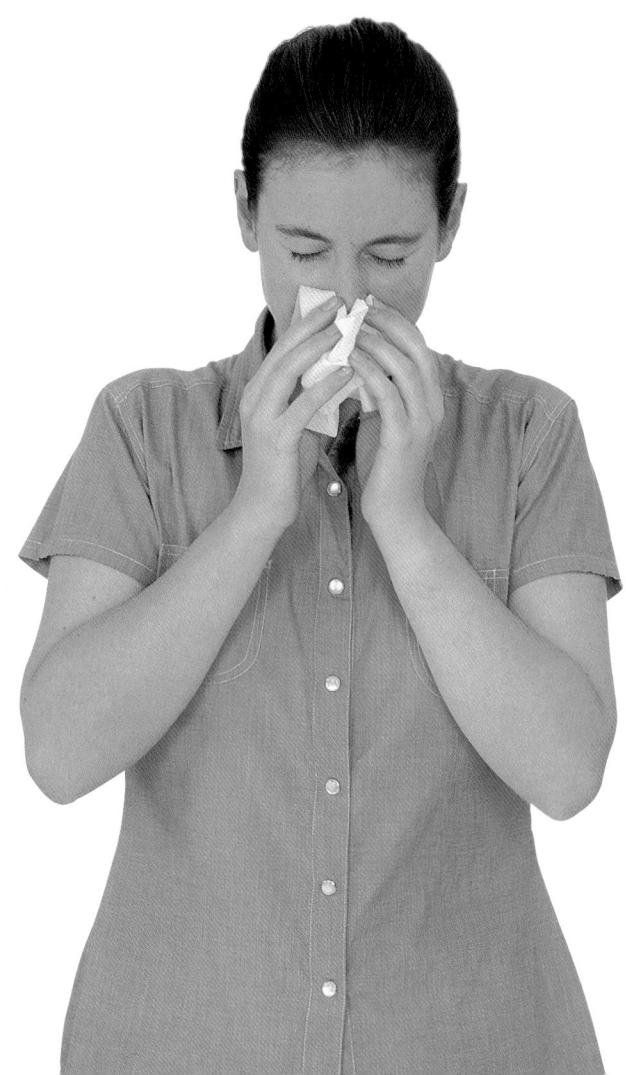

Sore Throat and Fever

At the first signs of a fever, lemon juice and honey or apple cider vinegar and honey diluted in plenty of warm water will help. Cold drinks of lemon juice, lemon barley water or fresh unsweetened fruit juices are all good remedies and will help to bring a temperature down.

Remedies for a Sore Throat

For a bad sore throat, make up a gargle with either salt, lemon juice or cider vinegar diluted with warm water. The salt helps to destroy the bacteria that cause the sore throat and helps to relieve the burning sensation. Squeeze the oil of a whole garlic clove

Salt, lemon juice or cider vinegar in a glass of warm water makes an effective gargle to ease a sore throat.

Hyssop, a herb belonging to the mint family, can provide a boost to the immune system in the form of a tea or tisane.

together with cayenne pepper and warm salt water and soak a clean cloth in the liquid. Wear the cloth around the throat for instant relief. Gargling with plain salt water can also be soothing.

Echinacea acts as a natural antibiotic by boosting the body's immune system and fighting infection and illness. Garlic and onions relieve congestion and infections by reducing the amount of mucus in the nasal cavities.

Blackcurrants, crushed up in boiling water, can help your body to fight infection and inflammation.

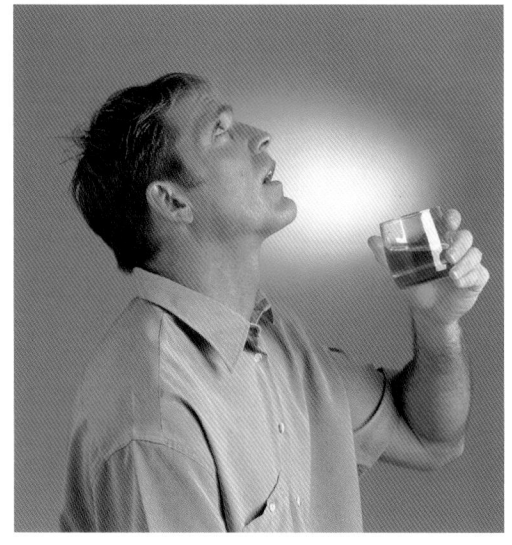

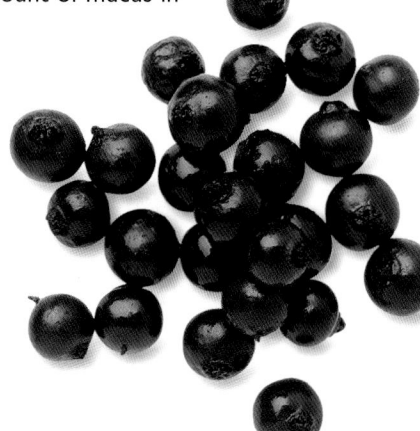

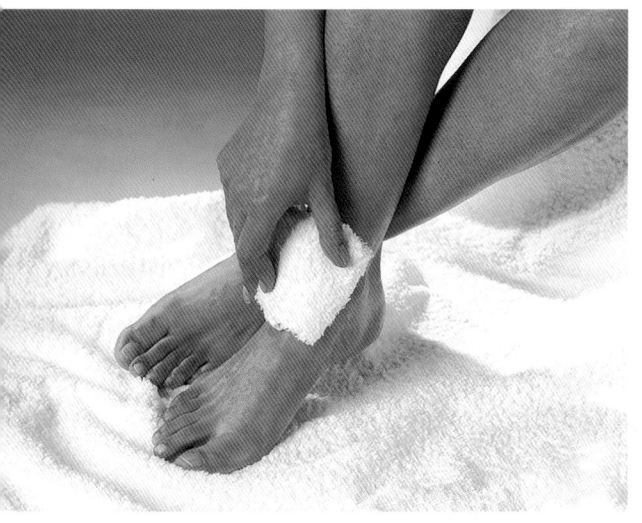

Try using a cool water compress applied to the legs and feet as a means of calming a fever.

Blackcurrants also counter infection and inflammation. Try a spoonful crushed into a cupful of boiling water and left to infuse for ten minutes – sip the drink slowly and chew the fruit. Red sage is the most famous remedy for sore throat – a tea made from the herb and drunk with a dash of cider vinegar will work wonders.

There is also a variety of teas and tisanes that help the immune system fight back. Some of the best remedies include hyssop, a member of the mint family. Lemon, which contains vitamin C, and any tea that contains

Boil angelica root in water to bring down a fever. You might need to add lemon, honey and brandy to make it more palatable.

Ancient Remedy for Fever

An ancient remedy for fever involved mixing cloves, cream of tartar and some cinnamon stick in a little tea with molasses or honey added. If you drank it every day of your life it was supposed to prevent fevers from occurring!

antioxidants will also help rid the body of free radicals which damage the cells in the body.

Remedies for Fever

You can calm a fever by applying cool water compresses to the legs and feet. Add some lavender or peppermint essential oils. Remove the compresses as soon as they warm up.

To combat infection you could use a cooled infusion of rosemary instead of cool water.

Angelica root boiled and infused in water will help to bring down a fever. Add the juice of two lemons, some honey and a drop of brandy to make it more palatable. Teas and tisanes that help to check a fever include hibiscus and basil.

For those with a cast-iron stomach, treat laryngitis with a syrup made up of grated horseradish root, lemon juice and honey which has been left to stand in hot milk or water, then strained.

Hay Fever and Asthma

Hay fever is an allergy to the pollen released by grasses, flowers and trees in spring and summer. The pollen causes cells to release histamine which results in streaming eyes, runny nose, sneezing and a sore itchy throat. Allergic reactions can also be caused by house-dust mites or the fur of animals or feathers of birds. Asthma is on the increase in the Western world – the jury is still out on the cause – but many people believe pollution to be a major factor.

Remedies for Hay Fever

In the old days people chewed natural honeycomb, which was supposed to protect them from allergies of every type. You can still find it in some health stores and it is worth a try. Eating plenty of garlic is also thought to counteract allergic reactions. Chamomile tea is a natural antihistamine – add honey to build up your immunity to pollen.

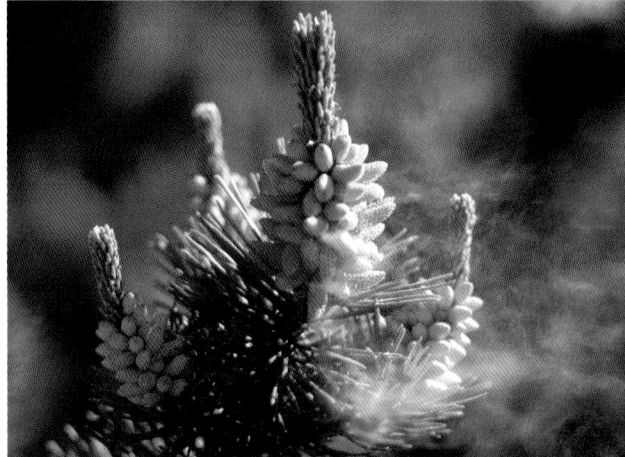

Pollen brings misery to many every year in the form of hay fever, which produces itchy eyes, runny nose and sneezing.

You could grate some horseradish and sniff it to help to clear out the sinuses as well as to stimulate breathing.

You could try taking a teaspoon of English mustard combined with a tablespoon of molasses first thing in the morning and last thing at night.

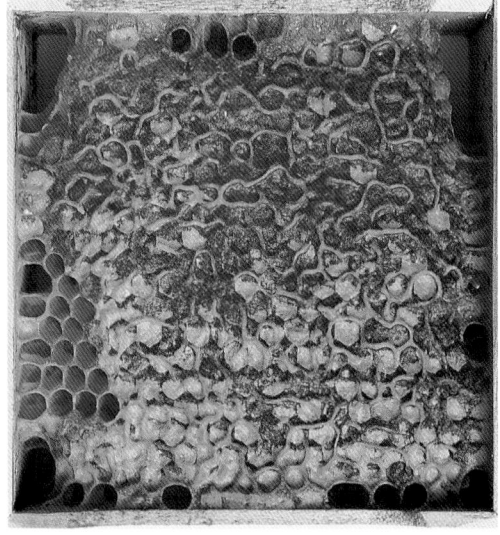

Natural honeycomb was once believed to protect people from all kinds of allergies.

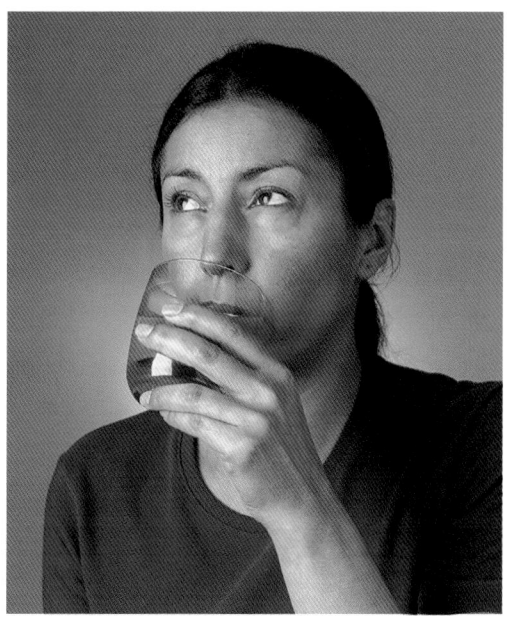

Fresh carrot juice is believed to help protect against asthma attacks. Drinking a glass a day could help to reduce the risk.

Elderflower tea or syrup drunk hot at bedtime will help keep the sniffles of hay fever at bay. Make your own syrup by mixing up elderflower heads, 450g (1lb) of brown sugar, three lemons and two sliced oranges. Add this to 1.7 litres (3 pints) of water and 55g (2oz) of tartaric acid. Steep it in a covered bowl for 24 hours, strain into a big pan and bring to the boil until the sugar is dissolved. Cool, then bottle or freeze and drink as needed.

Garlic is useful for both hay fever and asthma. Chop it and add it raw to salads. A Russian remedy recommends inhaling an infusion of two or three cloves of crushed garlic added to a basin of hot water.

Remedies for Asthma

Nettles and onions can protect against asthma. Or try soaking a fresh cabbage leaf in hot water until saturated and drink the liquid. Chew two cloves of garlic a day or make up a drink from three heads of garlic, 600ml (1 pint) of water, 300ml (½ pint) of cider vinegar and a spoonful of honey. Simmer the garlic cloves in the water for half an hour, add the vinegar and honey and simmer until it forms a syrupy consistency. Drink a sherry-glassful each day. Drink a small glass of carrot juice daily to reduce the risk of asthma attacks.

Irish moss is a jelly, which you can get from some health food stores. Combine it with half an onion, two cloves of garlic and half a cup of honey to make a syrup. It can be taken every couple of hours or as needed.

Hay fever symptoms can be relieved by several natural home remedies, including elderflower tea.

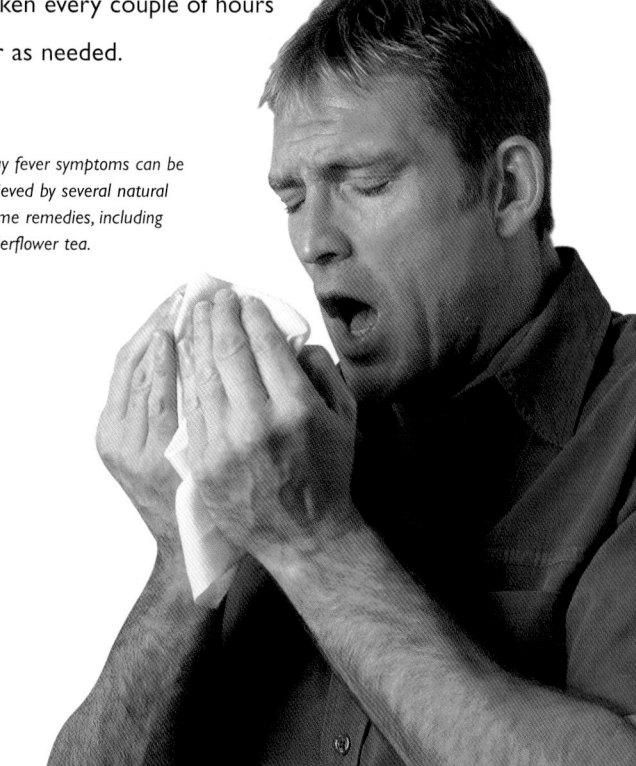

Back Pain

About 80 per cent of us will have some form of back pain at some time in our lives. Many people suffer in silence for years because they know there simply is no cure. Rest and warmth provide some comfort, but there is also a variety of remedies, particularly poultices, that can be applied to ease the pain – even if only temporarily. With any sort of back pain it is always best to consult a doctor.

Remedies for Lumbago

Massage is an excellent remedy for most kinds of back problem. Make up a soothing massage oil from peppermint or coriander oil in a tablespoon of almond oil. Massage it well into the muscles of the back.

Lumbago is a rheumatic pain in the lower region of the back and can be treated with similar remedies

Lumbago is rheumatic pain in the lower region of the back.

to those given for arthritis (see page 215). Some poultices may also be helpful. Cook up whole oats, then mash them with vinegar and apply them to the painful area as hot as possible.

Boil up cabbage leaves in milk until they become a jelly, spread this mixture on the affected area with a cloth and leave it on overnight, covered with gauze held in place with plaster. This helps to release toxins from the body and, although it may not endear you to your bed partner, you will feel rested after a good night's sleep!

Shake together a cup of vinegar and turpentine and add a dessertspoon of powdered camphor and a whole egg. Keep the mixture refrigerated and use as a back rub when necessary.

Remedies for Sciatica

Sciatica is an excruciating back condition caused by pressure on the sciatic nerve which

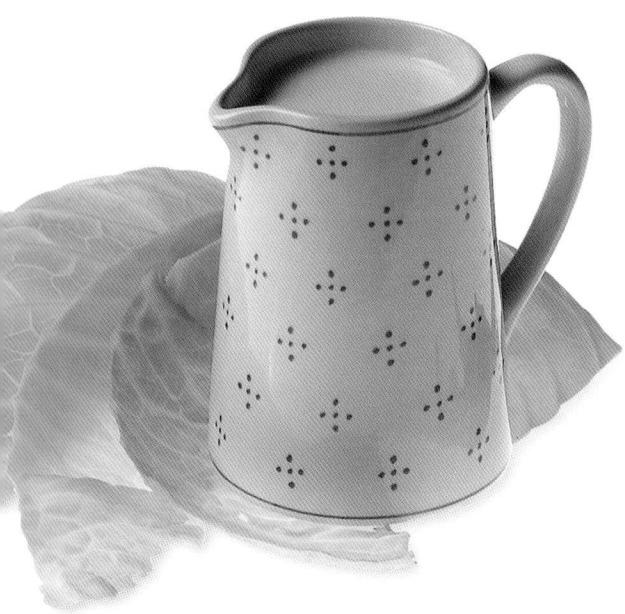

Cabbage leaves boiled up in milk turn into a kind of jelly that can be applied to the back to ease the pain of lumbago.

A cupful of Epsom salts added to a hot bath will ease the pain of sciatica, particularly if it is brought on by cold and damp. A daily supplement of seaweed extract is invaluable for back pain of any sort because of its iodine content. One dessertspoon of mustard or cayenne pepper in a hot bath will ease a bad back. You can also get relief from back pain by taking a warm bath infused with nettles and by having a lot of rest in a firm bed.

Make up a camphor rub from a quarter of a teaspoon each of camphor and mustard powder. Add 300ml (½ pint) of pure turpentine and 300ml (½ pint) of sunflower oil, mix with 300ml (½ pint) of rubbing alcohol and shake the ingredients together. Use it to massage an aching back or any other limbs that are seized up. Keep the area warm.

runs down the back of the leg to the knee. It is caused by pressure in the lower spine, inflammation of the nerve itself or by back strain or injury, which may need to be seen by a back expert.

Some people swear by ivy. Take two handfuls of ivy, chop well and mix with two handfuls of bran. Stir to a paste with 300ml (½ pint) of water and warm over a low heat for 10 minutes. Apply to the affected area using a cloth and leave for half an hour.

Ivy leaf is believed to make an excellent remedy for sciatica.

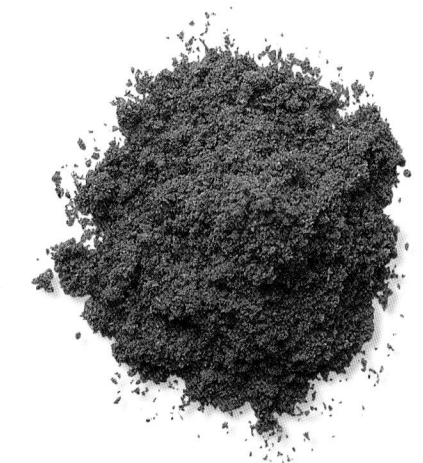

A dessertspoon of cayenne in a hot bath will help give some relief from most back problems.

Rheumatism and Arthritis

Arthritis affects the joints and bones and can be an extremely painful and debilitating condition. Rheumatism describes the swelling, soreness, stiffness and aching of joints and includes rheumatic fever and bursitis, a painful condition resulting from inflammation of the bursa, the fluid-filled sacs that cushion the joints.

Remedies for Rheumatism

Chillies and peppers are rich in capsaicin, an active chemical that desensitises nerves and controls pain. The Mayna Jivaro tribe of Peru still apply chilli fruits directly to their teeth to cure toothache, and this has prompted Western doctors to run trials to see if it may work as a pain reliever for rheumatic diseases.

Native Americans used to swear by a poultice of sage, tobacco, angelica and balsam

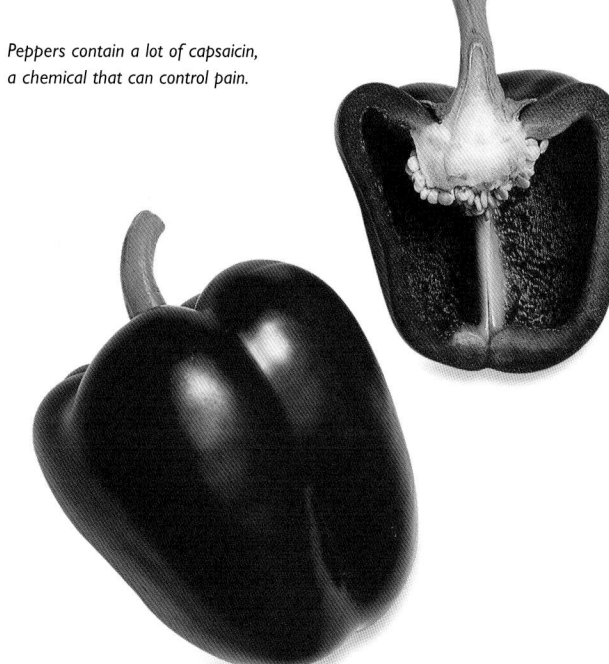

Peppers contain a lot of capsaicin, a chemical that can control pain.

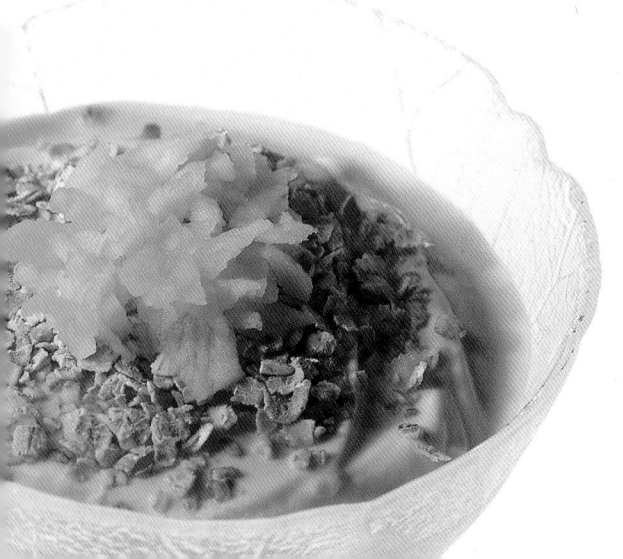

Yogurt with grated apple and raw oats can help to reduce joint pain.

for rheumatic aches and pains. A less dramatic remedy is Epsom salts added to a hot bath, which will ease the pain, or try mixing a dessertspoonful of dried mustard or cayenne pepper into your bathwater.

Eat plenty of onions and garlic – you can even make up a delicious onion drink by chopping up three unpeeled onions and boiling them gently in 600ml (1 pint) of water.

Garlic pounded in olive oil with parsley and eaten on coarse brown bread has been known to help, or a breakfast of grated apple with raw oats and yogurt is also good.

Remedies for Arthritis

Turmeric is a well-known cure for arthritis, so use plenty in your food. Drink warm milk with a teaspoon of ground turmeric mixed in three times a day. A back rub made from a dessertspoon of cayenne pepper in a cup of olive oil and applied to inflamed joints will bring a soothing heat to the aching area. Boil 600ml (1 pint) of apple cider vinegar with a dessertspoon of cayenne pepper, cool and use as a compress on the affected area. Cayenne can cause skin irritation, so make sure it heats the area but does not cause burning.

A good preventative measure is to mix a teaspoon of cider vinegar and honey in hot water and drink it first thing in the morning. Or try drinking the juice of one lemon in hot water sweetened with honey before breakfast.

Nettle soup, which is made with fresh nettle tops, chopped onion and garlic, or plain nettle tea, are both tried and tested remedies for arthritis.

Potatoes can provide pain relief for arthritis sufferers.

Potatoes have excellent anti-inflammatory properties and can relieve pain. To make a potato poultice, boil 450g (1lb) of potatoes in their skins until tender. Place them in some muslin and mash. Apply the sack to the affected area. Remove it only once it has cooled down completely.

Remedies for Bursitis

Make a poultice of cooked cabbage leaves, mashed and applied warm between layers of gauze or muslin. Linseed, marshmallow and slippery elm are other comforting herbs that can be taken as supplements. Boil up hot apple cider vinegar with cayenne pepper and apply as a compress, as for arthritis.

Turmeric can be used in many dishes and even drunk added to warm milk to counter the pain of arthritis.

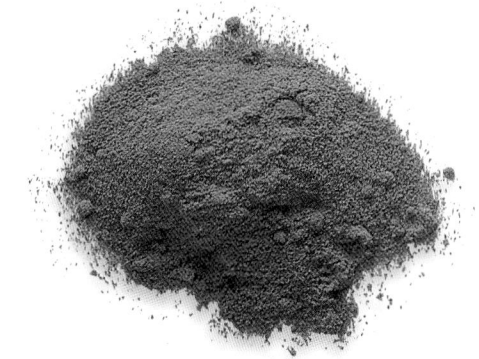

Hangovers

The best way to avoid a hangover is to avoid too much alcohol! However, that is little consolation if you are suffering the agonies of a banging head, parched throat and the constant threat of being sick. If you know you have drunk too much, you can prevent a hangover by drinking at least a litre (about two pints) of water before going to bed. This will help to flush out some of the toxins. Colas and fizzy drinks can also help your throbbing head because they alkalise the acid in the stomach.

Remedies for Hangovers

For some reason, eggs have always been a big feature of hangover cures across all cultures. And, in fact, eggs do contain a certain chemical now known to neutralise the effects of alcohol, so it seems that the old eggnog remedy or fried eggs the morning after may work well after all!

For an upset stomach or nausea, try grating some fresh ginger root into a mug of boiling water and sipping it slowly.

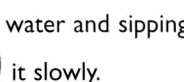

Colas and fizzy drinks alkalise the acid in the stomach and help to stop the banging sensation in your head.

Tea made from fresh ginger will soothe a queasy stomach when you have overdone it the night before.

Drinking ginger tea will also soothe your stomach, and it tastes delicious, too.

Umeboshi plums, available at Asian markets and health food stores, have long been reputed to cure hangovers. They may make some people want to vomit, but those people who have managed to keep them down swear by them.

One of the best herbal fixits for a hangover is peppermint tea. Adding organic honey will also ease your headache and begin the process of rehydration.

Replenish your lost vitamin C with a glass of fresh orange juice and add a teaspoon of lime juice or a dash of cumin powder to really get you back in gear. Drinking a cup of thyme

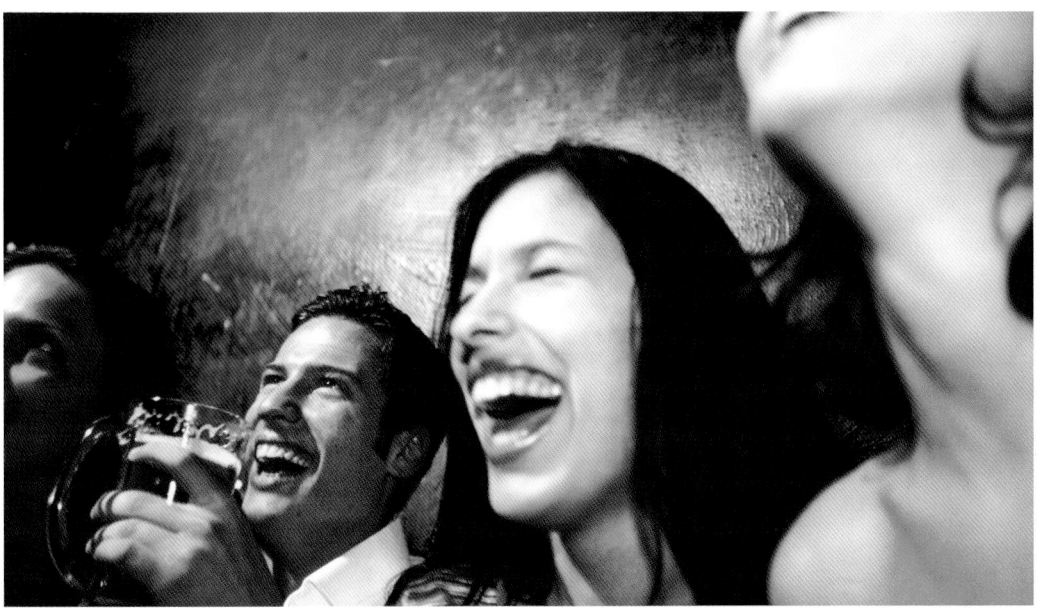

Eat, drink and be merry! But be prepared for the morning after the night before and have a natural hangover remedy to hand.

tea will ease your headache and queasy stomach more effectively and safely than many over-the-counter pain relievers.

Try the hair of the dog! Peel a whole head of garlic and put in a pan with 300ml (½ pint) of red wine. Bring to the boil and simmer for 20 minutes. Strain and drink slowly. It is the tannins, not the alcohol, that help to cure your banging head!

Once you can face food again, a vegetable broth which is high in potassium and natural minerals will help to replace fluid and mineral loss. Make it from celery, courgettes, beetroot or carrots. Try to avoid sulphur-containing vegetables such as broccoli, onions and cabbage. Replace intestinal flora with good bacteria from live yogurt.

Try a soothing bath with essential oils of eucalyptus, peppermint and sandalwood. A cup of peppermint tea will also help if you are feeling queasy. Soak a towel in icy cold water and wrap it around your forehead. The coldness should help to shrink away your headache.

Cook a healthy broth using vegetables to replace lost minerals and fluids.

Tummy Troubles

Indigestion is often known as heartburn, and as its name suggests it causes a feeling of discomfort just below the breastbone around the heart area. Eating too much, too quickly, is the main cause of indigestion, with symptoms varying from wind and rumblings in the stomach to pain or nausea.

Remedies for Indigestion

Ripe bananas are natural antacids and can soothe an inflamed stomach. If none is available, try cider vinegar or lemon juice in hot water, which alkalises an acid stomach. Ginger tea, made from fresh ginger root if possible, also warms and soothes an acid stomach. Drink an infusion

Infuse fresh mint and drink sweetened with honey for nausea.

of hot peppermint tea or try teas such as fennel, lemon balm or cinnamon. Slippery elm powder dissolved in hot water gives immediate relief.

Mix two tablespoons of bicarbonate of soda with one teaspoon of ground ginger in cold water and drink before sitting down to breakfast to prevent indigestion.

Tea made from peppermint helps combat feelings of nausea.

Remedies for Nausea

Peppermint is considered to be an excellent cure for nausea. Although it has long been associated with the relief of indigestion and travel sickness, how it works is little understood. It is believed to work by relaxing the

Water

- Avoid drinking water with a meal as it dilutes the gastric acid and leads to incomplete digestion.
- Water can also cause the fats and oils in the food to cling together, which stops them being absorbed properly.
- Drink water ten minutes before or three hours after eating.

oesophageal sphincter and equalising gastric pressures. Buy readymade peppermint tea bags or put four drops of peppermint oil, found with the cookery ingredients in the supermarket, in some hot water and let it cool. Drink slowly for quick relief from nausea. Infuse some fresh mint from the garden and drink sweetened with honey.

Remedies for Food Poisoning

Food poisoning can cause terrible vomiting, diarrhoea and stomach cramps. It is the body's way of getting rid of food that is bad or disagrees with it and is usually caused by germs that inflame the lining of the stomach and intestines. The main problem

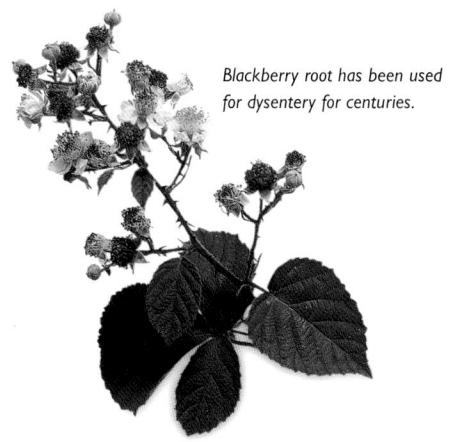

Blackberry root has been used for dysentery for centuries.

with food poisoning is fluid loss which causes dehydration, so it is important to keep up your liquid intake.

In the old days, remedies included a rather disgusting concoction of salt swiftly followed by a spoonful of castor oil. For mild food poisoning take raw garlic, which helps to fight the infection in the gut. Replace lost fluid by drinking plain water or diluted fruit juice.

Blackberry root has been used for years to combat the deadly form of dysentery so common in hot climates. During the American Revolution both sides accepted truces so that troops could go 'rooting' for blackberry roots and leaves. It is still one of the safest remedies for children's diarrhoea.

Stewed fennel, horseradish leaves or a strong dose of apple cider vinegar have all been used to help remove bad food from the digestive system.

Ripe bananas are believed to be natural antacids. They can provide relief from inflammation of the stomach.

Cystitis and Bladder Conditions

Cystitis is a painful condition caused by inflammation of the bladder. Symptoms include pain in the lower back and a stabbing pain when urinating. It is important to seek your doctor's advice if you have cystitis for any length of time, because if it continues it can lead to kidney infection. Cystitis has been called the 'honeymoon disease' as it often occurs after sex. Drinking water and urinating as soon after sex as possible may help to prevent an attack.

Remedies for Cystitis

Plain water flushes out the kidneys better than anything and will help to get rid of the bacteria that are causing the infection. Drink plenty and often. Make up 600ml (1 pint) of mild chamomile tea and drink it throughout the day to flush germs out of the bladder.

Try one teaspoon of bicarbonate of soda in a glass of tepid water every three hours. It makes the urine less acidic, which stops bacteria from breeding – it also relieves the burning sensation that so often accompanies cystitis.

Apply live yogurt to the affected area – its friendly bacteria can help to fight invading germs. Make up some home-made barley water by boiling up a cupful of barley in enough water to cover it. Add the rind of a lemon and simmer until the barley is soft. Strain off the barley, add some honey and sip slowly throughout the day.

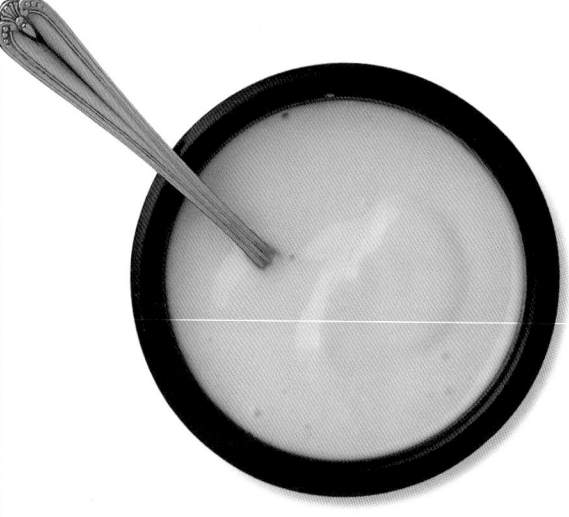

Plain live yogurt is a traditional natural home remedy used to combat the discomfort of cystitis.

Cranberry juice can reach the parts that other juices can't reach. A substance in cranberries appears to prevent bacteria from sticking to the walls of the urinary tract where they would normally proliferate. When you drink cranberry juice the bacteria lose their grip and are washed away.

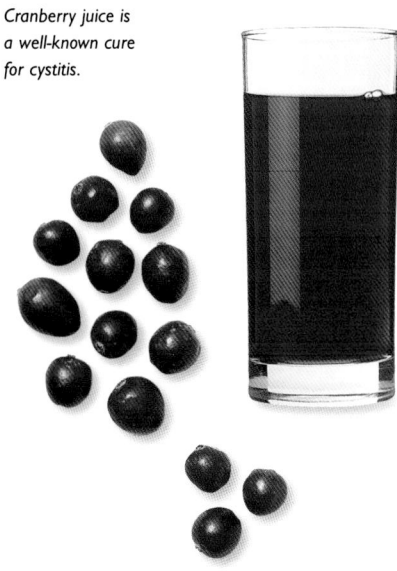

Cranberry juice is a well-known cure for cystitis.

Experts now believe the same component may also be present in blueberries. Eat the berries or pulp them with a little water in a food processor.

Turnips, celery, fennel and onions are all good diuretics; so are dandelion roots and stinging nettle leaves. Add any of these raw to salads.

Onions are a good diuretic, and can be added to many different dishes, including soups and salads.

Make an onion soup from three or four onions steeped in a litre (1¾ pints) of hot water. Drink it throughout the day – it tastes disgusting but does the trick. Horseradish also stimulates digestion and encourages the kidneys to flush through urine. Horseradish can be grated into foods or boiled up with mustard seed and water as a drink.

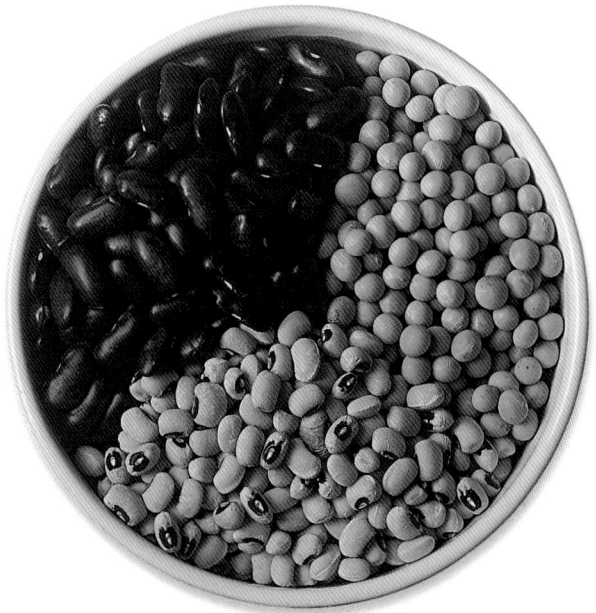

Cook up kidney beans, soya beans and black-eyed beans in an appetising dish which really benefits the kidneys.

Kidney beans are also helpful for any kidney or urinary tract infections. You can also try black soya beans or black-eyed beans. Cook them with garlic and use them to replace meat in the diet. Chinese herbalists swear by seaweed, fenugreek and saw palmetto for good results.

Bowel Problems

Constipation, diarrhoea, irritable bowel syndrome (IBS) and piles are four of the most debilitating conditions known to humankind – made all the worse because nobody wants to talk about them. Constipation occurs for many reasons, the most common of which is poor bowel habits learned from a young age, and can lead to piles. Medications including antidepressants can also cause constipation. Diarrhoea is often the result of food poisoning, and either constipation or diarrhoea can be symptoms of IBS.

Remedies for Constipation

Anyone who remembers syrup of figs from their childhood will not be at all surprised to learn that both figs and prunes are well-known laxatives.

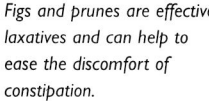

Figs and prunes are effective laxatives and can help to ease the discomfort of constipation.

laxative effect and are particularly useful when constipation is due to excessive meat or fat in the diet.

Drinking cooked cabbage or carrot juice can also help to ease constipation, or you could mash up raw apricots with a little honey in a bowl of yogurt.

Rhubarb stewed with honey will also have the desired effect. Strawberries have a mild

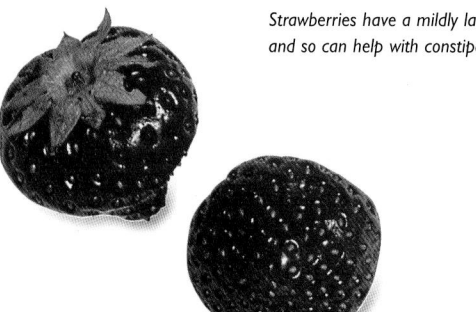

Strawberries have a mildly laxative effect and so can help with constipation.

Remedies for Diarrhoea

Rice pudding is one of the oldest remedies for diarrhoea. Make your own with one and a half cups of milk, a pinch of salt, six tablespoons of brown sugar, a teaspoon of vanilla extract, two to four eggs, grated lemon rind and two cups of cooked white rice. Add all the ingredients together and mix well. Spread the mixture in a buttered baking dish and cook for an hour. Sprinkle with cinnamon.

Boil rice in water for one and a half hours, then strain and drink the liquid to soothe an

Try grated apple that has gone brown – the oxidised pectin acts like an over-the-counter medicine to cure diarrhoea.

irritated bowel. You could also make a thick oatmeal drink by cooking together a cup of oats and 1.2 litres (2 pints) of water for five minutes. Strain and drink frequently. Oats also have a calming effect on the bowel, and starchy fluids tend to stop vomiting and reduce fluid loss.

Add a teaspoon of cornflour to a glass of water at room temperature – it tastes disgusting, so drink it down quickly and repeat the dose every three or four hours.

Blueberries contain compounds called anthocyanosides which control diarrhoea, so add them to your breakfast cereal.

Try eating a grated apple which has been allowed to go brown. The pectin oxidises and acts like many proprietary brands of diarrhoea remedies – slightly unripe bananas have the same effect.

Remedies for IBS

Peppermint has a well proven anti-spasmodic effect on the smooth muscle of the intestines – drink peppermint tea or, if you have mint growing in your garden, chew the fresh leaves or sprinkle them on salads. Potatoes can reduce stomach acid as they contain small amounts of atropine which has an anti-spasmodic effect. Wash and dice a large potato and steep it overnight in a cup of cold water with salt. Strain and drink the water every morning on an empty stomach. A two-day diet of potatoes will flush out toxins and waste from the body and help to purify the blood.

Remedy for Piles

Rub a small amount of either witch hazel or lemon juice into the affected area with a cotton wool swab before going to bed.

Rice pudding is one of the oldest remedies for diarrhoea.

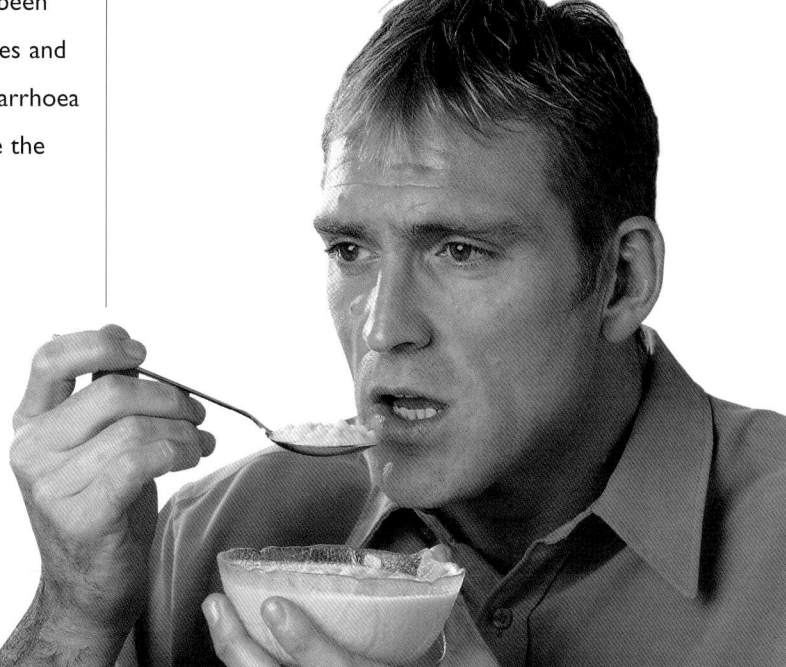

GENERAL AILMENTS
Skin Problems

Skin problems often reflect what is happening inside the body. Acne normally appears at adolescence and is believed to be caused by hormonal imbalances which produce too much of the oily substance in the skin known as sebum. Psoriasis occurs when skin cells reproduce up to a hundred times faster than normal. The skin then builds up in dry, flaky patches and causes itching and irritation.

Remedies for Acne

Avocado may be rich in fatty oils but it also contains plenty of vitamins A, C, E and B complex, which are all essential for good skin. It has strong anti-bacterial and anti-fungal properties, so it is excellent for acne or any other irritating skin conditions. Make up a paste of avocado pulp and apply to any dry skin rashes to soothe and moisturise.

Grate some horseradish, which is rich in sulphur, and infuse it in hot milk for half an hour. Strain it and use the liquid as a face wash. You can also

Avocados contain all the vitamins – A, B complex, C and E – needed for a healthy skin.

leave a teaspoon of the grated root to dissolve in a cupful of cider vinegar for a week and use it in the same way. It will sting badly but works a treat.

Remedies for Eczema

Make a paste from a teaspoon of powdered marshmallow root or slippery elm mixed with hot water. Spread it onto the affected area and leave for 20 minutes, then wash off with an infusion of comfrey. Comfrey leaves also make a wonderful facial wash and will promote growth of new tissue.

Make a rice-flour poultice and apply it hot to the affected area. Eat plenty of asparagus, which helps promote the elimination of toxins through urine and is also considered a liver

Eating a grapefruit a day is a routine that can help relieve the symptoms of psoriasis.

Comfrey leaves can be turned into a great facial wash for those affected by eczema.

tonic because of its high amino acid content. Drink the water of the asparagus after it has been steamed.

Beetroot was used by the Romans to relieve fever, but it also stimulates the immune system and helps to clear the blood. Drink the juice of cabbage, which contains anti-bacterial properties, to promote healing, and eat plenty of watercress, which contains sulphur.

Dandelions are a fantastic detoxifier of the liver, kidneys, blood and tissues. Use a tincture of dandelion roots for eczema or acne.

Remedies for Psoriasis

Make up an anti-fungal herbal tea from hops. Eat a grapefruit a day for breakfast. Drink cranberry juice, eat prunes and plums and avoid alcohol and smoking.

Make up a dandelion wine from a bunch of dandelion petals, 5 litres (9 pints) of water, two oranges and two lemons, cut into pieces, a pinch of yeast and 1.3kg (3lb) of sugar. Boil the dandelion petals for 20 minutes and pour over the orange and lemon pieces. Allow the mixture to cool, then add the yeast and let it stand for 48 hours. Strain the mixture through muslin and pour into a jug. Let the wine stand for around six weeks before bottling. Keep for at least six months before drinking.

Eating plenty of watercress, which contains sulphur, is recommended as a treatment for eczema.

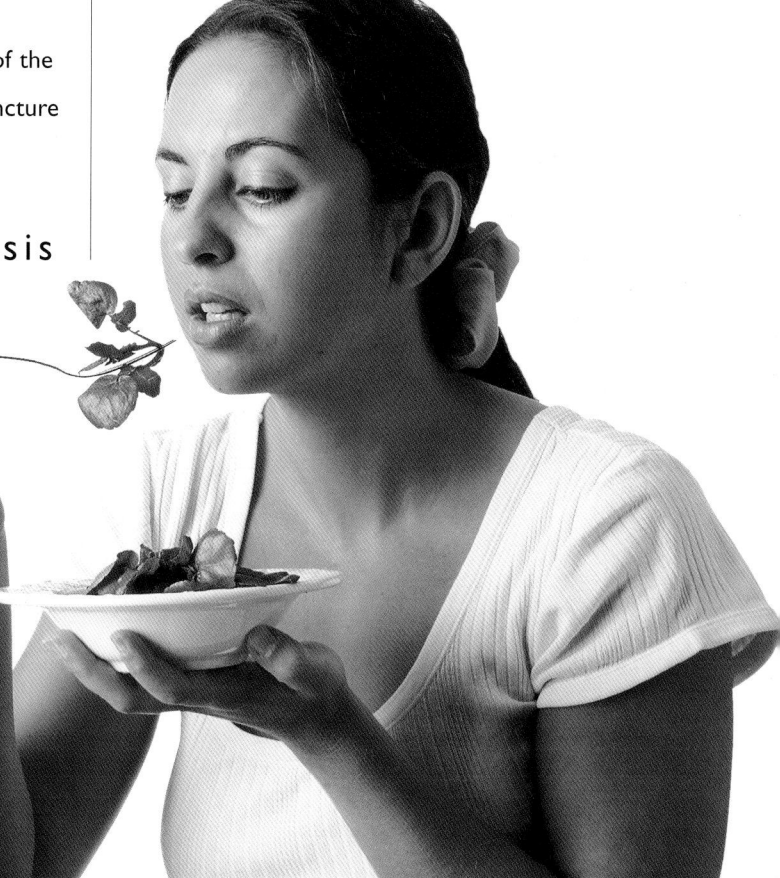

Toothache and Gum Disease

Unfortunately, toothache is an all-too-familiar condition in the Western world, and it is usually the result of poor care of the teeth and gums. Halitosis (bad breath) is often caused by sore gums or abscesses in the mouth.

Remedies for Toothache

Oil of cloves or a dried clove rubbed on to the gum around an aching tooth will help soothe it. Try chewing a clove over the offending tooth for instant relief, or pack dried hops or fresh peppermint into the tooth. In

Raw cloves rubbed onto the offending tooth can cure a toothache, or chew one whole to find instant relief.

Germany, dentists use a clove-based anaesthetic to eradicate the pain of toothache.

Native Americans used to apply the mashed green leaves or root of the willow as a poultice for toothache.

You could make a mouthwash of vinegar and salt to ease the pain. Apply ground black pepper and fresh ginger to a piece of gauze and pack the tooth with it.

If you are not worried about being antisocial, you could plug a cavity with cotton wool soaked in onion or garlic juice. It will disinfect the whole area and give some relief from the pain.

You could try putting a slice of lightly boiled apple between the teeth to help to relieve the pain of toothache.

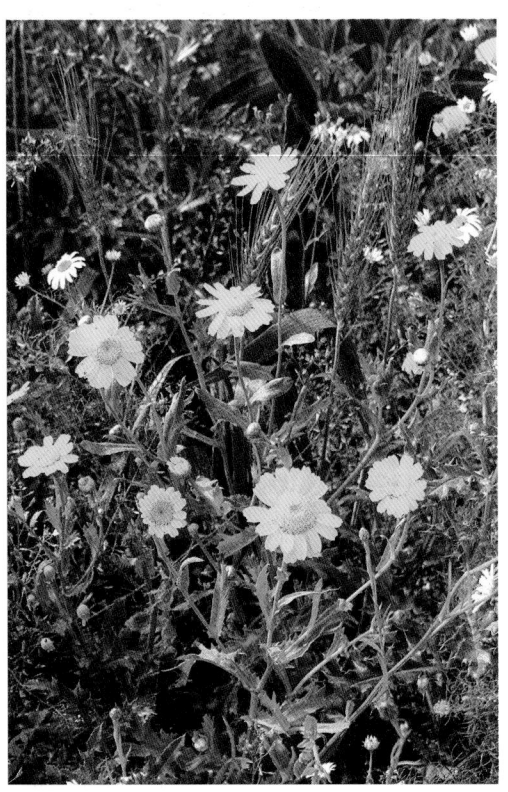

You can make a tincture of marigold that will help to ease the pain of a bad tooth or sore gums.

Remedies for Sore Gums

Cabbage is known for its anti-inflammatory properties, so you could dab a little white cabbage juice onto mouth sores.

Sore gums may be the result of vitamin B and C deficiency, so strengthen your gums by drinking plenty of rose hip or blackcurrant tea and tisanes.

Soak a small pad of cotton wool in tincture of marigold and press it to the sore gum or bad tooth.

Make a mouthwash out of marigold or agrimony, boiled in water and left to cool.

A tincture of lavender leaves rubbed onto the gums acts as an excellent antiseptic, or you could gargle with a cooled infusion of lavender leaves mixed with honey.

You can make your own natural toothpowder by mixing two parts of bicarbonate of soda to one part salt. If you have none to hand, you could even try cleaning your teeth with raw lemon.

Tincture of lavender leaves rubbed on the gum acts as an antiseptic.

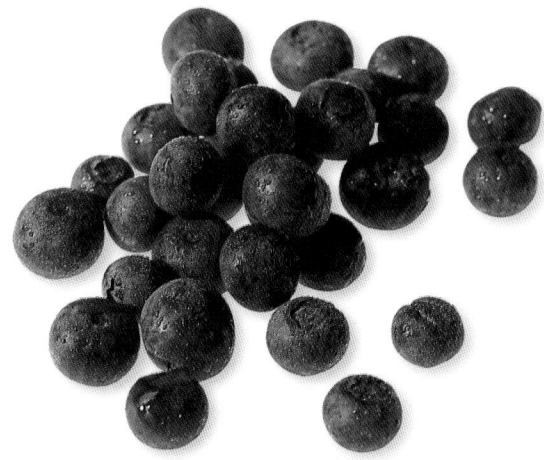

Blueberries are astringent and antiseptic and are therefore good for combating mouth ulcers and gum infection.

Remedies for Mouth Ulcers

Eat plenty of blueberries – they are astringent and act as a strong antiseptic, and so they can be useful for mouth ulcers or sores and infections of the gums.

Try mixing two teaspoons of sea salt and two teaspoons of hydrogen peroxide in a large glass of warm water as a mouthwash. (NB: Don't swallow.) Hot salt water held in the mouth over an abscess also helps to disperse it.

Mouth Fresheners

- Try chewing on a few sprigs of parsley to freshen the mouth.
- Crush cloves in a cupful of boiling water, cool for five minutes and then use as a mouthwash.

Migraine and Headache

Most people experience headaches at some time or another. Some are caused by tension or stress, others are the result of too much alcohol or may herald a cold or flu. Migraine is more than just a serious headache. It is actually a neurological disorder which includes a pounding headache along with visual disturbance, nausea and vomiting. If you have a headache that persists for any length of time, see a doctor.

Remedies for Headache

A warm cabbage leaf compress placed on the head can help to ease a headache, or try eating a crust of stale brown bread with butter and marmalade – a curious remedy, but very effective! A poultice of cucumber or raw potatoes placed on the brow can relieve a headache caused by too much sun.

Lavender will help to refresh and clear a muzzy head. You can make up your own

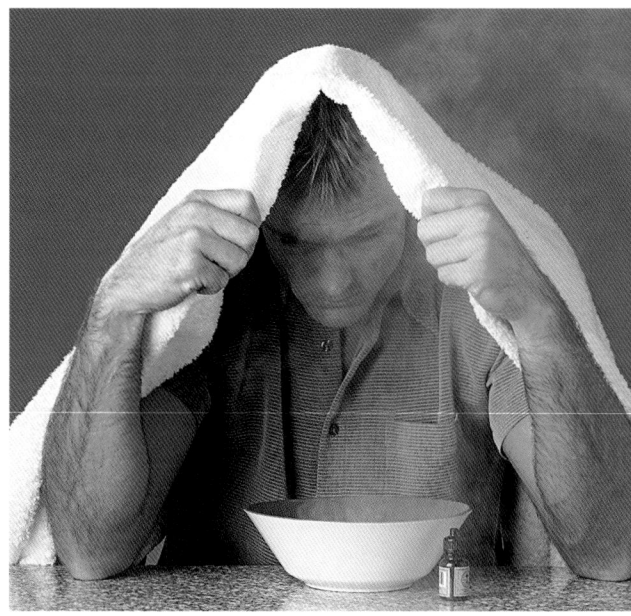

Steam inhalation is the best cure for a sinus headache. You can add various essential oils to help increase its efficacy.

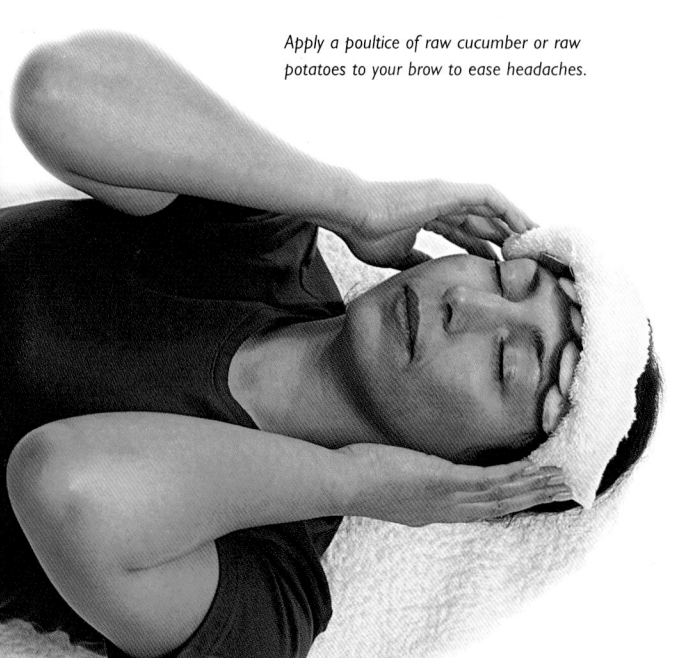

Apply a poultice of raw cucumber or raw potatoes to your brow to ease headaches.

lavender water with two tablespoons of dried lavender, two teaspoons of cinnamon, a pinch of grated nutmeg and a litre (1¾ pints) of surgical spirit. Breathe in the delicious fumes for instant relief. Headaches caused by hypertension can also be eased by eating garlic, which lowers blood pressure.

Remedies for Sinus Headache

Sinus headaches respond best to steam inhalations. Add the essential oils of pine, eucalyptus, rosemary or thyme, either on their own or in combination. Apply a hot compress of plain water to the forehead. You can also infuse the water with lavender or peppermint oils. Lie down and breathe in the aroma, keeping the compress hot.

Remedies for Migraine

Feverfew is the main herb proven to have an effect on migraine. Oregano has also been reported to be effective – the dried leaf can be used as snuff to clear a blocked head, or simmer the fresh leaf in olive oil and use it to massage the temples.

A drink made from fresh ginger root has been shown to be almost as effective at preventing migraines (when taken daily) as powerful prescription drugs.

Add ginger oil to almond oil and massage onto the temples during early warning signs. Or try soaking your feet in a footbath which has either fresh ginger or peppermint added, or their essential oil. The bath will draw the blood away from

The herb feverfew has been proven in clinical trials to have an effect on migraine.

the head to the heat and provide some relief.

Eating a bowl of tinned tomatoes simmered with basil and served with a dash of vinegar has been known to help migraine.

Make up an ointment out of oregano oil and vaseline and smooth onto the temples.

If you can get hold of feverfew, make up a tea from the herb. If not, try peppermint and rosemary. Use two parts peppermint leaves and one part rosemary and let them steep in a mug of hot water for at least ten minutes.

A crust of stale brown bread spread with butter and marmalade seems to work for headaches.

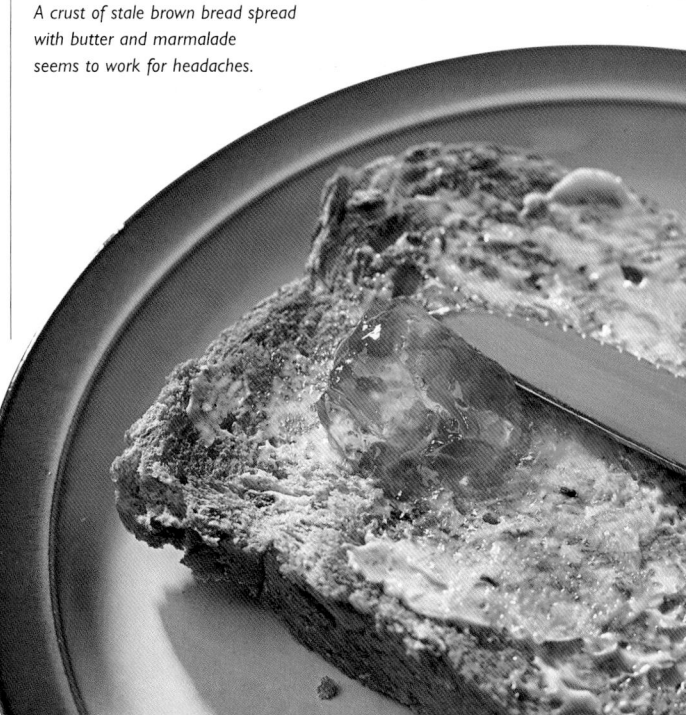

Earache and Neuralgia

Earache can be caused by a variety of things, from colds and catarrh to enlarged adenoids or an infection of the inner ear. Most home remedies are based on warmth and oil, but you should never poke the ear, no matter how bad the pain.

Any inflammation of the trigeminal nerve, which carries sensations into the skull near the ear, produces an excruciating spasmodic pain in one side of the face known as neuralgia. At one time, grated horseradish would have been applied to the

A lump of salt rolled in a hot, damp cloth and held against the ear can relieve earache.

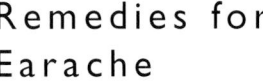

A hot water bottle wrapped in an old jumper can help soothe earache or neuralgia.

cheek until the pain subsided, but nowadays there are less harsh ways of curing the condition.

Remedies for Earache

Many earaches result from colds, flu or other types of congestion. If this is the case you can reduce the mucus and phlegm with a tea made from elderflowers or a cold elderberry drink.

One of the best remedies for earache is a hot water bottle covered in a warm jumper and held close to the ear. Put a few drops of warm olive oil in the ear and lie on the opposite side for about five minutes while the oil flows down into the inner ear.

Crush a clove of garlic and let it rest in some warm olive oil for fifteen minutes, then strain the liquid. Soak a cotton wool ball in the liquid and place it just inside the outer earlobe.

Remedies for Neuralgia

Massage the gums right at the back of the mouth with a clove. Sleeping with a hop pillow has been known to cure this most painful of conditions, or try holding a hot poultice of porridge oats wrapped in muslin against the area. Eating oats can also act as a stress reducer and excellent pain reliever.

Garlic, crushed and soaked in olive oil, can be an effective means of countering infection in the ear.

The garlic combats any possible infection. In the old days, a boiled onion placed on the affected ear was supposed to be a great cure. Some people used the juice of the onion in a warm oil. Heat up a teaspoon of almond oil and pour gently into the ear, then plug with a piece of cotton wool.

As a compress, try a lump of salt rolled in a cloth, steeped in hot water and wrung out, or a baked potato wrapped in wool — use both remedies as hot as you can stand it for the best effect.

Drink plantain tea to tone up the delicate membranes of the inner ear and prevent dizziness from ear inflammations.

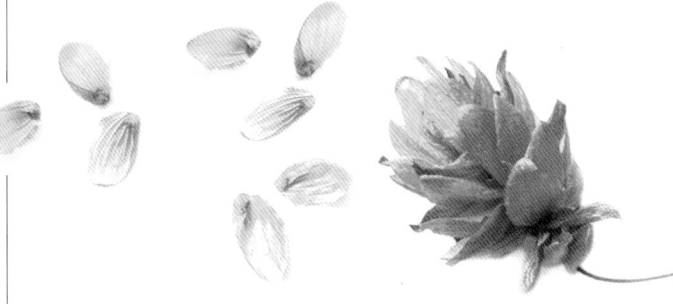

A hop pillow could provide just the solution you need for relief from painful neuralgia.

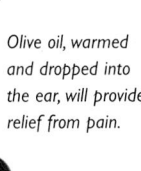

Olive oil, warmed and dropped into the ear, will provide relief from pain.

Period Pains and PMS

Period pains, also known as dysmenorrhoea, are the searing pains felt in the lower abdomen by more than half the female population during a period. About 15 per cent of those women say the pain interferes with their everyday lives. Period pains tend to start during adolescence and become less severe with age – particularly after having a baby.

Cramp-like pains in the lower abdomen at the start of a period are rarely a sign of illness but can cause great misery. Premenstrual syndrome (PMS) affects about 40 per cent of women and causes severe mood swings, headaches, bloating and sore breasts.

Remedies for Period Pains

Brown rice, wholemeal bread, oats, nuts and beans will all increase the magnesium, iron,

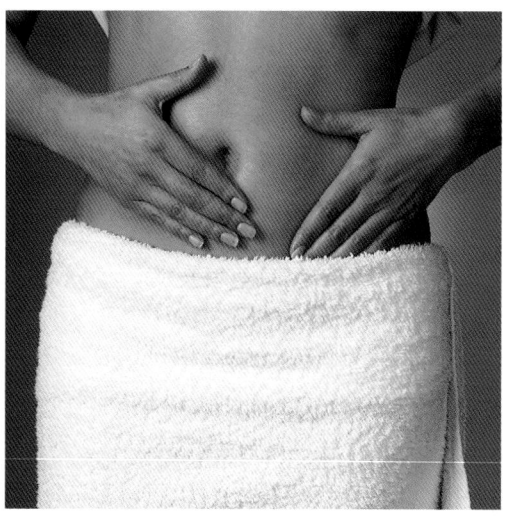

Massage warm castor oil over the lower abdomen to help to ease period pains and relieve the bloating of PMS.

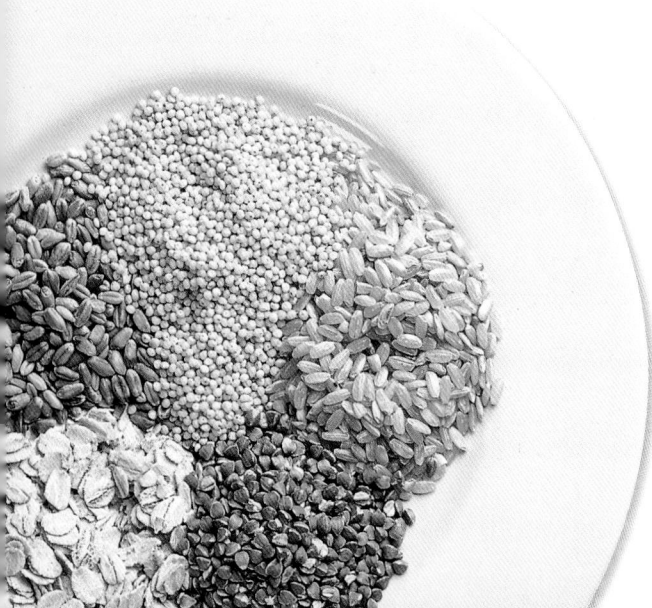

Oats and brown rice help to fight period pains.

zinc and vitamins in your body, which help you to fight pain. A warm bath with a few drops of chamomile or clary sage essential oils will ease tension and relax muscles. Geranium and rosemary essential oils counter fluid retention.

Angelica is a warming, stimulating herb suited to women who feel a chill during periods. To make a tea, add one part each of angelica, chamomile and ginger root to 600ml (1 pint) of water and simmer for 15 minutes.

Dandelion is a good source of iron and is one of the best diuretics, supplying plenty of potassium which helps to get rid of excess water. Add young dandelion leaves to a fresh green salad for an appetising remedy. Yarrow tea can help ease menstrual cramps and decrease menstrual bleeding.

Massage warm castor oil over the lower abdomen. Hot, fresh ginger tea or fresh ginger infused in milk is one of the oldest remedies for period pains. Boil up rhubarb roots into a tea, or try basil tea if you suffer with cramps and particularly heavy periods.

Remedies for PMS

Peppermint tea can help to ease the symptoms of PMS. Freshly cooked asparagus helps to control breast tenderness and bloating. Seaweed may also help – it's the natural iodine that relieves symptoms. Choose wakame, nori and kombu and use them in stews or soups.

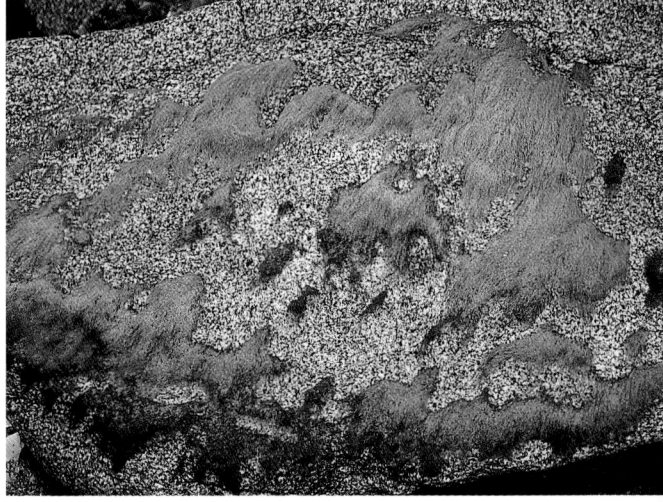

Seaweed contains natural iodine that is useful in relieving PMS. Edible seaweed is available for use in stews and soups.

A castor oil poultice placed on the lower abdomen will encourage the clearing of toxins through the lymphatic system. Soak an old hand towel in castor oil and place it over the abdomen, cover it with another towel and top it up with a hot water bottle.

Dandelion tea can help with bloating in the run-up to a period. It rids the body of excess fluids. Sage tea also helps, or you can eat either in a salad. Make up a cocktail of spinach, watercress, young nettle shoots, carrots and beetroot. Use the raw ingredients in a juicer if you have one, or cook the carrots and beetroot and process everything in a blender. This combination acts as a wonderful tonic at this time of the month.

Freshly cooked asparagus helps to alleviate the symptoms of breast tenderness and bloating associated with PMS.

Hot Flushes and Menopausal Problems

Hot flushes, night sweats and mood swings are all symptoms of the menopause, which, although not an illness, can cause untold misery to many women as they get older. Cutting out caffeine is particularly useful for most symptoms of menopause, and there is a range of teas and tisanes which can actively help to relieve symptoms.

Remedies for Hot Flushes

Mint is a famous cooler, so add fresh mint whenever you can to salads. Drink peppermint tea or add some peppermint essential oil to your bathwater.

Sage leaves can be made into a tonic wine that helps to relieve hot flushes.

Sage is known to be the herb of old age. Make up a sage tonic wine by taking a handful of fresh sage leaves and letting them stand in a bottle of good quality white wine for at least two weeks. Sweeten with honey and leave for another week. Strain the liquid through a cloth and bottle it. Drinking a glass before lunch and dinner is most beneficial.

Another great menopause tonic contains borage leaf, lemon balm, raspberry leaf, burdock root and plantain leaf. All you need to do is to steep the herbs in hot water and drink the liquid during the day in order to lift your spirits.

Celery contains oestrogen-stimulating substances that will help with menopausal symptoms.

Pumpkin seeds contain phytoestrogens, which can help with menopausal symptoms.

Remedies for Night Sweats

Drink two cupfuls of sage tea each day. Place three teaspoons of sage leaves in a pan and pour two cups of boiling water over. Cover and simmer for five minutes. Make it up in the morning and keep it in a thermos flask for drinking during the day. Ginseng tea is often recommended because it contains plenty of B vitamins and minerals. It also helps boost a flagging libido!

Try marigold tea made from an infusion of flower heads in a litre (1¾ pints) of boiling water, steeped for ten minutes. Drink it three or four times a day.

Place the leaves of lemon balm under your pillow at night, or drink a cup of lemon balm tea to soothe and revive you.

Remedies for General Symptoms

Calendula, hops, ginseng, sage and wild yam all have oestrogenic action which can be helpful – take these as an infusion or supplement. Eat plenty of rhubarb, oats and celery which contain similar oestrogen-stimulating substances.

Some foods have high levels of phytoestrogens (natural plant oestrogens), and these may have a beneficial effect on menopausal symptoms.

Many of these compounds, which are called isoflavones and lignans, are found in soya foods, flax seeds and some herbs.

In Asia, where women eat a diet high in soya foods, they report fewer menopausal symptoms and also have a lower incidence of breast cancer. Some trials have also shown that a diet high in soya decreases the incidence of hot flushes.

Other foods that contain phytoestrogens include mung beans, pumpkin seeds, tofu and tempeh, so try to include these foods in your diet.

Eat plenty of nettles, dandelion and plantain, which can all be added to salads.

As a general tonic, you could run yourself a hot bath and add essential oils of rosemary or lavender, and this will soothe and refresh you.

Lemon balm leaves, placed under your pillow at night, will soothe you and help you to counter night sweats.

Candida/Thrush

Stress, allergies, too much junk food and alcohol can all conspire to cause an imbalance in the flora of the gut, colon or vagina, causing the itching and soreness known as candida or thrush. Thrush is a fungal parasite, which can be stimulated by the contraceptive pill or by the use of antibiotics. Simple self-help includes avoiding synthetic underwear or tight jeans and avoiding sex while you have the infection. Oral thrush is more common in babies and children than in adults, and it can be caused by too much sugar in the diet.

Remedies for Vaginal Thrush

Thyme, in the form of a tea, can be used as a douche to ease the discomfort of thrush.

Eat a pot of live yogurt every morning or make up a breakfast of raw oats, live yogurt and orange juice. A weak solution of one teaspoon of hydrogen peroxide in a glass of warm water, dabbed gently onto the affected area with a swab of cotton wool, will ease the itching.

Live yogurt contains friendly bacteria known as acidophilus, which combat vaginal yeast and other infections caused by this fungus. Put some on a tampon and insert into the vagina (remove within two hours).

Drink honey in cider vinegar each morning, and if you are on a course of antibiotics eat as much raw garlic as you can take for up to a week – it counters most bacterial, fungal and viral infections. You can even place a peeled clove of garlic wrapped in a little gauze inside the vagina for a powerful local antiseptic effect – it stings like mad, so this one is not for the faint-hearted!

Live yogurt contains friendly bacteria which combat vaginal yeast.

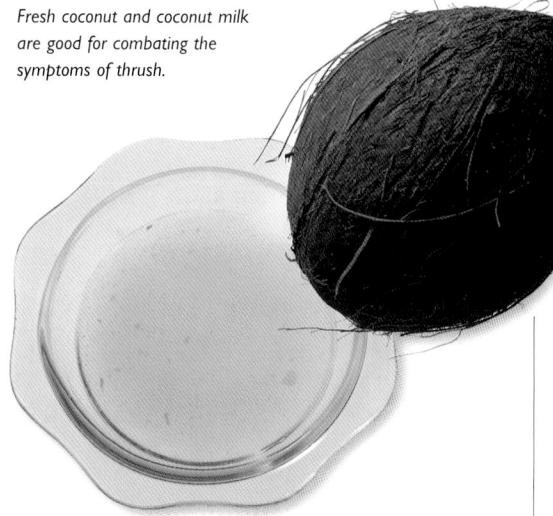

Fresh coconut and coconut milk are good for combating the symptoms of thrush.

You could make up a douche from 600ml (1 pint) of boiled, cooled water to which you have added two drops of lavender oil, or make a douche from chamomile or thyme tea. You can also use either of these mixtures in a shallow bath to ease the discomfort.

Use myrrh or tea tree oil diluted with a teaspoon of vodka and soak a tampon in the solution. Leave the tampon in for four to five hours once or twice a week.

Nasturtium is an age-old remedy for thrush because the flowers act as a natural antibiotic. You could make an infusion from the flowers and use it in a cool bath.

Remedies for Oral Thrush

The best remedies for oral thrush include eating plenty of garlic and lots of live yogurt. Rinse the mouth thoroughly with a solution of apple cider vinegar and warm water with a dash of salt.

Including plenty of foods such as onions, coconut and coconut milk in the diet is also particularly helpful.

The flowers of the nasturtium act as a natural antibiotic. Use them in an infusion or in a cool bath.

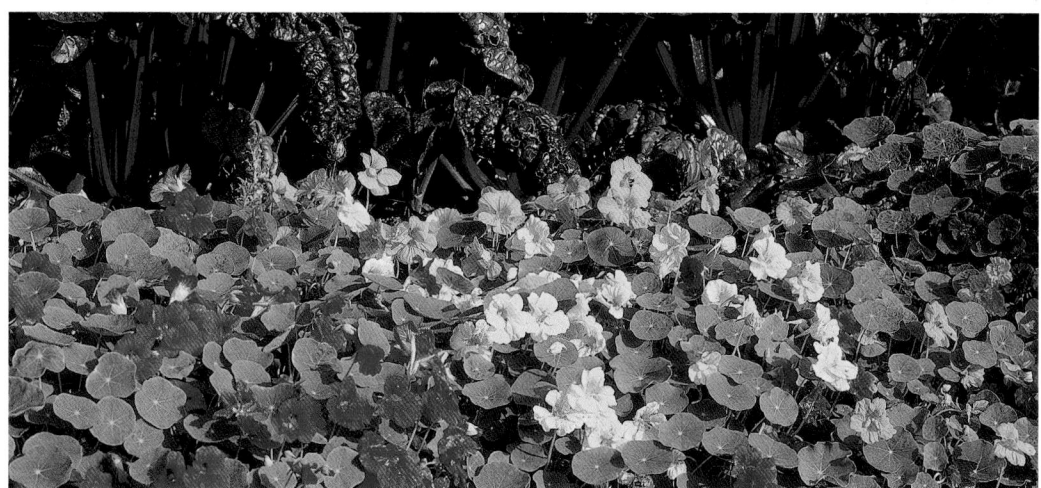

Chilblains, Cramp and Poor Circulation

Chilblains are actually a mild form of frostbite and are painful, itchy swellings that generally occur on the hands, feet or ears in response to cold weather. They are usually the result of poor circulation, which can be aggravated by smoking. Some naturopaths believe that cramps and poor circulation are also caused by low potassium or calcium levels.

Remedies for Chilblains

Whatever you do, resist the urge to put your feet on a radiator or a hot water bottle. Get the circulation going by rubbing the feet briskly with a towel.

As long as the skin is not cut or cracked, dust cayenne powder on the chilblains to stimulate blood circulation. If the skin is broken, rub in calendula ointment to promote healing.

One method is to chop up 450g (1lb) of turnips in their skins. Boil in three litres (about 5 pints) of water till soft. Soak the affected part in the water while it is still hot but bearable, rubbing pieces of turnip over the inflamed surfaces. The salts and essential oils present in the turnip act as an astringent while also improving circulation.

Celery contains compounds that lower blood pressure and help to improve circulation.

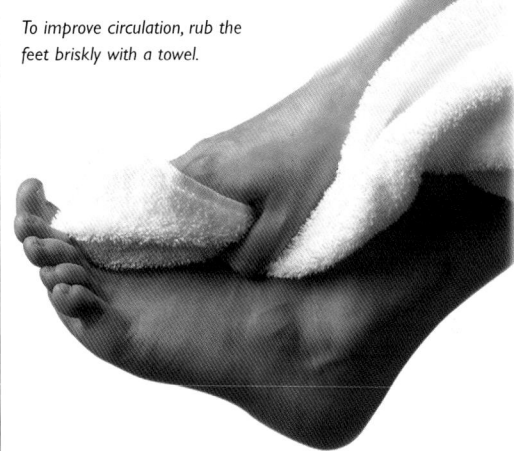

To improve circulation, rub the feet briskly with a towel.

Try fresh horseradish root, bandaged into place. Lemon, garlic or onion juice rubbed on the chilblains can be very effective, or bandage a piece of pithy lemon peel, garlic or onion in place overnight.

Celery is also a good remedy for chilblains. Simmer a bunch of stalks in a litre (1¾ pints) of water for an hour and then soak your feet in a bowl of the mixture for an hour. Make it as hot as you can stand it and try it first thing in the morning and before going to bed.

Remedies for Cramp

Celery contains compounds that reduce high blood pressure by relaxing the smooth muscle lining the blood vessels. The blood then flows more freely and pressure drops; this helps cramp symptoms.

Mix one tablespoon of apple cider vinegar and one teaspoon of honey in a glass of warm water. Gulp it down quickly and the discomfort will disappear after only a few minutes.

Much potassium may be lost in many of the commercial brands of vinegar now available, so look out for the unprocessed variety in a health store.

Almonds in the diet will help to reduce the incidence of cramp.

Drink teas that are rich in calcium such as dandelion, raspberry and plantain leaf. Eat plenty of almonds, sesame seeds, yogurt and most green vegetables.

'Restless legs' is cramp that causes pain and twitching in the legs. Add seed oils, avocados and wheatgerm to the diet to alleviate these symptoms. Reduce your meat, high-fat dairy produce and salt intake.

Soak your feet in a solution made from boiled celery stalks to ease chilblains.

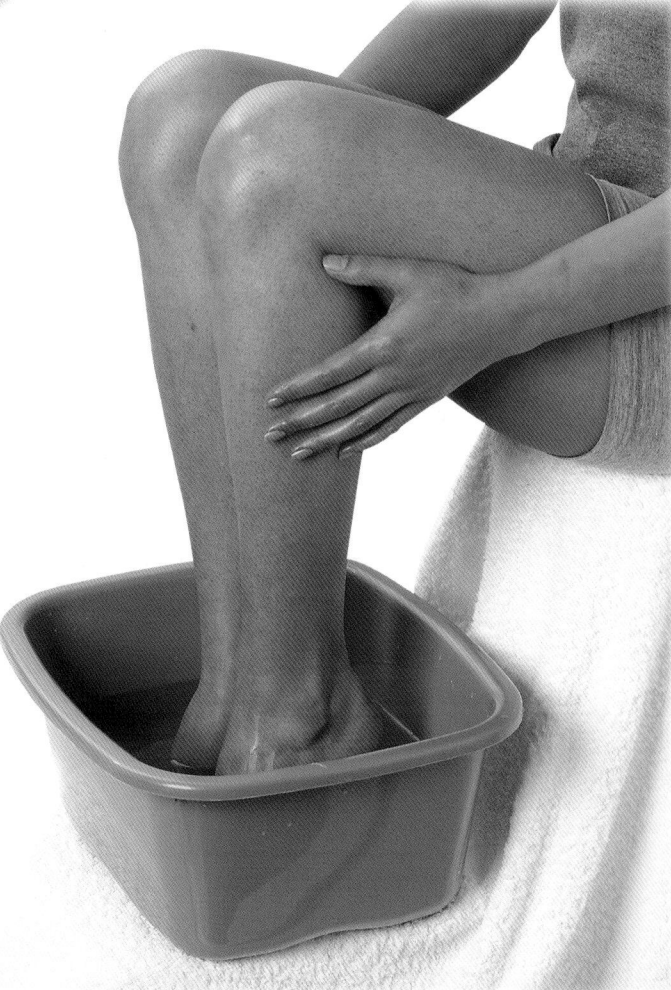

How to Make a Calcium Supplement

- Fill a jar halfway with crushed eggshells.
- Cover with vinegar and allow to sit for two weeks.
- Strain, then take one to three tablespoons daily.
- You can use it as salad dressing or in sauces.
- Sweetened with honey, it can be taken as a refreshing drink.

Eye Conditions

The eye is an incredibly delicate organ and yet it has been built to withstand a large amount of punishment. The anterior part of the eyeball is encased in a tough membrane called the cornea, which can survive and recover from even quite severe injuries. However, alcohol, smoky atmospheres and working too long at computer screens all conspire to harm, often resulting in sore, itchy or inflamed eyes.

Remedies for Tired Eyes

Rose petals are a traditional remedy for inflamed or irritated eyelids. Make up a cooling and soothing compress from two or three petals steeped in a glassful of boiling water for ten minutes. Soak some cotton wool or eyepads in the cooled and strained liquid and place over the eyelids.

Chamomile or marigold tea, used cold as a compress, can also be very healing. Witch hazel, ice-cold direct from the fridge, is a great refresher when your eyes feel tired or you have been staring at a computer all day. Eat plenty of fennel, which is another great food for tired eyes, or drink it as a tea.

Try an eyebath of three teaspoons of honey diluted in two cups of boiling water and left to cool. Or try a poultice of cabbage leaves,

Rose petals can soothe inflamed or irritated eyelids.

softened but not cooked in boiling water. You may look ridiculous with the leaves over your eyelids but it really does the trick.

A raw potato or cucumber placed over closed eyelids can have the same effect.

Borage was valued by the ancient Greeks for strengthening weak eyes and preventing cataracts. You are more likely to develop cataracts if your diet is lacking in beta-carotene, folic acid and vitamin C. Borage contains all three, so try to incorporate it in your diet.

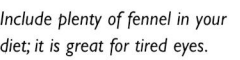

Include plenty of fennel in your diet; it is great for tired eyes.

Remedies for Styes

An eyebath of warm boracic lotion or a poultice of fresh, steamed cabbage leaves will disperse a stye. Or try a drop each of the essential oils of lavender and lemon with a teaspoon of cooled boiled water and bathe the eye with the solution. This will also ease the symptoms of conjunctivitis.

Second World War pilots were encouraged to eat plenty of carrots to improve their night vision.

Past Beliefs

Carrots were once believed to be a super-food for eyes, and pilots during the Second World War were officially encouraged to eat plenty. In the old days, anything golden was reputed to be benefit the sight, including gazing at marigolds during the day.

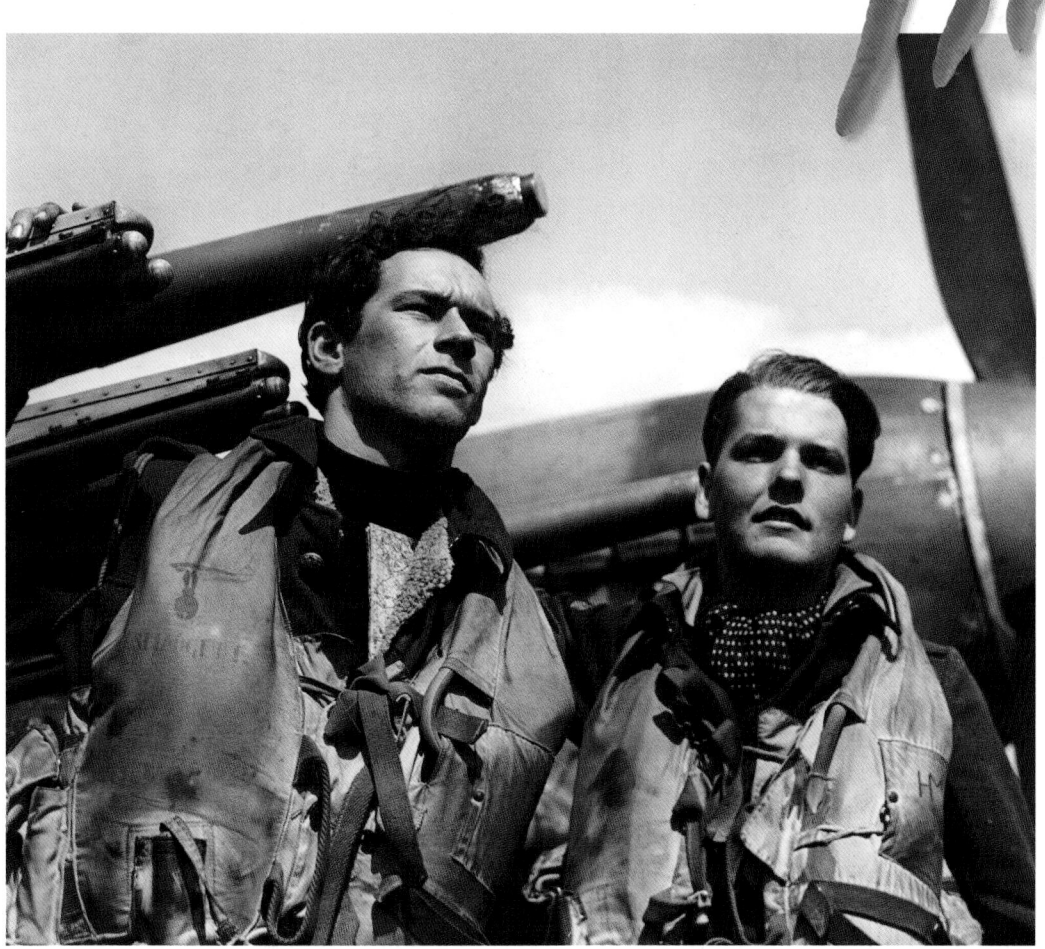

Insomnia

In these stressful times it is hardly any wonder that many people find it hard to get to sleep at night. However, there are certain things you can do to promote a good night's sleep. Try to relax before going to bed, and avoid coffee and alcohol, which tend to keep you awake rather than promote good sleep. Take a warm bath with Epsom salts or play some quiet music. Have a bedtime ritual, so your brain learns to slow down before you settle down to sleep.

Remedies for Insomnia

Natives of certain parts of Italy reputedly slept with cloves of garlic between their toes to ensure a good night's sleep! The Victorians, on the other hand, favoured washing the head with dill or placing dill on the pillow at night.

Adding two teaspoons of apple cider vinegar and two teaspoons of honey to a glass of hot water and drinking it at bedtime may seem a little more user-friendly. Try placing a few drops of lavender oil on the pulse points of the wrist and forehead before you go to bed – it

Eating plenty of lettuce will help you get a good night's sleep.

has a soothing and calming effect. Place celery seeds in a piece of muslin and inhale the fumes as you settle down for the night.

Lettuce is supposed to contain sleep-inducing compounds, so eat it raw or drink a lettuce infusion. Mandarin oranges also have

To help combat insomnia, place some drops of lavender oil on the wrists and forehead before settling down for the night.

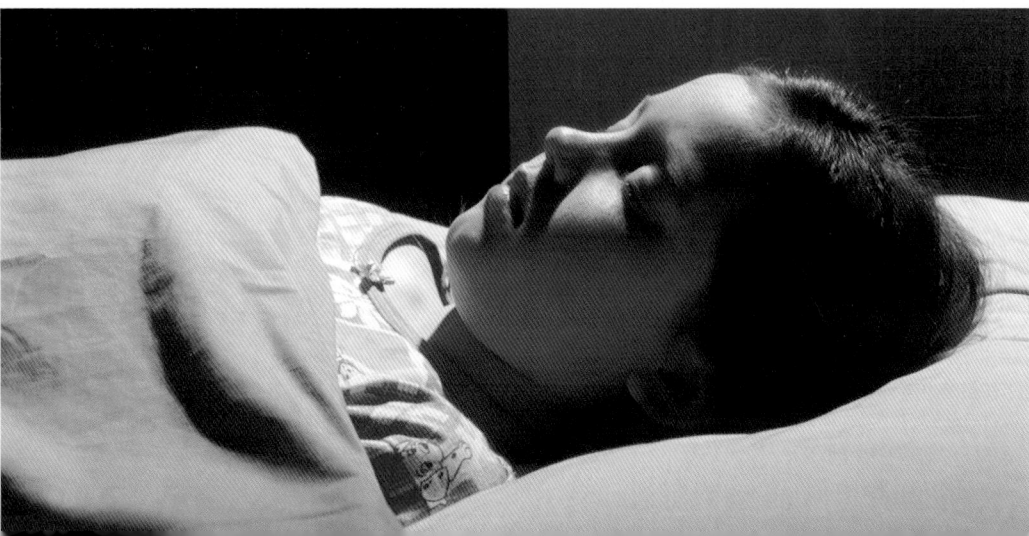

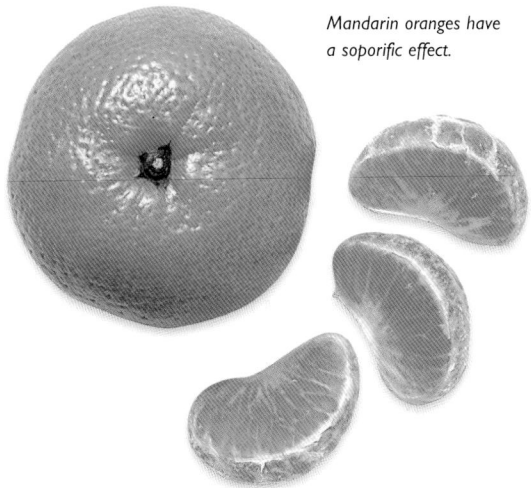

Mandarin oranges have a soporific effect.

a soporific effect – it is a good idea to eat one after your evening meal.

You could make up a tea from elderberry flowers, which are thought to relax the nerves and induce sleep.

Native Americans used to eat raw onions to get a good night's sleep. They also made a sleep potion from poppy heads infused in hot water. If this seems a little drastic, try valerian tea just before going to bed.

Make up this infusion: put the ground seeds from one cardamom pod, two drops of peppermint oil, one teaspoon of sugar and a pinch of bicarbonate of soda in a cup of boiling water and drink while it is still hot.

Add a teaspoon of honey to a cup of warm milk and sprinkle with cinnamon: this is a great drink for helping wakeful children go to sleep.

Orange flower water was a traditional cure for insomnia among English gentlewomen.

Make up your own version with the juice of two oranges in a little hot water sweetened with honey.

A footbath is a good way to bring on sleep because it encourages the blood to flow from the head to the feet. Mix up some lavender and rosemary essential oil and add to a bowl of warm water. A mustard footbath can work just as well.

Warm milk and honey sprinkled with a pinch of cinnamon helps prepare children for sleep.

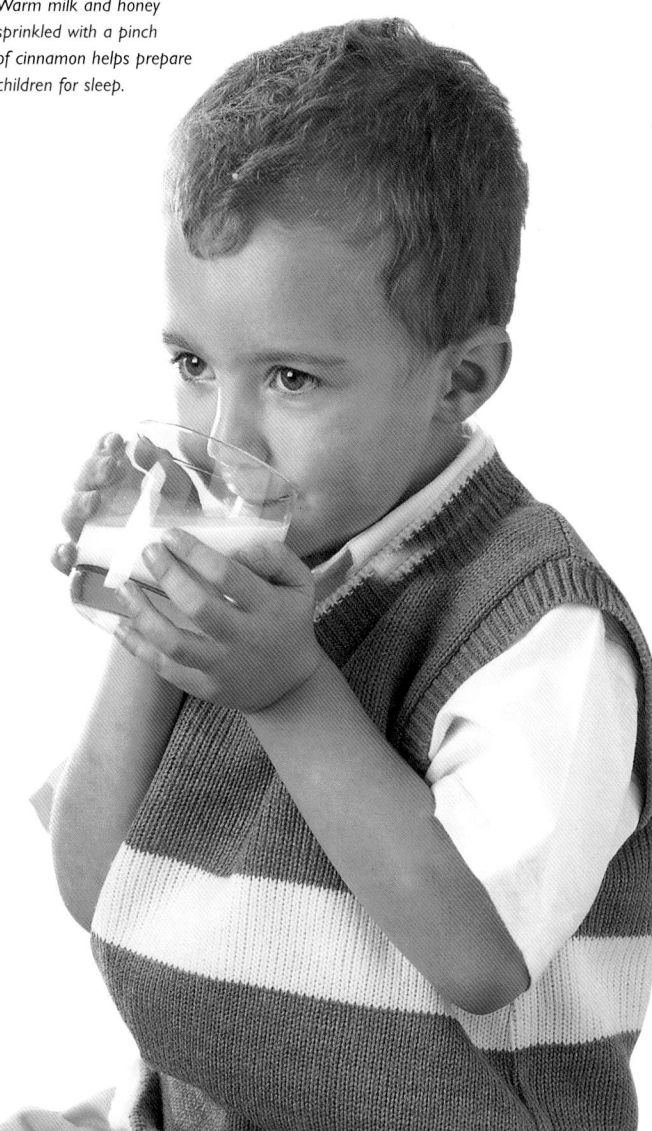

Foot and Hand Care

We have no respect for our feet – we cram them into badly fitting shoes, encase them in synthetic fabrics and demand they perform their task tirelessly, supporting us for hours on end. No wonder we suffer from all sorts of foot complaints, from bunions, callouses and corns to unpleasant fungal infections such as athlete's foot. Although we are kinder to our hands, we still think nothing of dipping them in and out of hot water all day, which can result in chapped skin or dry nails.

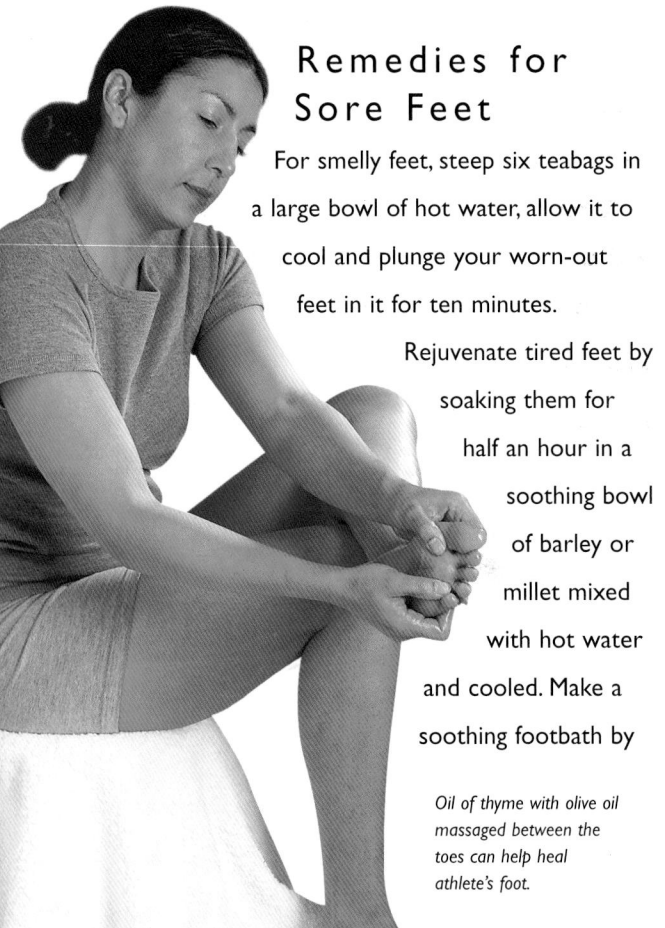

Remedies for Sore Feet

For smelly feet, steep six teabags in a large bowl of hot water, allow it to cool and plunge your worn-out feet in it for ten minutes.

Rejuvenate tired feet by soaking them for half an hour in a soothing bowl of barley or millet mixed with hot water and cooled. Make a soothing footbath by

Oil of thyme with olive oil massaged between the toes can help heal athlete's foot.

We need to have more respect for our poor old feet! Give them a soothing footbath or massage them with essential oils as a treat.

adding one tablespoon of sea salt to a basin of warm water. In cold weather add a teaspoon of mustard powder to really warm them up.

Remedies for Corns

Rub corns with castor oil daily for two weeks to get rid of them completely. Put a piece of lemon peel or raw tomato over the corn and cover with a bandage. The juice of the fruit will soften the corn overnight. The same can be done by soaking leeks in water or vinegar for 24 hours and then applying as a poultice. Make a soothing footbath by adding four or five drops of peppermint oil to a bowl of tepid water. You can also use a couple of peppermint teabags infused for ten minutes.

Remedies for Athlete's Foot

Make up a mixture of equal parts vinegar and warm water or surgical spirit and bathe the feet in a bowl. Massage between the toes with natural yogurt, leaving it to soak in overnight. Add a few drops of essential oil of thyme or rosemary to some olive oil and massage the feet carefully between the toes.

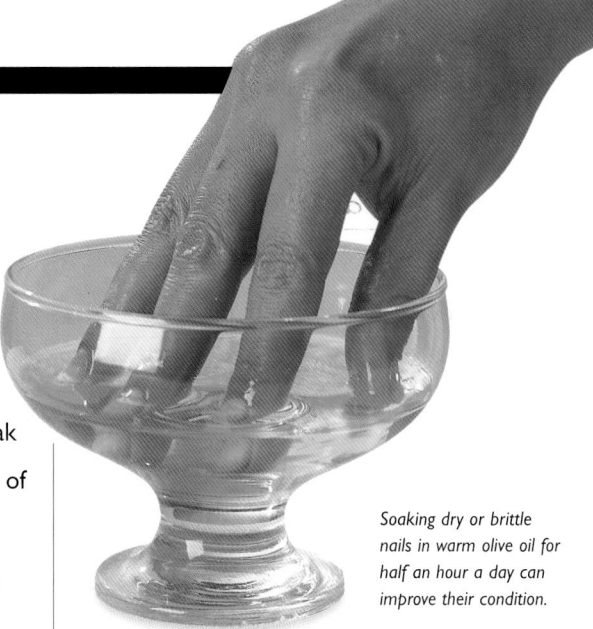

Soaking dry or brittle nails in warm olive oil for half an hour a day can improve their condition.

Remedies for Verrucas and Warts

Peel the skin of a potato as thinly as possible. Rub the inner side of the skin on the wart twice a day. Thanks to a chemical in the potato near the skin, the wart should turn black and drop off within a couple of weeks.

The milky juice squeezed from the stem of a dandelion or celandine can also be used as a balm. Smooth it onto the affected area and cover with a plaster. The next morning the wart or verruca should have disappeared.

Remedies for Brittle and Stained Nails

Immerse dry or brittle nails in warm olive oil for 30 minutes a day until you see an improvement.

To remove stains, rub the hands and nails with the pithy side of a piece of lemon peel, leave for a minute and then wash off.

A mixture of ground almonds, egg, comfrey and honey may be just the moisturiser your hands need.

Remedy for Dry Hands

Mix together 25g (1oz) of ground almonds, a beaten egg, a handful of comfrey root and a tablespoon of honey. Coat your hands with the mixture, pull on an old pair of leather or cotton gloves and wear overnight. Rinse your hands in the morning and repeat this for a week. Your hands will feel very soft and supple.

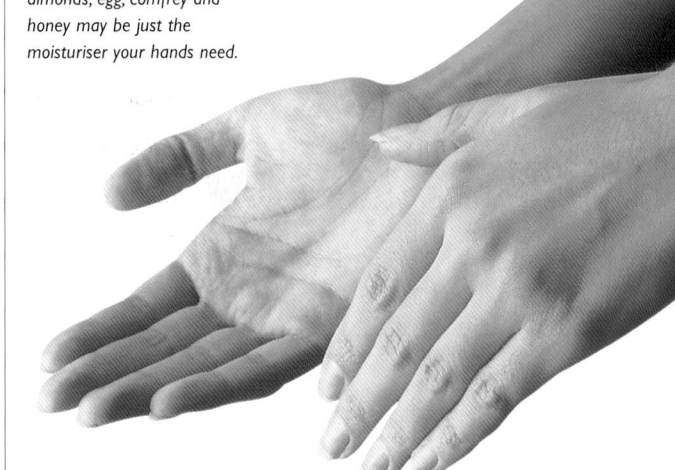

Shampoos, 'Feel Good' Treatments and Tonics

We tend to forget that many natural beauty treatments have been used through the ages for all sorts of cleansing creams and lotions. Cleopatra was reputed to have used aloe vera as a moisturiser, and today most proprietary brands of moisturising cream contain this substance. Almond oil is another great skin softener – you can add whatever essential oil you feel appropriate to smoothe and pamper your skin. The condition of your hair and scalp can be affected by your general state of health, so almost any stressful condition will cause your skin and hair to appear lifeless and dull. A balanced diet is the basis to good health, hair and skin, but here are some extra tips to give nature a helping hand!

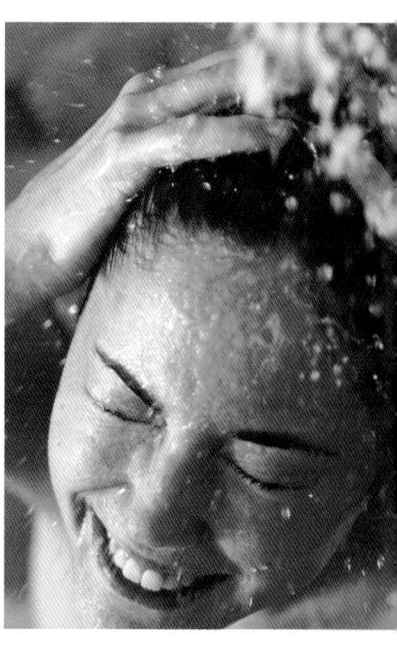

Pamper yourself with a natural, homemade shampoo or 'feel good' treatment and improve your general sense of well-being.

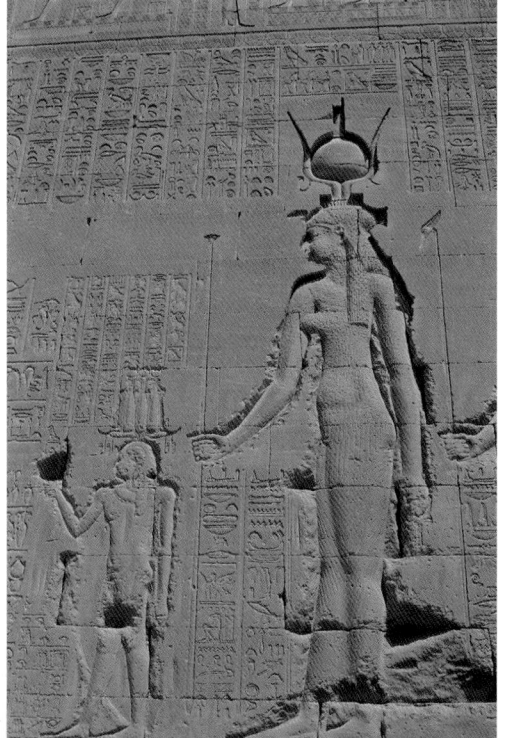

Remedies for Dry Hair

To keep your hair in tip-top condition, try massaging a few drops of oil of rosemary into the scalp then rinsing with an infusion of nettles. For very dry hair, warm two tablespoons of olive oil in a cup placed in a pan of hot water. Massage the oil into the scalp. Steep a towel in hot water, wring it out and wrap it around your head for about two

Even the ancient Egyptians needed a little help to stay beautiful! Cleopatra was reputed to have used aloe vera as a moisturiser.

hours. Rinse with a solution of one cupful of cider vinegar to 5 litres (9 pints) of water.

Make an egg shampoo for dry hair. Use 25g (1oz) of fresh rosemary, 600ml (1 pint) of hot water and one egg. Steep the rosemary in the water for 20 minutes and allow to cool. Beat in the egg. Massage into the hair and rinse well.

Aloe vera has been used in moisturisers through the ages and is still used today.

Then add half a cup of cider vinegar to 5 litres (9 pints) of cool water and rinse the mixture through your hair, followed by a cool rinse with clear water to remove all traces. For thinning hair, rinse your hair with flat beer.

Remedies for Dandruff

Cut a lemon in half and rub the two halves into the scalp. Leave for ten minutes, then wash the hair. Sour milk has the same effect but will not smell as nice.

Wrap one or two pieces of fresh ginger root in muslin. Boil it up in 600ml (1 pint) of water. After shampooing, rinse your hair with the liquid, massaging it into the hair.

Rinse your hair with cider vinegar, wrap your head in a towel and leave for half an hour. Rinse out completely. Repeat three times a week until the dandruff disappears.

Remedy for Split Ends

Comb in a mixture of equal quantities of warmed castor oil and olive oil. Follow this by shampooing with an egg yolk. Wrap your head up in a warm towel and let the egg yolk soak in for at least an hour.

'Feel Good' Tonics

Make yourself a natural tonic. Some people swear by drinking a teaspoon of apple cider vinegar and a teaspoon of honey in 225ml (6–8fl oz) of hot water mid-morning and mid-afternoon. It provides a boost of energy which carries them through to the next meal.

Or try making up a purifying tonic by mixing a tablespoon of crushed blueberries and a tablespoon of shredded watercress with 300ml (½ pint) of boiling water poured over. Cover the liquid and leave to cool, then strain it. Drink a cup twice a day. It's guaranteed to make you feel a million dollars.

You can make an egg shampoo with rosemary – it works wonders for dry hair problems.

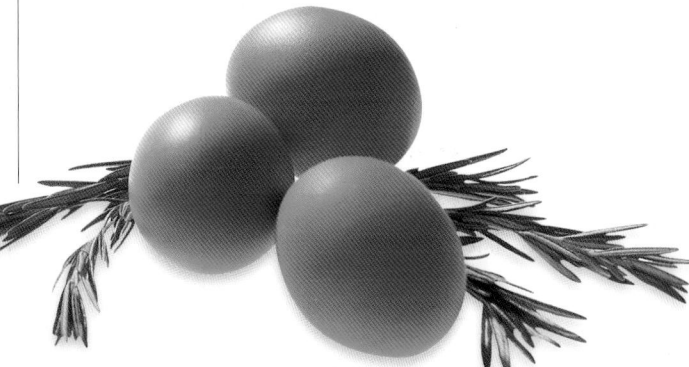

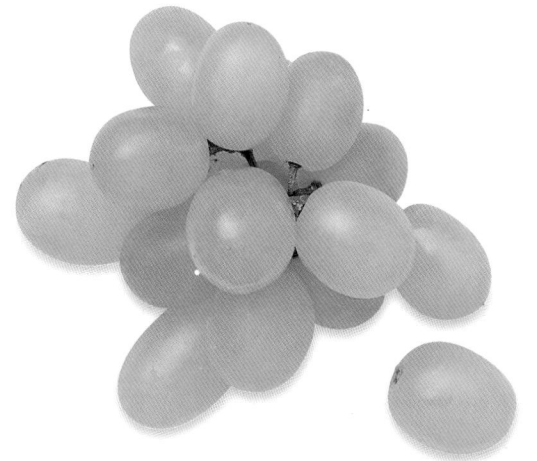

Green grapes can be used in a home-made facial cleanser.

For a dandelion tonic, pick enough dandelion flower heads to make 1.2 litres (2 pints) of petals. Cut off the stem and collar at the end of each flower. Rinse the dandelions in water before preparing the petals. Place the petals in a pan, cover with 2.5 litres (4½ pints) of water and boil for 20 minutes. Add two oranges and two lemons. Add a spoonful of baker's yeast and allow to stand for 48 hours before straining through muslin. Add 1.3kg (3lb) of sugar and stir well. Use as a feel good tonic whenever you need one.

For the Face

Make a natural cleansing cream with eight tablespoons of beeswax heated up with 425ml (¾ pint) of liquid paraffin. Add 300ml (½ pint) of water to the wax and oil mixture, stirring continuously. Leave it to cool and transfer it to jars for storage.

To make a cleanser, mix ten green grapes, two teaspoons of apple cider vinegar, one teaspoon of honey and a teaspoon of oatmeal in a blender until the liquid becomes sticky. Clean your face and neck in your usual way and apply the mixture, leaving it on for at least five minutes. Rinse with warm water and pat dry.

Lemons are great for greasy skin that is prone to blackheads – you can drink the juice and also apply it to the skin. Its high antioxidant content makes it an excellent treatment for wrinkles too. Dilute it with mineral water and massage it gently at the first sign of wrinkles, particularly around the mouth and eyes.

To make a face pack for greasy skin, seed and purée a large cucumber, add a teaspoon of lemon juice, a teaspoon of witch hazel, an egg white and two tablespoons of cream or plain yogurt and purée all the ingredients in a blender. Apply the mixture to the face and leave for 20 to 30 minutes until nearly dry, then rinse well with warm water.

For a great face mask, mix an equal

Make up a face pack for greasy skin from natural ingredients such as cucumber.

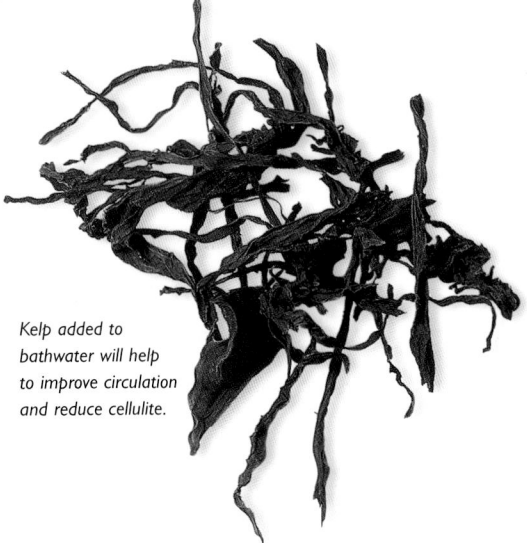

Kelp added to bathwater will help to improve circulation and reduce cellulite.

quantity of oatmeal and ground almonds into a paste by adding enough liquid to thicken the mixture and smooth onto the face and neck. Add one teaspoon of wheatgerm or brewer's yeast for dry skin, or kaolin to draw out spots and impurities.

If you have problem skin, Fuller's earth (a clay available at chemist's) will help an oily skin and stimulate the blood supply. Witch hazel, beaten egg white, yogurt or lemon juice will all help to dry up an oily skin. Egg yolk, honey, soured cream, pulped bananas or avocado will all benefit a dry skin. Rosemary or peppermint oil added to a base of oats and almonds will invigorate a tired, dull-looking skin.

You could use the pulp of the pawpaw fruit to rub over the face and this will help to slough off dead skin cells.

A tablespoon of castor oil mixed with two tablespoons of almond oil makes an excellent eye make-up remover.

For Cellulite

Cellulite is the term used to describe the puckered areas of fatty flesh, often referred to as 'orange peel skin', that generally occur around the tops of the thighs, hips, buttocks and upper arms, and is more common in women than men. No one really knows what causes cellulite, yet theories abound on how it can be treated.

Fresh parsley is a rich source of vitamin C, a good detoxifier, and a diuretic, so it helps the body eliminate excess water. Eat plenty of the raw herb in salads.

Boil up the rind of a lemon in water and leave it overnight. You then drink it first thing in the morning.

Use kelp in your bathwater – it boosts the circulation. Dandelion tea will rid the body of any excess fluid.

Chop two handfuls of ivy leaves and mix with four handfuls of bran and enough warm water to make a paste. This can then be applied to the affected areas as a poultice.

The pulp of the paw paw fruit will slough off dead skin cells.

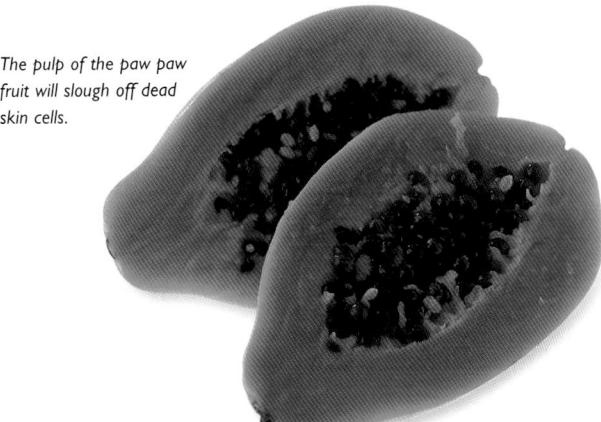

Useful Home Remedies

Almond oil: as a base for massage and rubs; for earache

Aloe vera: as a facial cleanser

Angelica: use the leaves or roots as a diuretic, expectorant, anti-spasmodic; digestive tonic for children's coughs and colds; for fainting fits; for a fever

Asparagus: for eczema

Avocado: as a hand cream; as a cleanser; for sunburn; for cuts and grazes; for acne

Bananas: for diarrhoea

Barley: for cystitis

Basil: as an antiseptic.

Beetroot: for fever; to clear the blood; for acne

Bicarbonate of soda: for sunburn; for cystitis

Blackberry leaves: for diarrhoea; for food poisoning

Blackcurrants: for infection and inflammation

Blueberries: for cystitis; for diarrhoea; for mouth ulcers and sore gums

Borage: for coughs; for constipation; as a diuretic

Buttermilk: for sunburn

Cabbage: for arthritis and rheumatism; as a poultice for back pain; as a detoxifier; for asthma; for constipation

Camphor oil: stimulant or sedative; antiseptic, can be used on cuts and grazes; for lumbago

Carrots: for stomach disorders; for cleansing the system; for eye problems; for asthma; for constipation

Castor oil: for food poisoning

Cayenne pepper: as a poultice for joint irritation; with garlic for a bad sore throat

Celandine: the juice is good for jaundice, throat infections, verrucas and warts, failing eyesight

Celery: for urinary tract infections

Chilli peppers: for rheumatism

Cider vinegar: can be used for practically anything. It cures fungal infections, stomach infections and can be used in a footbath for athlete's foot

Cinnamon: a warming digestive, antispasmodic and antiseptic; good for menstrual cramps and for diarrhoea; with ginger for a chesty cough

Cloves: as a painkiller for toothache and to ease wasp stings; can also help nausea; for a fever

Comfrey: for bruises and sprains

Cowslip: contains salicin which is like aspirin

Cranberries: the perfect answer to cystitis

Cream: for wounds

Cucumber: with glycerine for burns; for headaches

Dandelion: is a diuretic and can be used to cleanse the whole system of toxins; good for mosquito bites

Dock leaves: for nettle stings

Echinacea: an antibiotic; for colds and flu

Egg yolk: for a gravel graze; for a hangover; for lumbago

Elderberries: for burns and sunburn; for coughs; for earache; for fever; for headaches; for insomnia; for toothaches; for neuralgia

Epsom salts: for back pain; for infections; for menstrual pain

Fennel: for bad breath; for indigestion; for constipation; for colds and flu; as a diuretic

Feverfew: for migraine

Figs: for constipation

Friar's balsam: as an inhalant for allergies, eg, asthma and hay fever; for cuts and grazes

Fuller's earth: clay for use as a face pack to draw impurities from the skin

Garlic: as a natural antibiotic and antiseptic; for cleaning wounds; for stomach disorders; for cleansing the blood; for corns; for coughs; for earache; for diarrhoea; for hangovers; for thrush; for verrucas; as an insect repellent

Ginger: for arthritis and rheumatism; for colds and circulation problems; in a footbath for headaches and migraine; for insect bites; for nausea

Grapefruit: for psoriasis

Hibiscus: for a fever

Honey: for asthma and allergies; for constipation; for coughs, colds and fever; for sore throats; for cuts and grazes

Honeycomb: chewed for allergies

Hops: for insomnia; for headaches

Horseradish: for acne; for chilblains; for mosquito bites; for sinuses

Hyssop: in tea to support the immune system

Irish moss: for asthma

Ivy: for cellulite; for sciatica

Lavender: for acne; for burns; for coughs and colds; for earache; for a hangover; in a hair treatment; for menstrual cramps; for rheumatism; for the skin; for thrush; for sprains

Lemon: for colds; as a digestive; for fever; in hair and skin treatments; for teeth; for stings

Lemon balm: for burns

Lemon juice: for sunburn; for bites and stings

Linseed: in a poultice for bursitis

Marigold: for bruises and burns; for sore gums

Marshmallow: for bursitis; for eczema

Milk: in rice pudding for diarrhoea; with cinnamon for insomnia

Milk of magnesia: for indigestion; for sunburn

Mud and clay: for sunburn

Mustard: as a rub for bad backs; in a footbath for colds or flu

Nettles: as a diuretic; for cleansing the blood; for eliminating toxins; in soup for insomnia

Oats: for stress; for cleansing the blood; in a poultice for cellulite; for menopause and period pains

Olive oil: for food poisoning

Onions: for colds; for cystitis; to help digestion; for allergies

Oregano: for migraine

Parsley: for bad breath; as a diuretic

Pepper: for toothache

Peppermint: for nausea; for colds and fever; for headache; for menopause; as a mosquito repellent; for IBS

Plums: for psoriasis

Potato: for stomach disorders; for sore eyes; as an anti-inflammatory; for IBS

Prunes: for constipation; for psoriasis

Rice: for bowel disorders, especially diarrhoea

Rosemary: as a disinfectant; for fever; for headaches; in hair treatments; as a mouthwash; for rheumatism

Rose petals: as an eye treatment

Sage: for thrush; for menopause; for mouth/gums; for sore throats

Salt: as a gargle for sore throats; for fungal infections; in water for cuts and grazes

Sandalwood: in a bath for a hangover

Slippery elm: for indigestion; for bursitis

Soya: for menopausal symptoms

Strawberries: as a laxative for constipation

Thyme: for colds; as a disinfectant in a footbath; as an infusion for improving a hoarse voice

Tinned tomatoes: for migraine

Turmeric: for sprains; for rheumatism

Turnips: for coughs and colds; (boiled) for cystitis

Turpentine: for lumbago

Umeboshi plums: for food poisoning; for hangovers

Watercress: for acne

Willow: for toothache

Wine: for hangovers; garlic wine as a tonic

Witch hazel: first-line treatment for cuts and grazes; as a deodorant; for piles

Yogurt: for cuts and grazes; for thrush

Index